# Manual of Contemporary Otological Practice

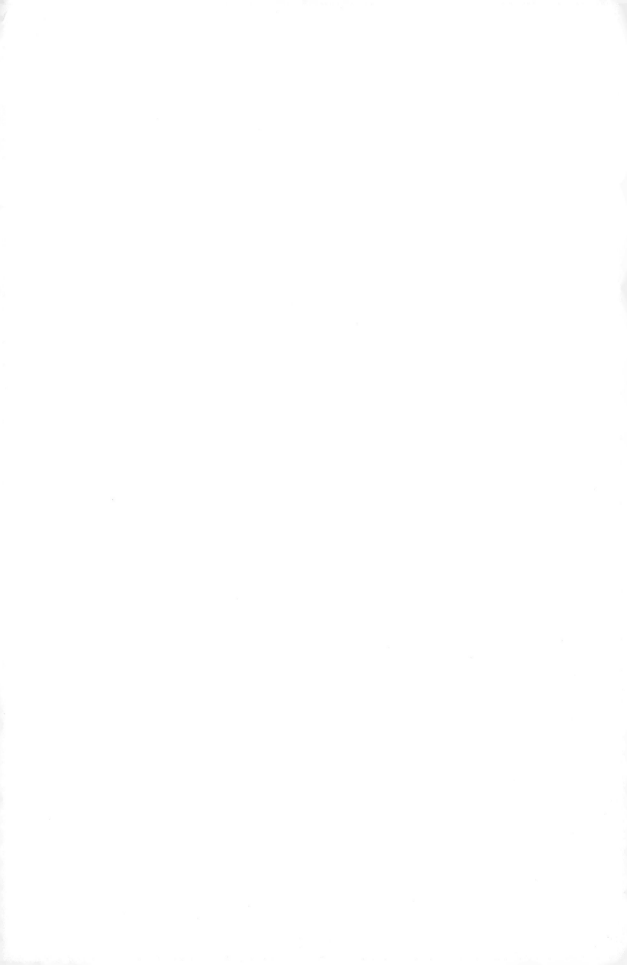

# Manual of Contemporary Otological Practice

**Chief Editor:**

**Dr Uma Patnaik**
*Professor and Head, Department of ENT*
*Command Hospital (SC)*
*Pune, Maharashtra, India*

**Executive Editors:**

**Dr Amit Sood**
*Assistant Professor (ENT)*
*Command Hospital (SC)*
*Pune, Maharashtra, India*

**Dr Dilip Raghavan**
*Professor and Head, Department of ENT*
*Armed Forces Medical College*
*Pune, Maharashtra, India*

**Dr Sabarigirish K**
*Professor, Department of ENT*
*Armed Forces Medical College*
*Pune, Maharashtra, India*

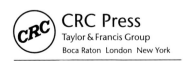

CRC Press
Taylor & Francis Group
Boca Raton London New York

CRC Press is an imprint of the
Taylor & Francis Group, an **informa** business

First edition published 2021
by CRC Press
6000 Broken Sound Parkway NW, Suite 300, Boca Raton, FL 33487-2742
and by Taylor & Francis Group
2 Park Square, Milton Park, Abingdon, Oxon, OX14 4RN

---

**Library of Congress Cataloging-in-Publication Data**

---

Names: Patnaik, Uma, editor. | Sood, Amit (Otolaryngologist), editor. | K., Sabarigirish (Kanjully),
editor. | Raghavan, Dilip, Professor, editor.
Title: Manual of contemporary otological practice / edited by Dr. Uma Patnaik, Wg Cdr Amit
Sood, Dr. Sabarigirish K., Surg Cmde Dilip Raghavan.
Description: First edition. | Boca Raton, FL : CRC Press, 2021. | Includes bibliographical references
and index. | Summary: "Practice of otology today, requires a contemporary knowledge base,
coupled with concurrent skill sets, and tempered with familiarity of the technological advances.
This manual has been designed to address these three domains, making it a ready reference to
guide specialists on the standards of care in practice. The chapters explore the current concepts,
with a background of past practices, touching upon the basics of anatomy and physiology before
dealing with clinical conditions and their management, covering specific clinical scenarios to
develop a patient-oriented approach in the readers using evidence-based guidelines"-- Provided
by publisher.
Identifiers: LCCN 2020051508 (print) | LCCN 2020051509 (ebook) | ISBN 9780367753184 (hard-
back) | ISBN 9780367489441 (paperback) | ISBN 9781003161974 (ebook)
Subjects: MESH: Ear Diseases--diagnosis | Ear Diseases--therapy | Diagnostic Techniques,
Otological
Classification: LCC RF291 (print) | LCC RF291 (ebook) | NLM WV 215 | DDC 617.8/075--dc23
LC record available at https://lccn.loc.gov/2020051508
LC ebook record available at https://lccn.loc.gov/2020051509

---

ISBN: 9780367753184 (hbk)
ISBN: 9780367489441 (pbk)
ISBN: 9781003161974 (ebk)

Typeset in Palatino LT Std
by KnowledgeWorks Global Ltd.

# Table of Contents

# List of Abbreviations

| | |
|---|---|
| **5 FU** | 5-Fluorouracil |
| **AABR** | Automated auditory brainstem response |
| **AAO-HNS** | American Association of Otolaryngology-Head & Neck Surgery |
| **AB Gap** | Air-bone gap |
| **ABI** | Auditory brainstem implant |
| **ABR** | Auditory brainstem response |
| **AC** | Air conduction |
| **ACE** | Angiotensin-converting enzyme |
| **AFB** | Acid fast bacilli |
| **AI** | Artificial intelligence |
| **ANA** | Anti-nuclear antibody |
| **ANCA** | Anti-neutrophilic cytoplasmic antibody |
| **ANN** | Artificial neural network |
| **ANSD** | Auditory neuropathy spectrum disorder |
| **AOAE** | Automated oto acoustic emissions |
| **AOM** | Acute otitis media |
| **AP** | Action potential |
| **APUD** | Amine precursor and uptake decarboxylase |
| **ASSR** | Auditory steady-state response |
| **AVS** | Acute vestibular syndrome |
| **BAAP** | Bone-anchored auricular prosthesis |
| **BAHA** | Bone-anchored hearing aid |
| **BC** | Bone conduction |
| **BCD** | Bone conduction device |
| **BCHD** | Bone-conducting hearing devices |
| **BERA** | Brainstem-evoked response audiometry |
| **BOA** | Behavioural observation audiometry |
| **BP** | Bell's palsy |
| **BPPV** | Benign paroxysmal positional vertigo |
| **BPVC** | Benign positional vertigo of childhood |
| **BTE** | Behind the ear |
| **CAD** | Computer-aided design |
| **CAEP** | Central auditory-evoked potential |
| **CAPD** | Central-auditory processing disorder |
| **CBCT** | Cone beam computed tomography |
| **CBT** | Cognitive behavioural therapy |
| **CCA** | Congenital canal atresia |
| **CE** | European conformity |
| **CEMRI** | Contrast-enhanced magnetic resonance imaging |
| **CERA** | Cortical-evoked response audiometry |
| **CI** | Cochlear implant |
| **CIC** | Completely in canal |
| **CISS** | Constructive interference in steady state |
| **CMV** | Cytomegalovirus |
| **CN** | Cranial nerve |
| **CNS** | Central nervous system |
| **CO₂** | Carbon dioxide |
| **COM** | Chronic otitis media |
| **COX** | Cyclo-oxygenase |
| **CP Angle** | Cerebellopontine angle |
| **CPA** | Conditioned play audiometry |
| **CROS** | Contralateral routing of signal |
| **CRP** | C-reactive protein |
| **CS** | Corrective saccades |
| **CSD** | Chronic subjective dizziness |
| **CSF** | Cerebrospinal fluid |
| **CT** | Computed tomography |
| **CVA** | Cerebrovascular accident |
| **CW** | Continuous wave |
| **CWD** | Canal wall down |
| **dB** | Decibel |
| **DBN** | Deep belief network |
| **DM** | Diabetes mellitus |
| **DNES** | Diffuse neuroendocrine system |
| **DP** | Directional preponderance |
| **DSA** | Digital subtraction angiography |
| **DWI** | Diffusion-weighted images |
| **ECochG** | Electrocochleography |
| **eABR** | Evoked auditory brainstem response |
| **EAC** | External auditory canal |
| **EBM** | Evidence-based medicine |
| **ECAP** | Evoked compound action potential |
| **EEG** | Electroencephalogram |
| **ELST** | Endolymphatic sac tumor |
| **EMG** | Electromyography |
| **EnoG** | Electroneuronography |
| **EPI** | Echo planar imaging |
| **ESR** | Erythrocyte sedimentation rate |
| **ESRT** | Elicited stapedial reflex threshold |
| **ET** | Eustachian tube |
| **EVA** | Enlarged vestibular aqueduct |
| **FDA** | Food and Drug Administration |
| **FDG** | Fluorodeoxyglucose |
| **FM** | Frequency modulation |
| **FN** | Facial nerve |
| **FNC** | Facial nerve canal |
| **FNH** | Facial nerve haemangioma |
| **FNS** | Facial nerve schwannoma |
| **GA** | General anaesthesia |
| **GAN** | Greater auricular nerve |
| **GBS** | Guillain-Barre syndrome |
| **GM** | Granular myringitis |
| **GORD** | Gastro-oesophageal reflux disorder |
| **GSA** | General somatic afferent |
| **GSPN** | Greater superficial petrosal nerve |
| **GTR** | Gross total resection |

| | | | |
|---|---|---|---|
| GVE | General visceral efferent | MML | Minimum masking level |
| HA | Hearing aids | MOE | Malignant otitis externa |
| HAT | Hearing-assistive technology | MPO | Myeloperoxidase |
| HBOT | Hyper baric oxygen therapy | MRI | Magnetic resonance imaging |
| HC | Horizontal canal | MRS | Melkersson-Rosenthal syndrome |
| HINTS | Head impulse, nystagmus, test of skew | NF | Neurofibromatosis |
| | | NIHL | Noise-induced hearing loss |
| HIT | Head impulse test | NLF | Nasolacrimal fold |
| HL | Hearing loss | NLP | Natural language processing |
| HRCT | High-resolution computed tomography | NO | Nitrous oxide |
| | | NOHL | Non-organic hearing loss |
| HST | Head shake test | NRR | Noise reduction rating |
| HSV | Herpes simplex virus | NSAID | Non-steroidal anti-inflammatory drugs |
| HTT | Head thrust test | | |
| IAC | Internal auditory canal | NTT | Neuromonics tinnitus therapy |
| IAD | Implantable auditory device | OAE | Oto acoustic emissions |
| IAM | Internal acoustic meatus | OCT | Optical coherence tomography |
| ICA | Internal carotid artery | OE | Otitis externa |
| ICU | Intensive care unit | OHC | Outer hair cell |
| ICVD | International Classification of Vestibular Disorders | OM | Otitis media |
| | | OMAAV | ANCA-associated otitis media |
| ICW | Intact canal wall | OME | Otitis media with effusion |
| IHC | Inner hair cell | OPD | Outpatient department |
| ILD | Inter-aural level difference | PA | Petrous apex |
| IPOG | International Paediatric Otolaryngology Group | PCHI | Permanent childhood hearing impairment |
| ISO | International Organisation for Standardisation | PCR | Polymerase chain reaction |
| | | PCS | Posterior circulation stroke |
| ISRS | International Stereotactic Radiosurgery Society | PET | Positron emission tomography |
| | | PFNS | Post-paralytic facial nerve syndrome |
| ISSNHL | Idiopathic sudden sensorineural hearing loss | PFP | Post-paralytic facial palsy |
| ITC | In the canal | PICA | Posterior inferior cerebellar artery |
| ITD | Inter-aural time difference | PLA | People Liberation Army |
| IVN | Inferior vestibular nerve | PONV | Postoperative nausea vomiting |
| JTP | Jugulotympanic paraganglioma | PORP | Partial ossicular replacement prosthesis |
| KTP | Potassium titanyl phosphate | | |
| LA | Local anaesthesia | PRRT | Peptide receptor radionuclide therapy |
| LCH | Langerhans cell histiocytoma | | |
| LCN | Lower cranial nerves | PSCC | Posterior semicircular canal |
| LLR | Low-power laser irradiation | PTA | Pure tone audiometry |
| LMA | Laryngeal mask airway | PTS | Permanent threshold shift |
| LMN | Lower motor neuron | QOL | Quality of life |
| LO | Labyrinthitis ossificans | RBC | Red blood cell |
| LPR | Laryngopharyngeal reflux | RCT | Randomized control trial |
| LSCC | Lateral semicircular canal | RF | Rheumatoid factor |
| LTBR | Lateral temporal bone resection | RHS | Ramsay Hunt syndrome |
| MAC | Monitored anaesthesia care | RMS | Rhabdomyosarcoma |
| MAV | Migraine-associated vertigo | ROS | Reactive oxygen species |
| MCF | Middle cranial fossa | RSV | Respiratory syncytial virus |
| MD | Ménière's disease | RTA | Road traffic accident |
| MDCT | Multi-detector computed tomography | SBO | Skull base osteomyelitis |
| | | SCC | Semicircular canal |
| MEP | Middle ear pressure | SDS | Speech discrimination score |
| MERI | Middle ear risk index | SLE | Systemic lupus erythematosus |
| MIBG | Metaiodobenzylguanidine | SMF | Stylomastoid foramen |
| ML | Machine learning | SNHL | Sensorineural hearing loss |
| MLP | Multilayer perception | SOM | Secretory otitis media |

| | | | |
|---|---|---|---|
| **SP** | Summating potential | **TORP** | Total ossicular replacement prosthesis |
| **SPECT** | Single-photon emission-computed tomography | **TQ Score** | Tinnitus quotient score |
| **SR** | Subtotal resection | **TRT** | Tinnitus retraining therapy |
| **SRS** | Stereotactic radiosurgery | **TTBR** | Total temporal bone resection |
| **SRT** | Speech reception thresholds | **TTO** | Tympanostomy tube-related otorrhoea |
| **SSCD** | Superior semicircular canal dehiscence | **TTS** | Temporary threshold shift |
| **SSD** | Single-sided deafness | **UHL** | Unilateral hearing loss |
| **SSNHL** | Sudden sensorineural hearing loss | **UMN** | Upper motor neuron |
| **SSRI** | Selective serotonin reuptake inhibitor | **UW** | Unilateral weakness |
| | | **VCN** | Vestibulo-cochlear nerve |
| **STBR** | Subtotal temporal bone resection | **VEMP** | Vestibular evoked myogenic potential |
| **SVA** | Special visceral afferent | | |
| **SVE** | Special visceral efferent | **VHL** | Von Hippel-Lindau |
| **SVM** | Support vector machine | **VM** | Vestibular migraine |
| **SVN** | Superior vestibular nerve | **VN** | Vestibular neuritis |
| **TA** | Transcranial attenuation | **VNG** | Video Nystagmography |
| **TBM** | Temporal bone malignancy | **VOR** | Vestibulo-ocular reflex |
| **TEES** | Transcanal endoscopic ear surgery | **VP** | Vestibular paroxysmia |
| **TFT** | Tuning fork tests | **VRA** | Visual reinforcement audiometry |
| **TIVA** | Total intra-venous anaesthesia | **VS** | Vestibular schwannoma |
| **TM** | Tympanic membrane | **VZV** | Varicella zoster virus |
| **TMS** | Transcranial magnetic stimulation | **WHO** | World Health Organisation |
| **TN** | Trigeminal nerve | **WRS** | Word recognition score |
| **TOM** | Tubercular otitis media | **YAG** | Yttrium aluminium garnet |

# Preface

"When you don't see the book you want on the shelf, write it."

**–Beverly Cleary**

Practice of otology today requires a contemporary knowledge base, coupled with concurrent skill sets, tempered with familiarity of the technological advances. This manual has been designed to address these three domains, so that it becomes a companion to guide specialists on the standards of care in otology. The seed for this manual was sown four years ago when the abject need for such a manual was realized and it took dedicated work of the team to conceptualize its focus and content. The immense task of collating the current data and compiling them into a reader-friendly format has indeed been onerous.

The art and science of otology has undergone metamorphosis in the last few decades with significant changes, not only in the evaluation and management of diseases, but also in the basic understanding of their pathology. Evolution of new age surgical microscopes, image-guided systems and endoscopy-assisted surgery techniques have been game changers in the practice of otological surgery, while advances in molecular biology and nanotechnology are beginning to gives us new perspectives on the disease processes. Add to this, the inroads made by artificial intelligence and machine learning are making a paradigm shift in the way we practice. This, we believed, was an appropriate juncture to provide an approach-based compendium in otology. The book is designed to be a confidant for the reader to refer to, in various clinical scenarios where sound clinical decisions will have a positive impact on the patient outcomes.

We express our sincere compliments to all the contributors for all their efforts, which I am sure, will be appreciated by the readers. I would also like to express my sincere gratitude to our executive editors, Amit Sood, Dilip Raghavan and Sabarigirish K, whose meticulous work of editing has substantially improved the quality of content. We also thank Taylor & Francis India for the determined support of the project, but in particular, Ms Shivangi Pramanik, the commissioning editor and Ms Himani Dwivedi, without whose patience and persistence, this project would not have seen the light of day.

Lastly, on a personal note, this mission would not have been possible without the blessings of my parents Saroja and R Jayaraman, unflinching cooperation of my spouse, Col S K Patnaik, and of course, my three-year-old angel, Ms Udisha, who ensured that the maternal nightouts were gainfully utilized for this academic effort.

Join us on this voyage, . . . "Read along, as the book starts when reader enters. . . . ."

*Uma Patnaik*

# Foreword

Otology has witnessed many advances over the last few decades. These include many exciting and headline grabbing advances such as cochlear implants and brainstem implants and also implantable hearing devices. Other advances seem mundane – such as the revolution in imaging – but they nevertheless have brought about an immense change in our practice and the quality of service we provide to our patients.

The *Manual of Contemporary Otological Practice* is a focused, very well-researched and referenced and a complete and comprehensive textbook on otology. It is a labour of love written with passion which brings out both the knowledge and the experience of the authors. In recent years, the focus of otology has moved from the basic concepts of middle ear pathology and surgery pertaining to chronic otitis media to the current hot topics relating to the inner ear and advances in implantation otology. This book stands out in detailing not only the contemporary topics, but also the basic concepts pertaining to middle ear disease which are less emphasized today. The experienced authorship has ensured that appropriate lessons pertaining to middle ear disease which are slowly being castigated to history continue to be listed and emphasized.

My congratulations to all authors and particularly to the chief editor, Dr Uma Patnaik, for bringing this challenging task to fruition and providing us a book which will serve as an informed and enjoyable read, and also a quick reference guide to the rapidly evolving science and craft of otology.

**Alok Thakar, MS, FRCSEd**
*Professor of Otolaryngology & Head-Neck Surgery*
*All India Institute of Medical Sciences, New Delhi*

## Contributors

**Dr Manikandan A, MS (ENT)**
Assistant Professor
Base Hospital
Guwahati, India

**Dr Dhanalakshmi B, MD (Radiodiagnosis)**
Assistant Professor, Department of Imaging
    and Intervention Radiology
Army Institute of Cardiothoracic Sciences
    (AICTS)
Pune, India

**Dr Sasikanth CM, MS (ENT)**
Assistant Professor
Base Hospital
Guwahati, India

**Dr Gunjan Dwivedi, MS**
Associate Professor, Department of ENT-HNS
Command Hospital (Southern Command)
Pune, India

**Dr Deepak Dwivedi, MS (Anaes)**
Associate Professor, Department of Anaesthesia
    and Critical Care
Command Hospital (Southern Command)
Pune, India

**Dr Sunil Goyal, MS**
Associate Professor, Department of ENT HNS
AHRR
Delhi Cantt, India

**Dr Atul Gupta, MS**
Assistant Professor ENT
153 General Hospital
Leh, India

**Dr Anandita Gupta, MS**
Assistant Professor ENT
Command Hospital (EC)
Kolkata, India

**Dr Mary John, MS, DNB, PhD**
Christian Medical College
Vellore, India

**Dr Anupam Kanodia, MS**
Senior Resident, Department of ENT and
    Head-Neck Surgery
All India Institute of Medical Sciences
New Delhi, India

**Dr Abha Kumari, MS**
Assistant Professor ENT
Command Hospital (SC)
Pune, India

**Dr Sabarigirish K, MS**
Professor ENT
Armed Forces Medical College
Pune, India

**Dr Virender Malik, MD (Radiodiagnosis)**
Assistant Professor, Department of Imaging
    and Intervention Radiology
Army Institute of Cardiothoracic Sciences
    (AICTS)
Pune, India

**Dr Smriti Panda, MS**
Assistant Professor, Department of
    Otolaryngology and Head and Neck
    Surgery
AIIMS
New Delhi, India

**Dr Uma Patnaik, MS, DNB**
Professor and Head of Department ENT
Command Hospital (SC)
Pune, India

**Dr N Ramakrishnan, MS**
Professor ENT
HQ 2 Corps
Ambala, India

**Dr Dilip Raghavan, MS**
Prof & HoD (ENT)
AFMC
Pune, India

**Dr SK Singh, MS (ENT), DNB (ENT)**
Professor, Deputy Director General (Medical)
Delhi Cantt, India

**Dr Roohie Singh, MS**
Associate Professor, Department of ENT HNS
Command Hospital (Air Force)
Bengaluru, India

**Dr Chirom Amit Singh, MS (ENT)**
Additional Professor, Department of
    Otolaryngology and Head and Neck
    Surgery
AIIMS
New Delhi, India

**Dr Rohit Singh, MS**
Senior Resident, Department of ENT
AFMC
Pune, India

**Dr Amit Sood, MS**
Assistant Professor ENT
Command Hospital (Southern Command)
Pune, India

**Dr Garima Upreti, MS**
Assistant Professor ENT
Christian Medical College
Vellore, India

**Dr Hitesh Verma, MS**
Associate Professor, Department of ENT and
   Head-Neck Surgery
All India Institute of Medical Sciences
New Delhi, India

## Editor Biography

**Dr Uma Patnaik** studied Otorhinolaryngology from Armed Forces Medical College, Pune. She further pursued her sub-speciality training in Neurotology under the aegis of Prof Mario Sana, Italy and AIIMS New Delhi. The focus of her work has been on neurotology, skull base and childhood hearing loss. She has been working on minimally invasive skull base surgery and hearing rehabilitation surgery.

Dr Uma's research work includes five funded projects. She has numerous research publications to her credit in various national/international journals. Her research has focused on clinical and applied aspects of otorhinolaryngological practice and has numerous awards for her research.

Outside of ENT, Dr Uma enjoys classical dance.

**Dr Amit Sood** is a graduate from Armed Forces Medical College and earned his MS (ENT) from Delhi University. He has a keen interest in skull base surgery and occupational hearing hazards. Dr Amit's research work includes funded research on effects of high-altitude and occupational noise exposure on hearing. He has various research publications to his credit. Dr Amit has a liking for adventure sports and has been involved in activities like parajumping and white water rafting.

**Dr Dilip Raghavan,** MS (ENT), is currently Professor & Head of the Department of Otorhinolaryngology at Armed Forces Medical College, Pune, India. He has been associated with Postgraduate Training of residents for close to two decades. He has a special interest in otology and paediatric hearing loss and has made numerous presentations and published many articles in his field of interest.

**Dr Sabarigirish K** is an officer in Armed Forces Medical Services of India, currently serving as Professor in the Department of ENT as well as the administrative head of graduate course at Armed Forces Medical College (AFMC), Pune. In his three decades of service, he has been in the teaching faculty at various tertiary care teaching hospitals of Armed Forces. He has been in the forefront for adoption of UNHS and has been credited for significant expansion of Cochlear Implant services in Armed Forces. With many major research projects and publications to his credit, he is an ardent proponent of the practice of evidence-based medicine in otolaryngology practice.

# SECTION I

# HEARING LOSS: APPROACH TO THE PATIENT AND MANAGEMENT

# 1 Hearing Loss in Children

*Mary John*

## CONTENTS

## INTRODUCTION

Hearing Loss (HL) in children is caused by a variety of conditions, of which congenital HL and Otitis Media (OM) are the most common. In recent times, otology has witnessed tremendous expansion with newer options for evaluation and management of HL. HL is one of the most common of all childhood disabilities where early identification and intervention provides better overall development and optimal performance of the child in the society (1, 2).

HL in newborns is a disability which can affect the speech and language acquisition and communication skills of the child. The estimated prevalence of congenital HL is 1–4/1000 population (3, 4). OM consisting of Acute Otitis Media (AOM), serous OM and Chronic Otitis Media (COM) is a common disease that causes HL in childhood.

Implementation of universal (newborn) hearing screening can help in early identification and rehabilitation of this correctable disability in children. The accessibility of imaging has revolutionized the diagnosis and follow-up of children with HL. The advancement in surgical techniques and implantable hearing devices has further improved hearing rehabilitation results.

This chapter summarizes the approach to a child with HL.

## REVIEW OF LITERATURE

### Paediatric Hearing Loss

Permanent Childhood Hearing Impairment (PCHI) is defined as confirmed permanent bilateral hearing impairment of ≥40 dB HL, averaged over the frequencies of 0.5, 1, 2 and 4 kHz in the better hearing ear. The prevalence of HL in children increases to 6% by the time the child starts primary school (5). As per WHO, disabling HL in children is termed more than 30 dB HL in the better ear. The classification according to the severity of the degree of HL is discussed in the section on adult HL.

### Workup of a Child with Hearing Loss

Since congenital HL is usually asymptomatic and early intervention is essential for the optimal performance of the child, history and examination should incorporate all details needed to identify various causes of HL. The onset of HL, pre-lingual or post-lingual, is an important factor in the management of the child. Conditions like microtia and anotia cause obvious deformity and are associated with conductive HL. AOM and middle ear effusion are more common causes of HL in children 5–8 years of age.

A detailed proforma including the relevant history for evaluation of a newborn with HL is provided in Figure 1.1. There are risk factors which increase HL in a child; however, nearly half of the times no risk factors are identified. The risk factors for HL in newborns adapted from the 2007 position statement of Joint Committee on infant hearing are given in Table 1.1 (6), the first three being considered as major risk factors (7, 8). Evaluation of a child with HL requires multiple specialty teamwork; the evaluation flowchart for a child with congenital HL is summarized in Figure 1.2.

Although autosomal recessive HL is the most common cause of genetic HL, HL can present in families with no history of HL. The prevalence of permanent Sensori Neural Hearing Loss (SNHL) will double by the second decade of life (9). Progressive HL can be associated with Pendred syndrome and congenital Cytomegalovirus (CMV) infection. Prematurity, hypoxia, sepsis and hyperbilirubinemia increase the risk of auditory neuropathy spectrum disorder. The risk of developing significant SNHL is 10% after meningitis and

it is considered as the most common cause of acquired HL (10, 11). Semicircular canal dehiscence, enlarged vestibular aqueducts, X-linked gusher and dilated internal auditory meati can cause third window effect and mixed HL. In countries with no rubella vaccine, congenital rubella syndrome is the most common cause of acquired congenital HL. CMV infection, especially in the first trimester, is considered a common cause of non-syndromic HL in western countries (12–14).

Vestibular function test is important in children with HL as 70% of children with profound HL can have some vestibular dysfunction (15, 16). Testing ability to stand on one foot with eyes closed for a minimum of 4 seconds in child with SNHL, aged 4 years and above, is a good screening test to detect bilateral vestibular impairment.

### Audiological Evaluation of Children with Hearing Loss

Assessment of hearing is crucial for management and can be challenging in young children. Hearing evaluation can be subjective or objective with the objective measurements more reliable in smaller children and children with learning disabilities (17). The audiological tests usually done for hearing assessment are summarized in Figure 1.3.

### Subjective Tests

*Behavioural Observation Audiometry* (BOA) assesses response of the infant less than 6 months of age to auditory stimuli such as warbled pure tones, narrowband noise and speech presented through speakers. However, BOA neither measures hearing thresholds accurately nor provides ear-specific information.

■ *Moros reflex:* Sudden movements of the limbs and extension of the head to 80–90 dB sound.

■ *Cochleo-palpebral reflex:* Blink to loud sounds.

■ *Cessation reflex:* Stops activity or starts crying for sound at 90 dB

*Visual Reinforcement Audiometry* (VRA) (18) is done for children between 6 months and 2 years of age to obtain frequency-specific testing of each ear. The child is required to turn to the sound source, usually at 90°, and is coupled with conditioned reinforcement like a lighted toy. Ear-specific information can be obtained by using insert earphones or headphones.

## Table 1.1: Common Risk Factors of Hearing Loss in Children

- Neonatal ICU stay more than 48 hours (major)
- Family history of childhood hearing loss (major)
- Craniofacial anomalies (major)
- In utero infection like CMV or toxoplasmosis
- Syndromes associated with hearing loss
- Neurodegenerative disorder
- Bacterial or viral meningitis
- Head trauma, especially skull base/ temporal bone fracture
- Chemotherapy
- Persistent otitis media for min 3 m
- Caregivers concerns regarding hearing or speech
- Birth weight less than 1500 g
- Hyperbilirubinemia requiring blood transfusion
- Others: respiratory distress syndrome, asphyxia, meconium aspiration, chromosomal abnormalities, drug / alcohol abuse by mother, maternal diabetes, prolonged ICU stay, APGAR score of 0–4 at 1 m, 0–6 at 5 m.

## HISTORY FOR CHILDREN WITH HEARING IMPAIRMENT

**CANDIDATE NAME:**    **HOSPITAL NO. :**

**DOB:**    **Age:**    **HANDEDNESS:** Right / Left / Ambidextrous

**INFORMANT:** Mother / Father / Adopted parents / Others    Date of examination: __/__/__

**INFORMANT EDUCATION STATUS:**    **SOCIOECONOMIC STATUS:** Low/Mid/Upper

**CHIEF COMPLAINTS:**
1. Hearing deficit
2. Delayed speech
3. Developmental. delay
4. Others

Duration: for _____

**HISTORY OF PRESENT ILLNESS / CONCERN:**

**MARITAL / FAMILY HISTORY:**

**PEDIGREE CHART**

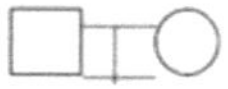

1. Non-consanguinity / Consanguinity ( I/II/III)
2. Contraceptive or fertility measures
3. Duration of marital life
4. Birth order / similar complaints in others

**ANTENATAL HISTORY:**

Antenatal check-ups / Antenatal scans / Gestational diabetes / Ecclampsia / Thyroid disorder / Immunization / TORCH infections / Exanthematous fever / HIV / Miscarriages / P/V bleeding / Trauma / Radiation / Environmental hazards / Exposure to teratogenic chemicals / Ototoxic medication / Alcoholism / Smoking / Others

**NATAL HISTORY:**

Full term / Preterm / Post term delivery    Weeks of Gestation _____

Delivery @ institutional / home    conducted by trained personnel or not

Mode of delivery – Normal vaginal delivery / Episiotomy / Forceps /

Caesarian section – indication _____

Birth weight – _____ kg  Normal / LBW / VLBW / Big baby    Cry at birth / asphyxia    APGAR score –

Congenital anomalies noted at birth – yes / no

**NEONATAL HISTORY:**

NICU /PICU stay / Breathing & feeding difficulty / Neonatal jaundice / Hyperbilirubinaemia / PUO / Phototherapy / Meningitis / Encephalitis / Septicaemia / Exanthematous fever / Seizures / Visual defects / Dysmorphic features / Trauma / ENT infections / Noise exposure / Transfusions / Hospital admissions / Ototoxic medications/ Noise trauma

**IMMUNIZATION:** Immunized: partial / complete    Not immunized

**MILESTONES:** normal / delayed globally

| GROSS MOTOR | months | FINE MOTOR | | Cognitive and Social Skills | | Speech and Language | |
|---|---|---|---|---|---|---|---|
| Neck Holding | 5 | Out reaching Hand | 4 | Recognition mother | 1 | Cooing | 2 |
| Sitting without support | 8 | Palmar grasp | 3.5 | Stranger anxiety | 7 | Monosyllables | 6 |
| Standing without support | 12 | Pincer Grasp | 9 | Says Bye Bye | 10 | Bisyllables | 10 |
| Walking | 14 | Scribbling | 13 | Self-feeding | 18 | 2 words | 12 |
| Running | 24 | Building blocks 6 cubes | 24 | Help to undress | 24 | 10 words | 18 |
| Climbing Stairs | 36 | Cooperates for dressing | 36 | Play simple games | 36 | 2 phrases | 24 |

Mode of communication – auditory verbal/ auditory oral/ lip reading/ sign language/ total/ nil

**SCHOOLING:** normal school / special school / do not go to school    performance- at par/ lagging

**HEARING LOSS:** Age when parents detected _____    Age when doctor consulted _____

Responds to loud sounds - Yes/ No

Intervention: investigated +/-: hearing aid  / wait

**SCREENING:** Yes/ not    **USE OF HEARING AID:** yes / no    Unilateral/Bilateral    duration -    Benefit

**SPEECH THERAPY:** given / not    duration -    benefit –

**OTHER SYSTEMS:** vision -    mental development / IQ -    syndromes –

**IMPRESSION:** Bilateral/Unilateral    Congenital Severe to Profound Hearing Loss

Syndromic/Non Syndromic _____

(Adapted from the hearing loss work up for children at Pediatric ENT Unit, Christian Medical College, Vellore.)

**Figure 1.1**  Proforma for Evaluation of Hearing Loss

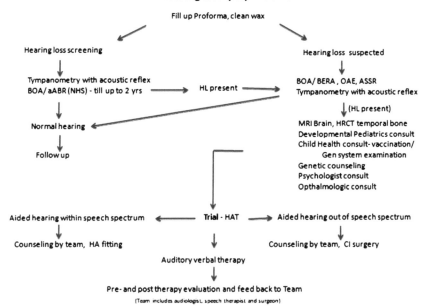

**Figure 1.2**  Flowchart for evaluation of children with hearing loss.

*Conditioned Play Audiometry* (CPA) is used for children from 2 years through 4–5 years. The aim of the testing is to obtain frequency and ear-specific information on both air conduction and bone conduction. Insert earphones are used for air conduction, whereas bone oscillators are used for bone conduction. The child is taught to listen to the sound and to perform an activity like putting a block in the box or pegs in a board as response.

*Pure Tone Audiometry* (PTA) can be done for children 4–5 years of age with average cognitive abilities. Ear-specific, air conduction and bone conduction thresholds can be measured using

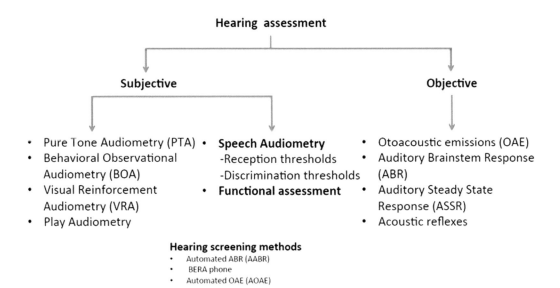

**Figure 1.3**  Tests of Hearing.

**Table 1.2: Examples of Speech Perception Tests Used in Assessment of Children with Hearing Loss and Children Fitted with Cochlear Implant**

| In Hearing Loss Children | | In Cochlear Implant Children | |
|---|---|---|---|
| Open-set | Closed-set | Open-set | Closed-set |
| Phonetically balanced kindergarten (PB-K) | Auditory numbers test (ANT) | Lexical neighbourhood test (LNT) | Monosyllabic trochee spondee (MTS) |
| | Pediatric speech intelligibility (PSI) | Hearing in noise test for children (HINT-C) | Early speech perception test (ESP) |
| | Word intelligibility by picture identification (WIPI) | Pediatric-AzBio sentence | auditory screening procedure (GASP) Glendonald |

pure tones with responses such as hand raising or button pushing.

*Speech audiometry* helps to understand the ability of the child to recognize and understand simple and complex sound stimuli. Sound field testing or testing for individual ears can be done. Speech detection threshold is the lowest intensity level the child is aware that a speech signal is delivered.

Speech Reception Threshold (SRT) is the minimum intensity at which the child can repeat 50% of the spondee words correctly. Pure tone averages and SRT correlates well within 6 dB. Speech perception threshold measures the ability of the child to discriminate speech at a suprathreshold level like conversational speech and detects the effect of HL in everyday conversation. The speech perception tests are done using closed-set tests and open-set tests; a few examples are given in Table 1.2.

*Objective Measurement*

Although the behavioural responses are the gold standard, objective measurement of hearing complements behavioural responses and can be done without the cooperation from the child, especially in smaller children.

*Otoacoustic Emissions* (OAE) are sound signals generated by outer hair cells of cochlea which are measured using a microphone kept in the ear canal. For clinical testing, two types of evoked OAEs are used: transient evoked OAE and distortion product OAE. OAE will be absent in HL more than 30 dB. A positive OAE response with absent ABR is suggestive of auditory neuropathy.

*Auditory Brainstem Response* (ABR) is the electrical potential recorded from a signal generated by the sound as it passes through the auditory pathway. In children, ABR is done under sedation or when the child is sleeping, using air conduction and bone conduction transducers. ABR report shows graphs with seven peaks representing specific areas of auditory pathway, with wave V being the most important one. The testing is started at the high intensity levels and then gradually

decreased to minimum intensity of sound needed to generate a reliable wave V.

*Auditory Steady-State Response* (ASSR) and *Cortical Evoked Response Audiometry* (CERA) are other audiological tests which can be done after routine objective investigations, especially for decision-making on surgical intervention like cochlear implant (CI) or brainstem implant. ASSR is an auditory-evoked potential which can assess the degree of HL.

**Functional Auditory Assessment**

Along with accurate diagnosis of the HL in a child, it is important to assess how the child functions in day-to-day life. There are various questionnaires designed for caregivers and teachers to obtain adequate information on the child's hearing and speech; some are summarized in Table 1.3 (19, 20).

**Table 1.3: Commonly Used Functional Auditory Assessment Tools**

| Tool | Age of the Child | Description |
|---|---|---|
| Infant toddler meaningful auditory integration scale (IT-MAIS) | Birth to 3 years | Parent questionnaire (10 Q) to assess the meaningful use of the sound |
| Little Ear: Auditory questionnaire | From birth | Parent questionnaire (35 Q) to assess the age appropriate auditory development |
| Auditory behaviour in everyday life (ABEL) | 2–12 years | 24-item questionnaire to assess the auditory behaviour in everyday life |
| Meaningful auditory integration scale (IT-MAIS) | 3 years and above | Parent questionnaire to assess the meaningful use of the sound |
| Children's home inventory for listening difficulties (CHILD) | 2–12 years | Questionnaire for both child and parents to rate speech understanding in 15 difficult situations |

Inconsistency between subjective and objective measurements can be due to Central Auditory Processing Disorder (CAPD), which is the inability of the brain to fully interpret and process sound with normal peripheral hearing.

### Neonatal Hearing Screening

Early identification and rehabilitation provide optimal results for congenital HL and can be achieved by neonatal hearing screening. Automated ABR (AABR) and OAE (AOAE) are two commonly used screening tools. Both have portable handheld screening devices, which use algorithms and display pass or refer to response during testing. The test and the protocol used depend on facilities available at each centre. Since 50% of the children diagnosed with HL do not have any risk factors, universal screening of all the newborns is recommended. AOAE is quick and cost-effective in terms of equipment and consumables compared to AABR, but it has high failure rate and can miss auditory neuropathy (21, 22).

The Joint Committee of Infant Screening 2007 Position Statement suggested all infants should have access to hearing screening by 1 month of age, confirmation of HL if present by 3 months of age and intervention by 6 months of age, which is termed as 1–3–6 rule (6).

### Radiological Evaluation of Children with Hearing Loss

A clear understanding of the osseous anatomy of the temporal bone can be obtained through high-resolution CT of the temporal bones.

However, MRI provides better soft tissue details, including membranous labyrinth and central auditory pathway along with identification of the intracranial pathologies (23, 24). MRI is costlier and needs sedation in younger children.

HRCT temporal bone is recommended for children with cholesteatoma (25). CT shows pneumatization of the mastoid air cell – variations in position of structures embedded in temporal bone. It will identify scutum erosion – an early sign of squamous COM, erosion of air cells, bony labyrinth, facial canal and tegmen tympani (26). Diffusion-weighted MRI (DW MRI) can differentiate cholesteatoma from inflammatory tissue and brain tissue; hence, it is useful in detecting recurrent or residual cholesteatoma after surgery (27, 28).

In congenital profound HL, morphologically only 20% of the malformations are bony which can be picked up by HRCT and the rest 80% will have a normal imaging. Jackler et al. in 1987 classified the congenital malformations of the inner ear as malformations of osseous and membranous labyrinth and malformations limited to membranous labyrinth (29). With the advances in imaging, especially HRCT, Sennaroglu et al. added more details to the classification and surgical approach to various anomalies (30, 31), which are summarized in Table 1.4.

Enlarged Vestibular Aqueduct (EVA) is the most common inner ear malformation (84%) detected in patients with SNHL (32). HL is often bilateral, progressive and fluctuating, though it can present as sudden SNHL also. The common syndromes associated with HL are described in

## Table 1.4: Classification of Inner Ear Malformations (IEM) and Their Characteristics

| Type of IEM | Radiological Findings | Type of Implant | Surgical Implications |
|---|---|---|---|
| Complete labyrinthine aplasia | Absent labyrinth | Brainstem implant | CI contraindicated, facial nerve anomalies may be present |
| Rudimentary otocyst | Remnant of otic capsule | Brainstem implant | CI contraindicated, facial nerve anomalies may be present |
| Cochlear aplasia | Absent cochlea | Brainstem implant | CI contraindicated |
| Common cavity | Fused cochlea and vestibule forming ovoid cystic structure | CI | Transmastoid labyrinthotomy or double labyrinthotomy lateral wall placing electrode |
| Cochlear hypoplasia | Smaller cochlea; type1-4 | CI or HA as per HL | If CI, short compressed electrode |
| Incomplete partition (IP) type 1 | Cystic cochlea | CI with a stopper | 50% CSF gusher, facial nerve abnormalities may be present |
| Incomplete partition (IP) type 2 | Basal turn normal; fused middle and apex turns | CI with a stopper | CSF oozer, 10% CSF gusher |
| Incomplete partition (IP) type 3 | Modiolus absent with interscala septa present | CI with a stopper | 100 % CSF gusher, lateral wall placing electrode |
| Enlarged vestibular aqueduct | Cochlea normal enlarged VA | CI/ HA | Varying degree of HL, progressive HL |
| Cochlear aperture abnormalities | Narrow or absent cochlear aperture | CI/ ABI | ABI in cochlear naplasia, CI in cochlear N hypoplasia |

Table 1.6 (33–38). The most common cause for bilateral postnatal acquired SNHL is meningitis (39). Cochlear ossification can be picked up by T2-weighted MRI, whereas fibrosis and earlier cochlear changes preceding ossification can be seen in T1-weighted MRI (40). Post-meningitic scarring and labyrinthine ossification following meningitis are concerns during cochlear implantation.

## DIFFERENTIAL DIAGNOSIS OF HEARING LOSS IN CHILDREN

HL in children can be congenital or acquired and progressive or fluctuant according to its onset and progression. It can also be classified according to the aetiology and severity of the HL. The management varies according to the cause, the age of the child, pre-lingual/post-lingual and the severity of HL.

### Congenital Hearing Loss

In nearly 45% of newborns with HL, the cause remains unknown. Among the remaining, nearly 60%, have a genetic cause and 70% of children with a genetic cause are non-syndromic (41). Nearly 80% of the non-syndromic HL is autosomal recessive and usually presents prelingually. Autosomal dominant type is around 20%, which is usually progressive and post-lingual, and 1% is X-linked recessive/mitochondrial inheritance (42). GJB2 mutation, the gene that encodes the protein Conexin 26, accounts for nearly 50% of non-syndromic severe to profound HL (43) and can be screened with Sanger sequencing. The differential diagnosis of PCHI is summarized in Table 1.5.

In autosomal recessive type, the hearing-impaired child has normal parents and relatives; there is 25% chance for siblings to develop HL. The genes identified are enumerated by letters "DFN" followed by "A" if gene is dominant and by "B" if the gene is recessive. The mutation of gene OTOF encoding the protein otoferlin, a protein needed for synaptic transmission, and expressed in inner hair cell also causes autosomal recessive HL (auditory neuropathy).

The common syndromes causing HL are summarized in Table 1.6.

*Management of Congenital Hearing Loss:* Management of HL in children needs multi-disciplinary approach, including otolaryngologist, audiologist, speech therapist, paediatrician, child psychiatrist and ophthalmologist. It also

## Table 1.5: Aetiology and Classification of Hearing Loss in Children

**Congenital Hearing Loss**

| | | |
|---|---|---|
| Genetic | Syndromic | Autosomal recessive (AR) |
| | | Autosomal dominant (AD) |
| | | X-linked |
| | | Mitochondrial |
| | Non-syndromic | Autosomal recessive (AR) |
| | | Autosomal dominant (AD) |
| | | X-linked |
| | | Mitochondrial |
| Non-genetic | | Congenital rubella syndrome, CMV infection, congenital syphilis, toxoplasmosis |
| | | Drugs during pregnancy – aminoglycosides, antiepileptic drugs, cytotoxic drugs, antimalarial drugs, diuretics |
| | | Maternal substance abuse – alcohol, drugs |
| | | Maternal endocrine disorder – thyroid dysfunction, DM |
| | | Third window effect caused by SSC dehiscence, EVA, X-linked gusher syndrome, enlarged IAM |

**Acquired Hearing Loss**

| | |
|---|---|
| Perinatal | Hypoxia |
| | Hyperbilirubinaemia |
| | Low birth weight |
| | Birth asphyxia |
| | Birth trauma – intracranial haemorrhage |
| Postnatal | Infections – meningitis, measles, mumps, COM, Herpes, HIV |
| | Ototoxic drugs |
| | Trauma and noise exposure |
| | Neoplastic disorder, immune system disorder, foreign body EAC |
| Idiopathic | |

*Source:* Adapted from Scott-Brown, 8th edition; Chapter 10: Management of the hearing impaired child.

**Table 1.6: Summary of Common Syndromes Causing Hearing Loss**

| Syndrome | Chromosomal Abnormality | Ear Abnormality | Other Abnormalities | HL-related Radiological Findings |
|---|---|---|---|---|
| Down's syndrome | Trisomy 21 | Small low set pinna, narrow EAC, IAC stenosis, ossicular and vestibular malformation, OME Conductive or mixed hearing loss | Brachycephaly, upslanting palpebral fissures, flat facial profile with epicanthal folds and brushfield spots, upper airway obstruction with macroglossia and increased risk for atlanto-occipital subluxation during intubation, mental retardation, single palmar crease, heart disease, wide sandal gap | Narrow external and internal ear canals with ossicular abnormalities |
| Treacher Collins | TCOF1 gene mutations First and second arch abnormalities | Bilateral microtia, CCA, ossicular abnormalities Conductive hearing loss | Micrognathia, cleft palate, mandibular hypoplasia and flat malar region, down slanting palpebral fissures, coloboma of the lower eyelids, sparse eye lashes | Narrow or absent external ear canals with ossicular abnormalities, absent mastoid pneumatization, a bony cleft in the lateral aspect of the temporal bone |
| Goldenhar | Several chromosomal abnormalities U//L first and second arch abnormalities | Unilateral microtia, preauricular appendages, ossicular abnormalities, abnormal facial nerve | Hemifacialmicrosomia, epibulbardermoid, congenital heart disease and vertebral abnormalities | Unilateral smaller external ear with ossicular abnormalities and abnormal facial canal |
| CHARGE | CHD7 gene mutations Autosomal dominant | Dysplastic (short, wide) pinnae, various middle and inner ear abnormalities, facial nerve palsy Sensorineural /mixed/conductive hearing loss of varying degree | Coloboma, **Heart** defects, **A**tresia choanae, **R**etarded growth and development, **G**enital abnormalities, **E**ar abnormalities | Hypoplasia of SCC, abnormalities of ossicular chain and facial nerve |
| Branchio-oto-renal | EYA1, SIX1 and SIX5 gene mutations Autosomal dominant | Preauricular sinuses or tags, ossicular abnormalities WVA malformed cochlea and vestibular apparatus | Branchial cleft abnormalities and renal malformations | Malformed ossicles, tapered basal turn and hypoplasia of the middle and apical turns of cochlea – "unwound appearance" |
| Alports syndrome | Gene mutation that codes for collagen 1V | Sensorineural hearing loss – varying and progressive | Nephropathy, lenticonus and macular flecks | |
| Pendred syndrome | Autosomal recessive | Congenital sesorineural hearing loss | Hypothyroidism and goiter. perchlorate testing replaced by genetic testing | Mondini malformation and EVA |
| Usher syndrome | Autosomal recessive | Hearing loss | Progressive retinitis pigmentosa. Three types depending on the degree of hearing loss and vestibular dysfunction | |
| Waardenburg syndrome | Autosomal dominant | Congenital HL | Synophrys, heterochromia iridium, white forlock, dystopia canthorum, heterochromicirides | Aplasia of the posterior semicircular canal, poorly developed vestibule and EVA |
| Jervell Lange-Neilson syndrome | Autosomal recessive | Profound hearing loss | Syncopal attacks, prolonged QT interval, ventricular tachycardia of ventricular fibrillation | |
| Congenital rubella syndrome | | Congenital hearing loss | Growth retardation and mental retardation, cataracts and pigmentary retinopathy; patent ductus arteriosus, peripheral pulmonary artery stenosis | |

requires ongoing monitoring to detect progressive or late-onset HL. Exposure to consistent and meaningful sounds during the early years of the child is required for the development of auditory neural pathways. Hence, early identification and management is required. Auditory-oral communication assisted by hearing aids (HAs) or CI results in highest levels of educational achievements and job opportunities for a child.

*Hearing Aids:* HAs provide the child with audible broad frequency range of speech at soft to loud levels. Air conduction HAs are commonly used, which amplify the sound transmitted via the ear canal to the tympanic membrane (TM). In chronically draining ears, atresia of the ear canal where HA cannot be used or in patients with severe conductive/mixed HL, bone conduction HAs are beneficial. Behind the ear type is the most common HA used in children. The ear mould should snugly fit in the ear canal to reduce acoustic feedback and help retention of the device. In younger children, regular follow-up is required as the ear canal volume increases, requiring changes in ear mould.

*Implantable Auditory Devices (IADs):* IADs are active implants and can be acoustic or electrical implants. Acoustic implants transduce acoustic sound energy to the perilymph through one of the pathways – ossicular chain, skull vibration or direct stimulation. The electrical implants, the CI and auditory brainstem implants (ABI) stimulate the cochlear nerve or brain stem nuclei electrically.

Acoustic implants work using various principles and include bone-conducting devices, active middle ear implants and direct acoustic cochlear stimulators and can be partially or fully implantable (44–47). The summary of the acoustic implants is given in Table 1.7.

*Bone-Anchored Hearing Aid (BAHA):* BAHA works by transmitting sound through the bone using an osseo-integrated abutment, which can be percutaneous or transcutaneous. The

## Table 1.7: Summary of the Middle Ear Implants Used in Children

| Type | Examples | Indications and Age | Features | Disadvantages |
|---|---|---|---|---|
| *Bone conduction devices (BCD)* | | | | |
| Skin drive | Baha Attract Sophono | SSD, mild to moderate CHL, chronic discharging ear, CCA >5 years of age (FDA) | Osseointegration – external processor with internal magnet fixed to mastoid bone Short surgery | Transcutaneous energy loss MRI incompatible |
| Direct drive | Baha Connect Ponto | SSD, mild to moderate CHL, chronic discharging ear, CCA, radiated bone >5 years of age (FDA) | Osseointegration – external processor on percutaneous abutment fixed to mastoid bone Short surgery | Abutment visible Skin infection and reaction MRI compatible |
| Direct drive (active) | Bonebridge | SSD, mild to moderate CHL, chronic discharging ear, CCA >5 years of age (EU, FDA not approved in children) | External processor magnetically attaches to the internal transducer fixed to mastoid bone | MRI incompatible Need favourable mastoid anatomy – pre-op CT and planning |
| *Active middle ear implants* | | | | |
| Partially implantable | Vibrant sound bridge | Moderate-severe to severe CHL/mixed HL, CCA, advanced otosclerosis 5 years (EU, FDA not in children) | External processor with internal floating mass transducer (FMT) FMT couple to ossicular chain | MRI incompatible Need favourable mastoid anatomy – pre-op CT and planning Surgery challenging CI in active ME disease, radiation and tumour |
| Fully implantable | Carina | Moderate-severe to severe CHL/mixed HL, cosmetic reasons, poor tolerance to HA | Internal sensor and transducer couple to ossicular chain | MRI incompatible Need favourable mastoid anatomy – pre op CT and planning Surgery challenging CI in active ME disease, radiation and tumour Reoperation for battery change |

common indications are when conventional HA cannot be fitted and in single-sided deafness (48). BAHA soft band can be used in children till there is reasonable skull thickness to fix the abutment, which is usually at 5 years of age. Soft tissue complications are more common in children and include soft tissue reactions, implant infections, soft tissue overgrowth of the abutment and failure of osseointegration (49, 50).

*Cochlear Implants:* CI has revolutionized hearing rehabilitation in pre-lingually deaf children with the aim to restore the hearing for adequate speech and language development (51). It replaces the non-functional transducer system of the hair cells of cochlea by converting the sound signals into electronic signals, thus directly stimulating the cochlear nerve. According to the latest NICE guidelines, the candidacy for CI has been expanded with revision of hearing thresholds for CI candidacy. Children with hearing level less than 70 dB and with poor aided speech understanding are considered for CI as per the revised criteria (73). Children with profound HL implanted as early as less than 1 year with bilateral CI develop better binaural skills, better language skills and thus more chance of attending normal school (52).

*Cochlear Implant in Congenital Malformations*: The facial nerve course can be altered in cochlear hypoplasia and common cavity deformities. When the basal turn of the cochlea is not well-formed, electrode insertion through facial recess approach may be difficult and alternative methods such as transmastoid labyrinthotomy, scala vestibular insertion, canal wall down (CWD) with blind sac closure, trans-canal approach are planned (53, 54). In common cavity, an electrode with complete contact rings and hypoplastic cochlea, shorter electrode, will be more beneficial. Cerebrospinal fluid (CSF) gusher is the main complication, especially in incomplete partition type 3, which can be managed by using tissue threaded through the electrode as stopper or using electrode with a stopper. Radiologically, when cochlear nerve aplasia/cochlear aperture stenosis is suspected, electrically evoked ABR (eABR) is a useful tool; if present, it indicates the favourability for CI. However auditory outcome after CI in cochlear nerve hypoplasia is poor (55). CI is contraindicated in cochlear aplasia and absent cochlear nerve and is an indication for ABI.

Auditory neuropathy spectrum disorder (ANSD) patients can benefit with CI in selected cases like OTOF gene mutation (56, 57). However, children with associated hypoplastic cochlear nerve and abnormal electrically evoked compound action potential (ECAP) have poorer outcomes (58, 59). In case of COM, staged surgery can be performed with clearing of the disease and making the ear dry at the first stage, followed by implantation at a later stage.

The electrode can be inserted through the round window (60) after drilling the round window niche or extended round window or through a cochleostomy. Insertion via cochleostomy provides more favourable angle and thus can be less traumatic (60); however, round window insertion decreases the risk of traumatizing basilar membrane and acoustic/mechanic trauma to the cochlea from drilling a fenestram (61). However, studies have not shown much difference in the audiological outcome (62) and hearing preservation (63). Atraumatic insertion techniques include minimal manipulation of the ossicles, minimizing cochlear bony drilling, avoidance of perilymph suctioning and slow insertion of the electrode (64). Soft insertion technique minimizes cochlear reaction to the implant, which also includes avoidance of bone dust and blood entering the cochlea and topical application of the steroids just before the electrode insertion (65). A small amount of hyaluronic acid will act as a barrier to bone dust and blood, decreases the electrode insertion force by lubrication and hence may be beneficial for hearing preservation (66). Early age of implantation, use of peri-operative steroids, electrode length and insertion depth also contribute to success of hearing preservation techniques (67, 68).

Postoperative measurements of impedance and neural responses along with check X-ray (modified Stenver's view) confirm the optimal placement of the electrodes. After 2–3 weeks, the CI is switched on, mapping is done, an optimal programme for the CI made and auditory verbal therapy is commenced. Complications are usually rare with the incidence less than 3%; however, increased incidence is noted in malformed cochleae (69, 70). Wound infection, facial/chorda tympani nerve (71) injury, CSF fistula, device failure and cholesteatoma are the possible complications of CI surgery.

Multiple factors, including age of the implantation, residual hearing, prior use of HAs, consistent use, family support and motivation and rehabilitation, will affect the outcome of implantation. In children with complex needs, the results can be obtained by quality of life measurement parameters (72). CI technology is rapidly progressing with newer less traumatic electrode designs, research and animal model studies looking at gene therapy and delivery of drugs to cochlea and development of totally implantable CI.

*Auditory Brainstem Implants:* ABI directly stimulate the cochlear nuclei electrically. ABI surgery was introduced in children after it was successfully done in adults (74). Along with cochlear/cochlear nerve aplasia, severe cochlear ossification and advanced cochlear otosclerosis are the indication for ABI (75). Labyrinthine and retrosigmoid approach have been used for ABI placement. Cerebral oedema, CSF leak, meningitis, bleeding and facial nerve palsy are the usual complications (76). Only few children will develop open-set speech discrimination after ABI (77, 78).

*Assistive Listening/Alerting Devices:* For optimum listening in noisy environment, a signal-to-noise ratio of 20 dB is advisable, which helps those with hearing impaired to listen efficiently in the background noise, over telephone and in auditoriums or theatres. Frequency modulation (FM) devices, induction loops, amplitude modulation system and infrared signals are used. In older children, in a daily situation like doorbell or an alarm, an extra loud signal is relayed to alert the child; vibrations or flashing lights can also be used for assistance. Devices fitted to the telephone like a telephone amplifier which amplifies the telephone sound or a telephone coupler which allows the signals from the telephone to be picked up by the HAs can also be used.

## Congenital Abnormalities of External and Middle Ear

Abnormalities of the external ear canal cause obstruction of air conduction mechanism and thus HL. Severe external ear deformity is usually associated with middle ear ossicular chain deformity; many of them with named syndromes are summarized in **Table 1.6**.

Congenital Canal Atresia (CCA) can cause conductive HL and is commonly associated with severe degree of microtia. The prevalence of microtia is 1/10,000. CCA and microtia are graded according to the increasing severity of deformity, which is summarized in Table 1.8 (79, 80).

*Management:* The Management of Microtia and CCA should consider auditory rehabilitation and cosmesis. Nearly 90% of the patients have normal cochlear function. Bone conduction hearing device (BCHD) is a good option for Hearing Rehabilitation in Children (81). For the pinna deformity, the options available will include no treatment, autologous ear reconstruction using cartilage, Bone-Anchored Auricular Prosthesis (BAAP).

Isolated middle ear abnormalities are rare and usually are minor malformations with delay in diagnosis. Minor malformation was classified by Cremer and modified by Tos into four subtypes: isolated stapes ankylosis, stapes

## Table 1.8: Common Grading and Description of Microtia and Congenital Canal Atresia (CCA)

|  | Grading System | Grades Description and Significance | | | |
|---|---|---|---|---|---|
| Microtia | Weerda (according to surgical management) | 1° dysplasia Most structures of pinna present | 2° dysplasia some structures of pinna present | 3° dysplasia none of the structures of pinna are clear | Anotia or absence of the ear |
|  |  | No additional skin/cartilage for reconstruction | Partial reconstruction – some skin/ cartilage | Total construction: lot of skin/ cartilage | |
|  | Marx (According to clinical appearance) | Grade 1 Small pinna, all features present | Grade 2 Some features recognizable | Grade 3 Rudiment of skin and cartilage | Grade 4 Absent pinna/ear canal |
| CCA | Weerda (According to clinical appearance) | Type A Marked narrowing with intact skin layer | Type B Partial patency lateral wall with medial atretic plate | Type C Complete atresia of the ear canal | |
|  | Jahrsdoefer (According to imaging) | Parameters – points Stapes present – 2 Open oval window – 1 Middle ear space – 1 Mastoid well pneumatized – 1 Malleus/ incus complex normal – 1 Round window normal – 1 Incus /stapes connection – 1 External ear appearance – 1 | Rating for surgery 10 – excellent for surgery 9 – very good 8 – good 7 – fair 6 – marginal <5 – poor | | |

ankylosis with other ossicular anomaly, isolated ossicular anomaly and aplasia/dysplasia of oval widow or round windows. Unilateral or bilateral conductive HL, normal TM and normal middle ear status are the usual findings, which can be misdiagnosed as OM. HRCT temporal bone along with middle ear endoscopy assist diagnosis (82, 83). Auditory rehabilitation can be achieved by HA or BAHA, according to severity of the condition. Surgical reconstruction should be attempted only by experienced surgeons due to the expertise required and the chance of SNHL.

### Acquired Abnormalities of External and Middle Ear

Local irritation of the external auditory canal by trauma, inflammation or burns can cause acquired EAC stenosis. It can be of two types – solid or membranous – with solid being more common (84) and can be complicated by canal cholesteatoma. During the wet/discharging phase, regular ear cleaning and topical treatment is required. HL can be addressed by bone conduction or air conduction HAs. Long-term success after surgery requires expertise (85). Exostosis are multiple bony swellings in the EAC with strong association with cold water exposure and are usually asymptomatic (86). Osteomas are single bony swellings of EAC. However, if the EAC is significantly obstructed, it can cause conductive HL and will require surgical removal (87, 88).

### Otitis Media

Otitis Media (OM), the most common cause of acquired HL in children, can be classified as Acute Otitis Media (AOM), Serous Otitis Media (SOM) or Chronic Otstis Media (COM).

Any factor predisposing to eustachian tube (ET) dysfunction, which includes recurrent upper respiratory infections, exanthematous fever, nasal allergy, adenoid hypertrophy causing obstruction in the tubal end of ET, tumours of the nasopharynx, palatal paralysis and anomalies like cleft palate causing impaired function of the tensor palati muscle, increases the chances of OM (89). There are multiple risk factors for the OM, which include genetic, ethnicity, defect in the immunity and environmental factors such as day care attendance, poor socioeconomic status and passive smoking (90).

### Acute Otitis Media

It is one of the commonest illness of the childhood with the highest incidence at the first year of life (91, 92). AOM can be defined as inflammation of the middle ear cleft of acute onset and infective origin associated with middle ear effusion and varied signs and symptoms.

According to the nature of the AOM, it can be divided into four subgroups: sporadic, resistant, persistent and recurrent. It usually starts as a viral infection, which later becomes secondarily infected with bacteria. The predominant clinical features are due to presence of inflammation, although HL is also a symptom.

The most common route of spread of infection from upper airway is via the eustachian tube either through the lumen or along the subepithelial peritubal lymphatics. The eustachian tube is shorter, wider and more horizontal in children and some ethnic populations (93), thus making them more prone for OM. Infection can also reach the middle ear via a perforation in the TM or through blood (rare).

*Aetiology:* The most common organisms that cause AOM are *Streptococcus pneumoniae*, *Moraxella catarrhalis* and *Haemophilus influenzae*. In 60–90% of the children with AOM, respiratory viruses, especially respiratory syncytial virus (RSV), have been detected (94).

*Clinical features:* The child usually presents with otalgia and fever. Examination may reveal a mild conductive HL along with findings of a retracted/hyperaemic/red bulging TM, which clinches the diagnosis (95). Otalgia may be relieved with onset of otorrhoea, which is initially bloodstained and later becomes muco-purulent.

*Treatment:* In uncomplicated AOM, watchful waiting can be considered as two-thirds of children will recover in 24 hours with or without treatment. Antibiotic is recommended for AOM in children less than 6 months, if more than 6 months with severe symptoms (pyrexia [>39°C], severe otalgia), recurrent episodes in less than 2 years and not responding after watchful waiting for 2 days. Children who are at high-risk OM also require antibiotics. Amoxicillin 80–90 mg/kg/day is the dose recommended for 10–14 days. For persistent or resistant AOM, higher dose of amoxycillin will help in treating resistant pneumococcal infection. However, *Haemophilus* being beta-lactam producing may require broad-spectrum antibiotics. If allergic to penicillin, cefdinir, cefuroxime or ceftriaxone is advised (95, 178).

Systemic analgesic either acetaminophen or ibuprofen is recommended for pain management, though topical analgesics may provide short-lived benefit (96). Decongestant nasal drops, oral anti histamine and corticosteroids (97) are supportive measures for which the level of evidence is debatable. Modification of the risk factors (day care attendance, parental smoking, absence of breastfeeding, usage of pacifier use, supine bottle feeding) (98) and antibiotic prophylaxis during winter months are also recommended. Vaccination against causative organism like *S. pneumoniae* has proven beneficial (99).

Myringotomy is indicated to release the tension of the pus accumulation if the TM is still bulging after a week of antibiotics or incomplete resolution with persistent HL or when effusion persists beyond 12 weeks. Ventilation tubes were shown to reduce the number of episodes of AOM by 50%, though cautious interpretation of the study is required (100).

### Serous Otitis Media

**(OM with effusion (OME)/secretory OM/glue ear)** Serous otitis media is termed as accumulation of fluid in the middle ear cleft, which is usually thick and viscid. OME is termed chronic, if it persists for a minimum of 3 months (101). Nearly 80% of the children will have at least one episode of OME before the age of 3 years (102). Boys are more affected and those with less pneumatized mastoids are more prone for OME. A review of multiple studies showed that the distribution of OME showed two peaks: one at around 2 years, when the social contact of the child increases, and another at 5 years, the time when child enters preschool (103). Though OME is not considered to have infective aetiology, positive bacteriological culture has been observed in the middle ear aspirate of children with OME. In another study, biofilms were demonstrated from middle ear mucosal biopsy in 92% of patients undergoing grommet insertion. In the temperate climates, the incidence of OME was twice in winter months as compared to summer months (104, 105). Unilateral OME is twice as common as bilateral OME.

Eustachian tube dysfunction and increased secretory activity of the middle ear mucosa are the two major mechanisms in the pathogenesis of OME (106, 107). Unresolved otitis media due to inadequate treatment and other factors can lead to increase in mucous production and OME. Allergy and upper respiratory viruses can cause increased secretory activity of the middle ear mucosa. Gastroesophageal reflux disease (GORD) and craniofacial anomalies can also be associated with OME (108).

*History:* HL is usually mild (less than 25 dB) and can be the only symptom, which may pass unnoticed in nearly 80% cases (109). Difficulty in understanding in a noisy environment is more evident in children. Seasonal fluctuation of HL may be observed. Behavioural issues along with inattention may be noticed by children attending day care by the teachers (110). Delayed speech and language development may occur secondary to the HL. Child may also have symptoms of associated pathology like upper respiratory infection, allergy, adenoid hypertrophy etc.

*Examination:* Otoscopic examination of small children can be challenging; however, otomicroscopy has an accuracy more than 90% in diagnosing OME (111). On examination, the TM appear dull and lustreless with varying shades of yellow, grey or blue in colour. The position of the TM can be retracted or bulged out due to fluid with the restriction of mobility, fluid level or air bubbles.

*Investigations:* Tuning fork test results are confirmed with audiometry and shows conductive HL usually within 25–30 dB. Audiometry also helps to rule out associated causes of HL, including SNHL. The "B"-type tympanogram is suggestive of middle ear fluid. The combined sensitivity of type "B" tympanogram with otoscopic findings is 98%. When HL is confirmed, active monitoring of HL for 3 months are advised (112).

*Management:* The aim of the treatment is removal of fluid and prevention of recurrence. In half the children, it resolves in 3 months, but in 5% it can persist even after 1 year. In more than 90% of the patients, the OME resolves in 9 months, but there is a chance of recurrence.

*Medical:* Topical decongestants in the form of drops or spray help to relieve the mucosal oedema. Antihistamine and topical steroid spray will be beneficial in allergy (113). Antibiotics have been found to be beneficial in treating upper respiratory infection. However, according to studies, none of the above medications have significant effect in improving OME (114). Amoxycillin-clavulanic acid combination was found to be beneficial in short term. Auto-inflation methods like Valsalva's manoeuvre (115), repeated swallowing and using chewing gum can improve the ventilation of the middle ear cleft. Hib immunization have also shown to have positive effect on resolution of OME.

*Surgical:* In children with documented HL with bilateral OME for a minimum of 3 months, recurrent AOM, and at-risk children with unilateral or bilateral OME, myringotomy and grommet insertion are recommended (116). At-risk children are prone to developmental difficulties due to physical, sensory or cognitive disorder (117). Myringotomy is done by placing a radial incision in the antero-inferior quadrant of the TM. The radial incision can prevent excessive damage to the middle layer and hold the grommet in place. When the mucous is thick, saline or mucolytic agents can be used to thin out the mucous before aspiration. Continued aeration of the middle ear is obtained by grommet insertion, which can be long stay or short stay ones, individualized depending on the pathology. Short-term tubes such as Shah tubes and Paparella tubes usually extrude between 6 and 14 months, whereas long-term tubes can stay up to 2 years (115). Titanium or gold or silver oxide coated grommets prevent biofilm formation. Antibiotic-coated grommet was shown to prevent biofilm formation in vitro. Adenoidectomy/ tonsillectomy may be combined with grommet insertion to treat the causative factor.

*Sequelae:* The long-standing nature of the disease can cause dissolution of the fibrous layer of the TM leading to atrophic changes and atelectasis of the TM. Ossicular necrosis though rare can also occur, mostly affecting long process of the incus causing the HL to worsen. Tympanosclerosis, cholesterol granuloma, retraction pockets (RPs) and cholesteatoma can also be sequelae of OME.

### Chronic Otitis Media

The term COM comprises varied pathology resulting from chronic middle ear inflammation. The incidence of COM is estimated to be 31 million cases globally, with the highest incidence occurring in the first year of life and the highest percentage of affected people occurring geographically in Oceania (118). Environmental factors and population characteristics play a role in the prevalence of COM, with American Indians, Australian Aborigines and Eskimos having the highest incidence in the developed countries, probably due to genetic predisposition (119, 120).

Continuous inflammation in COM causes submucosal cellular infiltration, increased vascularity and increase in goblet cell production. There is osteitis with bone destruction, to which the body react with healing and repair. COM can be active with ongoing inflammation or can be inactive where there is no active inflammation, but there is a chance to become active. Healed COM (Figure 1.4) is resolved inflammation with time or by medical or surgical intervention. The description and clinical features of mucosal and squamosal COM are given in Table 1.9.

The prevalence of COM is more in lower socioeconomic group of people. Nutritional and environmental factors, including lack of hygiene, predisposes children to COM (121). COM has much higher incidence in children with cleft

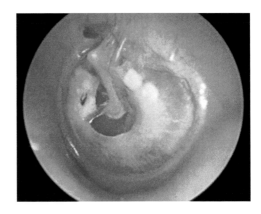

**Figure 1.4** Left healed tympanic membrane. (Courtesy of *Scott-Brown's Otorhinolaryngology Head and Neck Surgery*; Chronic Otitis Media; George G Browning, Justin Weir, Gerard Kelly, Iain R C Swan; Paediatrics, The Ear, Skull Base; Eighth Edition; Volume 2; 2018; Page 992, Chapter 83: Figure 83.17; reproduced with permission.)

**Table 1.9: Summary of the Types of Chronic Otitis Media (COM)**

| Types | Description | Findings |
|---|---|---|
| COM mucosal inactive | Permanent perforation in the pars tensa, with non-inflamed ME mucosa | Central dry perforation |
| COM mucosal active | Permanent perforation in the pars tensa, with inflamed ME mucosa and discharge | Discharge – mucoid, profuse, non-foul smelling, non-blood stained Pale polyps, granulation uncommon |
| COM squamosal inactive | Retraction of the pars tensa or pars flaccida with a potential to become active | Retraction pocket with visible fundus |
| COM squamosal active | Retraction of the pars tensa or pars flaccida with retained squamous epithelial debris, with inflammation, discharge | Discharge is scanty, foul smelling and purulent. Inflamed polyps, granulation common |
| COM healed | Thinning of pars tensa (local/ generalized) with or without thickened opaque TM | Dimeric drum/ tympanosclerosis |

palate – at 10 years follow-up, 20% developed pars tensa retraction (122) and 2% developed cholesteatoma (123). Biofilms are also associated more commonly with COM (124). Tympanosclerosis is found in 25% of the ears undergoing surgery. *Pseudomonas aeruginosa*, *Proteus mirabilis* and *Staphylococcus aureus* are the common organisms isolated from patients with COM (125).

### COM Mucosal

COM mucosal presents with TM changes, like perforation, tympanosclerosis or atrophy, and ossicular changes, including erosion or fixation. It develops as a sequela to AOM with perforation of pars tensa. The margin of the perforation epithelializes making it permanent, thus permitting repeated infection from the ear canal. The middle ear mucosa gets exposed to the external environment and is sensitized to airborne allergens causing persistent otorrhea.

*Diagnosis:* Ear discharge and HL are the most common symptoms. HL is usually conductive type. Otoscopic examination will show a central perforation with sizes varying from small to subtotal (Figure 1.5). Ear findings are confirmed by examination under microscope, after clearing the discharge if present. Audiogram is done to assess the type and severity of the HL. The degree of HL depends on the size of the perforation, erosion of the ossicles especially long process of the incus and tympanosclerosis obstructing ossicular mobility (126).

*Treatment:* Aural toilet is done usually using microscope and suction clearance. Topical

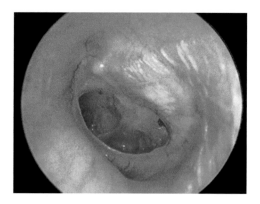

**Figure 1.5** Left COM mucosal inactive type showing tympanic membrane with central perforation. (Courtesy of *Scott-Brown's Otorhinolaryngology Head and Neck Surgery*; Chronic Otitis Media; George G Browning, Justin Weir, Gerard Kelly, Iain R C Swan; Paediatrics, The Ear, Skull Base; Eighth Edition; Volume 2; 2018; Page 992, Chapter 83: Figure 83.19; reproduced with permission.)

antibiotics drops are more effective compared to systemic antibiotics (127–129). Quinolone antibiotics (ciprofloxacin/ofloxacin) are the preferred topical agents used in active COM (130). Supportive measures like treatment of the underlying infective and allergic focus in the upper respiratory tract is done. The aim of the surgery is to reduce the hearing disability and to prevent recurrent ear infection. Most surgeons prefer to do myringoplasty at 7 years of age as ET function improves at 7 years. The success rate of tympanoplasty in expert hands is around 95% (131); though longer follow-up showed recurrent perforation (132). The failure rate is higher in larger perforation and anterior perforations, which can be overcome by tucking the anterior margin beneath the annulus (133). The success rate is reduced after revision surgery (132).

In patients with air-bone gap more than 35 dB, ossicular erosion or fixation due to tympanosclerosis is expected and requires ossiculoplasty (126). The most common ossicle to be affected is long process of incus. If the handle of the malleus is also eroded, then prosthesis sitting over the stapes head (PORP – partial ossicular replacement prosthesis) connecting to TM can be used. Prosthesis over footplate (TORP – total ossicular replacement prosthesis) is used, if stapes suprastructure is also absent. The choice of the prosthesis depends on the diseased ear, availability of the prosthesis and surgeon's expertise. An analysis done by Lurato et al. showed that when malleus and stapes suprastructure were present, the postoperative air-bone gap of 0–10 dB was achieved in experts hand only in 50% of the cases (134).

Ossiculoplasty results are significantly affected by the status of the middle ear along with prosthesis design and surgical technique. The materials used for reconstruction are autograft (incus most commonly used), alloplastic materials (Table 1.10) and to a less extent homograft. Meaningful analysis of the results of ossiculoplasty can be done by various classifications proposed by Austin (135, 136), Belluci (137) and Kartush (138) and Middle

### Table 1.10: Materials Used for Ossiculoplasty

| Material | Examples |
| --- | --- |
| Solid plastics | Polytetrafluoroethylene, polyethylene |
| Solid metals | Stainless steel, gold, titanium |
| Porous sponge-like plastics | Proplast®, Plasti-Pore® |
| Ceramics | Aluminium oxide, hydroxyapatite |

## Table 1.11: Various Classifications of Ossicular Chain Defects and Middle Ear Status

**Austin Classification with Absent Incus**

| Group 1 | Malleus handle (M)+ ; Stapes suprastructure (S)+ |
| Group 2 | M+ S– |
| Group 3 | M– S+ |
| Group 4 | M– S– |

Middle Ear Risk Index (MERI)

| Otological factor | Maximum score |
| --- | --- |
| Otorrhoea | 3 |
| Perforation | 1 |
| Cholesteatoma | 2 |
| Ossicular status | 4 |
| Middle ear granulations | 2 |
| Previous surgery | 2 |
| Smoking | 2 |

**Kartush Modification of Ossicular Status**

| Group O | Intact ossicular chain |
| Group E | Ossicular head fixation |
| Group F | Stapes fixation |

Belluci classification of otorrhoea

| Otorrhoea | Risk value |
| --- | --- |
| Dry ear | 0 |
| Occasionally wet | 1 |
| Persistently wet | 2 |
| Persistently wet + cleft palate | 3 |

Ear Risk Index (MERI) (139), which are summarized in Table 1.11.

### COM Squamous

"**Cholesteatoma** is a mass formed by keratinizing squamous epithelium in the middle ear/mastoid, sub-epithelial connective tissue and by the progressive accumulation of the keratin debris with or without surrounding inflammatory reaction" (140). It can be congenital or acquired.

Congenital cholesteatoma (Figure 1.6) is an expanding cystic mass with keratinizing squamous epithelium, located medial to the intact TM, assumed to be present at birth, but usually diagnosed during infancy or in early childhood in patients with no prior history of otorrhea, perforation or previous ear surgery (140). The most accepted theory of congenital cholesteatoma is persistence of epidermoid cell that rests in anterior epitympanum (141). A four-point staging system was used by Potsic (142) to describe the extent of the spread of cholesteatoma.

Acquired cholesteatoma can be primary or secondary. Primary acquired cholesteatoma develops with in-growth of keratin epithelium through the perforation of the TM or due to trauma or can be iatrogenic.

The pathogenesis of secondary acquired cholesteatoma is not clear and there are four theories – metaplasia theory/retraction theory, immigration theory and the basal hyperplasia theory. The RP can develop either in pars tensa or pars flaccida; when the pocket cannot self-clean, it will cause slow invasion. The RPs can be present in pars tensa (143) (Figure 1.7) or pars flaccida (144)

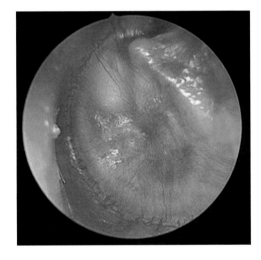

**Figure 1.6** Left ear congenital cholesteatoma. (Courtesy of *Scott-Brown's Otorhinolaryngology Head and Neck Surgery*; Chronic Otitis Media; William P L Hellier; Paediatrics, The Ear, Skull Base; Eighth Edition; Volume 2; 2018; Page 158, Chapter 15: Figure 15 .2; reproduced with permission.)

(Figure 1.8) and can be graded into four types, as is described in Table 1.12.

Paediatric cholesteatoma is more aggressive and extensive (145) with higher recurrence rate (146), due to immaturity of the ET function, and thus need long-term follow-up. Eustachian tube dysfunction leading to negative middle ear pressure and retraction of the TM is the most widely accepted theory.

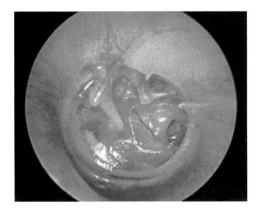

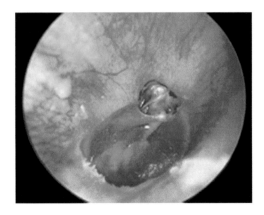

**Figure 1.7** Grade 4 retraction pocket of the pars tensa. (Courtesy of *Scott-Brown's Otorhinolaryngology Head and Neck Surgery;* Chronic Otitis Media; George G Browning, Justin Weir, Gerard Kelly, Iain R C Swan; Paediatrics, The Ear, Skull Base; Eighth Edition; Volume 2; 2018; Page 994, Chapter 83: Figure 83:29; reproduced with permission.)

**Figure 1.8** Retraction pocket in the pars flaccida. (Courtesy of *Scott-Brown's Otorhinolaryngology Head and Neck Surgery;* Chronic Otitis Media; George G Browning, Justin Weir, Gerard Kelly, Iain R C Swan; Paediatrics, The Ear, Skull Base; Eighth Edition; Volume 2; 2018; Page 995 Chapter 83: Figure 83: 33; reproduced with permission.)

*Diagnosis:* HL and ear discharge are the common symptoms and on examination the presence of RP with keratin pearls is diagnostic of COM squamous active. Inactive squamous type will present with RPs without keratin debris. However, in smaller children, eliciting the history and examination remain a challenge. Diagnosing unilateral disease or congenital cholesteatoma is even more challenging.

*Treatment: Retraction Pockets:* Self-cleaning RPs have to be closely monitored in children. Small RPs can be regularly cleaned. Surgical treatment is to prevent discharge, prevent progression of RP and improve hearing. This also includes management of TM and ventilation of the middle ear. Excision of RP and grafting of the TM is a good option in most of the cases (147, 148).

Ventilation tubes do not have long-term effect on TM RPs (149, 150).

*Cholesteatoma:* The primary treatment modality is surgery with the aim of eradication of all cholesteatoma and any complication, thus making the ear dry and self-cleaning and preventing further recurrence. The surgical procedure can be broadly divided into CWD surgery or less invasive canal wall up (CWU) procedures. CWD procedures include inside-out surgery like atticotomy +/− reconstruction, modified radical mastoidectomy and subtotal petrosectomy for extensive diseases, which can be combined with cavity obliteration techniques. CWU procedures are mastoidectomy, combined approach tympanoplasty and tympanoplasty. The advantages of CWU procedure over CWD are it does not need

### Table 1.12: Classification of Retraction Pockets in Pars Tensa and Pars Flaccida

| Pars Tensa Retraction Pocket (Sade et al.) 140 | | Pars Flaccida Retraction Pocket (Tos et al.) 141 | |
|---|---|---|---|
| Grade 1 | Minimal retraction of pars tensa | Grade 1 | Dimple in PF, not attached to malleus |
| Grade 2 | Retraction touching the long process of the incus | Grade 2 | RP attached to malleus neck, full extent visible |
| Grade 3 | Retraction touching the medial wall but can lift up | Grade 3 | RP full extent not visible, minimal erosion of bony attic wall |
| Grade 4 | Retraction adherent to medial wall | Grade 4 | Definite erosion of bony attic wall with extent of RP not visible |

repeated cleaning of cavity and HA can be fitted if HL warrants; however, there is more chance for recurrence. Studies support better audiological outcomes with CWU procedures (151, 152). However, the procedure is technically more demanding and requires a second look surgery. In the recent times, endoscopic ear surgery has become adjuvant to microscopic ear surgery (153, 154), the efficacy and safety of this technique are validated in paediatric cholesteatoma (155, 156).

In OM, if not treated appropriately, patients can develop extracranial complications such as acute mastoiditis, abscesses in relation to pinna, labyrinthitis, facial palsy, petrositis and intracranial complications such as extradural abscess, subdural abscess, meningitis, brain abscess, lateral sinus thrombosis and otitic hydrocephalus (157).

### Other Causes of Hearing Loss in Children

**Unilateral Hearing Loss**: It is one condition which is under-diagnosed, but it has a prevalence of 0.6 per 1000 (8) among neonatal screening and 1 per 1000 among school-age children. Children with unilateral HL showed lower oral language scores, manifested behavioural issues and some required academic assistance; the maximum effect is seen in children with profound HL (162). Preferential seating, frequency modulating system, conventional HAs and contralateral routing of signal (CROS) aids are found to be beneficial (163). **Single-sided deafness** (SSD) is defined as severe to profound HL with minimal benefit with hearing amplification and normal hearing in contralateral ear (164). CI is the available option for the SSD which can provide binaural auditory input (165, 166).

**Ototoxicity:** The common drugs causing ototoxicity are aminoglycosides – amikacin, streptomycin and tobramycin, antitumour agents – cisplatin, antimalarials – quinine, chloroquine, and loop diuretics – frusemide; these medications need to be used with caution with serial audiogram to document hearing level.

**Sudden sensorineural hearing loss**: It is an otological emergency with HL of 30 dB or more developing in three consecutive frequencies in less than 72 hours (167). The possible causes can be infectious, traumatic, metabolic, neurologic, circulatory, toxic or others; immediate management mainly consists of anti-inflammatory such as steroids (168) and antivirals.

### DISCUSSION

The WHO lists HL as one of the leading causes of disability and one of the leading causes of burden of disease globally. For any disability, prevention can be primary, secondary or tertiary. Genetic counselling (158), immunization, avoidance of trauma and ototoxic medications (159) constitute primary prevention of HL. Hearing screening (68, 160) and treatment of HL are considered secondary prevention and early rehabilitation of HL (161), the tertiary prevention. Newer and improved methods are added rapidly to all these areas, thus making management options for children with HL better every day.

### RECENT ADVANCES

The advancement made in genetics in recent years, for example, whole genome sequencing, has helped to map deafness and other associated traits to specific chromosomes, thus helping to identify the causes of various syndromic and non-syndromic HL. In bilateral SNHL, genetic testing proves to be high yielding with identification of cause in 44% cases (169, 170).

The introduction of smaller diameter endoscopes with high definition has expanded the field view and improved resolution of endoscopic ear surgery as compared to microscopic ear surgery (171). Angled endoscopes enable to visualize areas which are difficult to assess such as sinus tympani and epitympanum (172). Incorporation of flexible fibre $CO_2$ laser (173) and ultrasonic bone curette (174) has broadened the endoscopic ear surgery indications. Ear-specific 3D printed temporal bones with add-on details of external and middle ears will be highly beneficial for skills training of paediatric otologists. Robotic-assisted and robotic-performed otological surgery that has potential to decrease the morbidity and improve the outcomes is still under development stage.

Medical therapy for SNHL targets inner ear for novel gene therapy, RNA-based therapy and stem cell therapy. It aims at modification of hair cells or auditory neurons at cellular level through gene therapy to augment protein production that may protect or regenerate hair cells (175); RNA-based therapy to inhibit protein that causes hair cell damage (176) and stem cell therapy to replace damaged or dead hair cells or auditory neurons (177).

### CONCLUSION

In the formative years of childhood, HL caused by a variety of reasons can go unnoticed affecting the overall development of the child and suboptimal performance in the society. Early detection and tailor-made treatment is highly rewarding owing to the recent advances which are rapidly evolving and redefining the diagnosis and management. Research in this field, especially gene therapy and stem cell therapy, are promising and hopefully will bring better answers to this disability of HL.

## REFERENCES

1. Korver AM, Konings S, Dekker FW, et al. Newborn hearing screening vs later hearing screening and developmental outcomes in children with permanent childhood hearing impairment. JAMA. 2010;304(15):1701–8.

2. Ching TY, Dillon H, Marnane V, et al. Outcomes of early- and late-identified children at 3 years of age: findings from a prospective population-based study. Ear Hear. 2013;34(5):535–52.

3. Cunningham M, Cox EO, Committee on Practice and Ambulatory Medicine and the Section on Otolaryngology and Bronchoesophagology. Hearing assessment in infants and children: recommendations beyond neonatal screening. Pediatrics. 2003;111(2):436–40.

4. John M, Balraj A, Kurien M. Neonatal screening for hearing loss: pilot study from a tertiary care centre. Indian J Otolaryngol Head Neck Surg. 2009;61(1):23–6.

5. WHO. Addressing the Rising Prevalence of Hearing Loss. Geneva: World Health Organization, 2018.

6. American Academy of Pediatrics, Joint Committee on Infant Hearing. Year 2007 position statement: principles and guidelines for early hearing detection and intervention programs. Pediatrics. 2007;120(4):898–921.

7. Davis A, Wood S. The epidemiology of childhood hearing impairment: factor relevant to planning of services. Br J Audiol. 1992;26(2):77–90.

8. Controlled trial of universal neonatal screening for early identification of permanent childhood hearing impairment. Wessex Universal Neonatal Hearing Screening Trial Group. Lancet. 1998;352(9145):1957–64.

9. Fortnum HM, Summerfield AQ, Marshall DH, Davis AC, Bamford JM. Prevalence of permanent childhood hearing impairment in the United Kingdom and implications for universal neonatal hearing screening: questionnaire based ascertainment study. BMJ. 2001;323(7312):536–40.

10. Drake R, Dravitski J, Voss L. Hearing in children after meningococcal meningitis. J Paediatr Child Health. 2000;36(3):240–3.

11. Wellman MB, Sommer DD, McKenna J. Sensorineural hearing loss in postmeningitic children. Otol Neurotol. 2003;24(6):907–12.

12. Dahle AJ, Fowler KB, Wright JD, Boppana SB, Britt WJ, Pass RF. Longitudinal investigation of hearing disorders in children with congenital cytomegalovirus. J Am Acad Audiol. 2000;11(5):283–90.

13. Barbi M, Binda S, Caroppo S, Ambrosetti U, Corbetta C, Sergi P. A wider role for congenital cytomegalovirus infection in sensorineural hearing loss. Pediatr Infect Dis J. 2003;22(1):39–42.

14. Foulon I, Naessens A, Foulon W, Casteels A, Gordts F. Hearing loss in children with congenital cytomegalovirus infection in relation to the maternal trimester in which the maternal primary infection occurred. Pediatrics. 2008;122(6):e1123–7.

15. Cushing SL, Papsin BC, Rutka JA, James AL, Gordon KA. Evidence of vestibular and balance dysfunction in children with profound sensorineural hearing loss using cochlear implants. Laryngoscope. 2008;118(10):1814–23.

16. Cushing SL, Papsin BC, Rutka JA, James AL, Blaser SL, Gordon KA. Vestibular end-organ and balance deficits after meningitis and cochlear implantation in children correlate poorly with functional outcome. Otol Neurotol. 2009;30(4):488–95.

17. Rupa V. Dilemmas in auditory assessment of developmentally retarded children using behavioural observation audiometry and brain stem evoked response audiometry. J Laryngol Otol. 1995;109(7):605–9.

18. Gravel JS, Traquina DN. Experience with the audiologic assessment of infants and toddlers. Int J Pediatr Otorhinolaryngol. 1992;23(1):59–71.

19. Robbins AM, Renshaw JJ, Berry SW. Evaluating meaningful auditory integration in profoundly hearing-impaired children. Am J Otol. 1991; 12(Suppl): 144–50.

20. Purdy SC, Farrington DR, Moran CA, Chard LL, Hodgson SA. A parental questionnaire to evaluate children's Auditory Behavior in Everyday Life (ABEL). Am J Audiol. 2002;11(2):72–82.

21. Benito-Orejas JI, Ramirez B, Morais D, Almaraz A, Fernandez-Calvo JL. Comparison of two-step transient evoked otoacoustic emissions (TEOAE) and automated auditory brainstem response (AABR) for universal newborn hearing screening programs. Int J Pediatr Otorhinolaryngol. 2008;72(8):1193–201.

22. Doyle KJ, Burggraaff B, Fujikawa S, Kim J, Macarthur CJ. Neonatal hearing screening with otoscopy, auditory brain stem response, and otoacoustic emissions. Otolaryngol Head Neck Surg. 1997;116(6):597–603.

23. Bamiou DE, Phelps P, Sirimanna T. Temporal bone computed tomography findings in bilateral sensorineural hearing loss. Arch Dis Child. 2000; 82(3):257–60.

24. Mafong DD, Shin EJ, Lalwani AK. Use of laboratory evaluation and radiologic imaging in the diagnostic evaluation of children with sensorineural hearing loss. Laryngoscope. 2002;112(1):1–7.

25. Ayache D, Darrouzet V, Dubrulle F, et al. Imaging of non-operated cholesteatoma: clinical practice guidelines. Eur Ann Otorhinolaryngol Head Neck Dis. 2012;129(3):148–52.

26. Yildirim-Baylan M, Ozmen CA, Gun R, Yorgancilar E, Akkus Z, Topcu I. An evaluation of preoperative computed tomography on patients with chronic otitis media. Indian J Otolaryngol Head Neck Surg. 2012;64(1):67–70.

27. Li PM, Linos E, Gurgel RK, Fischbein NJ, Blevins NH. Evaluating the utility of non-echo-planar diffusion-weighted imaging in the preoperative evaluation of cholesteatoma: a meta-analysis. Laryngoscope. 2013;123(5):1247–50.

28. Muzaffar J, Metcalfe C, Colley S, Coulson C. Diffusion-weighted magnetic resonance imaging for residual and recurrent cholesteatoma: a systematic review and meta-analysis. Clin Otolaryngol. 2017;42(3):536–43.

29. Jackler RK, Luxford WM, House WF. Congenital malformations of the inner ear: a classification based on embryogenesis. Laryngoscope. 1987;97(3 Pt 2 Suppl 40): 2–14.

30. Sennaroglu L. Cochlear implantation in inner ear malformations: a review article. Cochlear Implants Int. 2010;11(1):4–41.

31. Sennaroglu L, Bajin MD. Classification and current management of inner ear malformations. Balkan Med J. 2017;34(5):397–411.

32. Madden C, Halsted M, Benton C, Greinwald J, Choo D. Enlarged vestibular aqueduct syndrome in the pediatric population. Otol Neurotol. 2003;24(4):625–32.

33. Morzaria S, Westerberg BD, Kozak FK. Systematic review of the etiology of bilateral sensorineural hearing loss in children. Int J Pediatr Otorhinolaryngol. 2004;68(9):1193–8.

34. Madden C, Halsted MJ, Hopkin RJ, Choo DI, Benton C, Greinwald JH, Jr. Temporal bone abnormalities associated with hearing loss in Waardenburg syndrome. Laryngoscope. 2003;113(11):2035–41.

35. Huang BY, Zdanski C, Castillo M. Pediatric sensorineural hearing loss, part 2: syndromic and acquired causes. AJNR Am J Neuroradiol. 2012;33(3):399–406.

36. Robson CD. Congenital hearing impairment. Pediatr Radiol. 2006;36(4).309–24.

37. Jahrsdoerfer RA, Aguilar EA, Yeakley JW, Cole RR. Treacher Collins syndrome: an otologic challenge. Ann Otol Rhinol Laryngol. 1989;98(10):807–12.

38. Gruen PM, Carranza A, Karmody CS, Bachor E. Anomalies of the ear in the Pierre Robin triad. Ann Otol Rhinol Laryngol. 2005;114(8):605–13.

39. Lalwani AK, Castelein CM. Cracking the auditory genetic code: nonsyndromic hereditary hearing impairment. Am J Otol. 1999;20(1):115–32.

40. Isaacson B, Booth T, Kutz JW, Jr., Lee KH, Roland PS. Labyrinthitis ossificans: how accurate is MRI in predicting cochlear obstruction? Otolaryngol Head Neck Surg. 2009;140(5):692–6.

41. Shearer AE, Smith RJ. Genetics: advances in genetic testing for deafness. Curr Opin Pediatr. 2012; 24(6):679–86.

42. Hilgert N, Smith RJ, Van Camp G. Function and expression pattern of nonsyndromic deafness genes. Curr Mol Med. 2009;9(5):546–64.

43. Angeli S, Utrera R, Dib S, et al. GJB2 gene mutations in childhood deafness. Acta Otolaryngol. 2000; 120(2):133–6.

44. Agterberg MJ, Frenzel H, Wollenberg B, Somers T, Cremers CW, Snik AF. Amplification options in unilateral aural atresia: an active middle ear implant or a bone conduction device? Otol Neurotol. 2014;35(1):129–35.

45. Verhaert N, Fuchsmann C, Tringali S, Lina-Granade G, Truy E. Strategies of active middle ear implants for hearing rehabilitation in congenital aural atresia. Otol Neurotol. 2011;32(4):639–45.

46. Frenzel H, Hanke F, Beltrame M, Steffen A, Schonweiler R, Wollenberg B. Application of the Vibrant Soundbridge to unilateral osseous atresia cases. Laryngoscope. 2009;119(1):67–74.

47. Siegert R, Mattheis S, Kasic J. Fully implantable hearing aids in patients with congenital auricular atresia. Laryngoscope. 2007;117(2):336–40.

48. Tjellstrom A, Hakansson B, Granstrom G. Bone-anchored hearing aids: current status in adults and children. Otolaryngol Clin North Am. 2001; 34(2):337–64.

49. McDermott AL, Williams J, Kuo M, Reid A, Proops D. The Birmingham pediatric bone-anchored hearing aid program: a 15-year experience. Otol Neurotol. 2009;30(2):178–83.

50. Kiringoda R, Lustig LR. A meta-analysis of the complications associated with osseointegrated hearing aids. Otol Neurotol. 2013;34(5):790–4.

51. Kral A, O'Donoghue GM. Profound deafness in childhood. N Engl J Med. 2010;363(15):1438–50.

52. Semenov YR, Yeh ST, Seshamani M, et al. Age-dependent cost-utility of pediatric cochlear implantation. Ear Hear. 2013;34(4):402–12.

53. Yiin RS, Tang PH, Tan TY. Review of congenital inner ear abnormalities on CT temporal bone. Br J Radiol. 2011;84(1005):859–63.

54. McElveen JT, Jr., Carrasco VN, Miyamoto RT, Linthicum FH, Jr. Cochlear implantation in common cavity malformations using a transmastoid labyrinthotomy approach. Laryngoscope. 1997;107(8): 1032–6.

55. Zanetti D, Guida M, Barezzani MG, et al. Favorable outcome of cochlear implant in VIIIth nerve deficiency. Otol Neurotol. 2006;27(6):815–23.

56. Gibson WP, Sanli H. Auditory neuropathy: an update. Ear Hear. 2007;28(2 Suppl):102S–6S.

57. Wu CC, Hsu CJ, Huang FL, et al. Timing of cochlear implantation in auditory neuropathy patients with OTOF mutations: our experience with 10 patients. Clin Otolaryngol. 2018;43(1):352–7.

58. Walton J, Gibson WP, Sanli H, Prelog K. Predicting cochlear implant outcomes in children with auditory neuropathy. Otol Neurotol. 2008;29(3):302–9.

59. Teagle HF, Roush PA, Woodard JS, et al. Cochlear implantation in children with auditory neuropathy spectrum disorder. Ear Hear. 2010;31(3):325–35.

60. Hamamoto M, Murakami G, Kataura A. Topographical relationships among the facial nerve, chorda tympani nerve and round window with special reference to the approach route for cochlear implant surgery. Clin Anat. 2000;13(4):251–6.

61. Meshik X, Holden TA, Chole RA, Hullar TE. Optimal cochlear implant insertion vectors. Otol Neurotol. 2010;31(1):58–63.

62. Adunka OF, Dillon MT, Adunka MC, King ER, Pillsbury HC, Buchman CA. Cochleostomy versus round window insertions: influence on functional outcomes in electric-acoustic stimulation of the auditory system. Otol Neurotol. 2014;35(4):613–8.

63. Havenith S, Lammers MJ, Tange RA, et al. Hearing preservation surgery: cochleostomy or round window approach? A systematic review. Otol Neurotol. 2013;34(4):667–74.

64. Kiefer J, Gstoettner W, Baumgartner W, et al. Conservation of low-frequency hearing in cochlear implantation. Acta Otolaryngol. 2004;124(3):272–80.

65. Friedland DR, Runge-Samuelson C. Soft cochlear implantation: rationale for the surgical approach. Trends Amplif. 2009;13(2):124–38.

66. Skarzynski H, Lorens A, D'Haese P, et al. Preservation of residual hearing in children and post-lingually deafened adults after cochlear implantation: an initial study. ORL J Otorhinolaryngol Relat Spec. 2002;64(4):247–53.

67. Nguyen Y, Mosnier I, Borel S, et al. Evolution of electrode array diameter for hearing preservation in cochlear implantation. Acta Otolaryngol. 2013;133(2):116–22.

68. Robinshaw HM. Early intervention for hearing impairment: differences in the timing of communicative and linguistic development. Br J Audiol. 1995;29(6):315–34.

69. Ramsden JD, Papsin BC, Leung R, James A, Gordon KA. Bilateral simultaneous cochlear implantation in children: our first 50 cases. Laryngoscope. 2009;119(12):2444–8.

70. Broomfield SJ, Murphy J, Wild DC, Emmett SR, O'Donoghue GM, Writing for the UK National Pediatric CI Surgical Audit Group. Results of a prospective surgical audit of bilateral paediatric cochlear implantation in the UK. Cochlear Implants Int. 2014;15(5):246–53.

71. Leung RM, Ramsden J, Gordon K, Allemang B, Harrison BJ, Papsin BC. Electrogustometric assessment of taste after otologic surgery in children. Laryngoscope. 2009;119(10):2061–5.

72. Rafferty A, Martin J, Strachan D, Raine C. Cochlear implantation in children with complex needs: outcomes. Cochlear Implants Int. 2013;14(2):61–6.

73. Carlson ML, Sladen DP, Haynes DS, et al. Evidence for the expansion of pediatric cochlear implant candidacy. Otol Neurotol. 2015;36(1):43–50.

74. Colletti V, Carner M, Fiorino F, et al. Hearing restoration with auditory brainstem implant in three children with cochlear nerve aplasia. Otol Neurotol. 2002; 23(5):682–93.

75. Sennaroglu L, Colletti V, Manrique M, et al. Auditory brainstem implantation in children and non-neurofibromatosis type 2 patients: a consensus statement. Otol Neurotol. 2011;32(2):187–91.

76. Colletti V, Carner M, Miorelli V, Guida M, Colletti L, Fiorino F. Auditory brainstem implant (ABI): new frontiers in adults and children. Otolaryngol Head Neck Surg. 2005;133(1):126–38.

77. Teagle HFB, Henderson L, He S, Ewend MG, Buchman CA. Pediatric auditory brainstem implantation: surgical, electrophysiologic, and behavioral outcomes. Ear Hear. 2018;39(2):326–36.

78. Sung JKK, Luk BPK, Wong TKC, Thong JF, Wong HT, Tong MCF. Pediatric auditory brainstem implantation: impact on audiological rehabilitation and tonal language development. Audiol Neurootol. 2018; 23(2):126–34.

79. Weerda H. Classification of congenital deformities of the auricle. Facial Plast Surg. 1988;5(5):385–8.

80. Jahrsdoerfer RA, Yeakley JW, Aguilar EA, Cole RR, Gray LC. Grading system for the selection of patients with congenital aural atresia. Am J Otol. 1992;13(1):6–12.

81. Alasti F, Van Camp G. Genetics of microtia and associated syndromes. J Med Genet. 2009;46(6):361–9.

82. Nakasato T, Sasaki M, Ehara S, et al. Virtual CT endoscopy of ossicles in the middle ear. Clin Imaging. 2001;25(3):171–7.

83. Karhuketo TS, Ilomaki JH, Dastidar PS, Laasonen EM, Puhakka HJ. Comparison of CT and fiberoptic videoendoscopy findings in congenital dysplasia of the external and middle ear. Eur Arch Otorhinolaryngol. 2001;258(7):345–8.

84. Becker BC, Tos M. Postinflammatory acquired atresia of the external auditory canal: treatment and results of surgery over 27 years. Laryngoscope. 1998; 108(6):903–7.

85. Magliulo G. Acquired atresia of the external auditory canal: recurrence and long-term results. Ann Otol Rhinol Laryngol. 2009;118(5):345–9.

86. Graham MD. Osteomas and exostoses of the external auditory canal: a clinical, histopathologic and scanning electron microscopic study. Ann Otol Rhinol Laryngol. 1979;88(4 Pt 1):566–72.

87. Fenton JE, Turner J, Fagan PA. A histopathologic review of temporal bone exostoses and osteomata. Laryngoscope. 1996;106(5 Pt 1):624–8.

88. House JW, Wilkinson EP. External auditory exostoses: evaluation and treatment. Otolaryngol Head Neck Surg. 2008;138(5):672–8.

89. Bluestone CD, Swarts JD. Human evolutionary history: consequences for the pathogenesis of otitis media. Otolaryngol Head Neck Surg. 2010;143(6):739–44.

90. Kong K, Coates HL. Natural history, definitions, risk factors and burden of otitis media. Med J Aust. 2009;191(S9):S39–43.

91. Stangerup SE, Tos M. Epidemiology of acute suppurative otitis media. Am J Otolaryngol. 1986;7(1):47–54.

92. Pukander J, Luotonen J, Sipila M, Timonen M, Karma P. Incidence of acute otitis media. Acta Otolaryngol. 1982;93(5–6):447–53.

93. Casselbrant ML, Mandel EM. The genetics of otitis media. Curr Allergy Asthma Rep. 2001;1(4):353–7.

94. Greenberg DP. Update on the development and use of viral and bacterial vaccines for the prevention of acute otitis media. Allergy Asthma Proc. 2001;22(6):353–7.

95. Lieberthal AS, Carroll AE, Chonmaitree T, et al. The diagnosis and management of acute otitis media. Pediatrics. 2013;131(3):e964–99.

96. Foxlee R, Johansson A, Wejfalk J, Dawkins J, Dooley L, Del Mar C. Topical analgesia for acute otitis media. Cochrane Database Syst Rev. 2006(3):CD005657.

97. Ranakusuma RW, Pitoyo Y, Safitri ED, et al. Systemic corticosteroids for acute otitis media in children. Cochrane Database Syst Rev. 2018;3:CD012289.

98. Schilder AG, Chonmaitree T, Cripps AW, et al. Otitis media. Nat Rev Dis Primers. 2016;2:16063.

99. Zhao AS, Boyle S, Butrymowicz A, Engle RD, Roberts JM, Mouzakes J. Impact of 13-valent pneumococcal conjugate vaccine on otitis media bacteriology. Int J Pediatr Otorhinolaryngol. 2014;78(3):499–503.

100. Venekamp RP, Mick P, Schilder AG, Nunez DA. Grommets (ventilation tubes) for recurrent acute otitis media in children. Cochrane Database Syst Rev. 2018;5:CD012017.

101. Rosenfeld RM, Shin JJ, Schwartz SR, et al. Clinical practice guideline: otitis media with effusion executive summary (update). Otolaryngol Head Neck Surg. 2016;154(2):201–14.

102. Teele DW, Klein JO, Rosner B. Epidemiology of otitis media during the first seven years of life in children in greater Boston: a prospective, cohort study. J Infect Dis. 1989;160(1):83–94.

103. Zielhuis GA, Rach GH, van den Bosch A, van den Broek P. The prevalence of otitis media with effusion: a critical review of the literature. Clin Otolaryngol Allied Sci. 1990;15(3):283–8.

104. Rovers MM, Straatman H, Ingels K, van der Wilt GJ, van den Broek P, Zielhuis GA. The effect of ventilation tubes on language development in infants with otitis media with effusion: a randomized trial. Pediatrics. 2000;106(3):E42.

105. Midgley EJ, Dewey C, Pryce K, Maw AR. The frequency of otitis media with effusion in British preschool children: a guide for treatment. ALSPAC Study Team. Clin Otolaryngol Allied Sci. 2000;25(6):485–91.

106. Paradise JL, Rockette HE, Colborn DK, et al. Otitis media in 2253 Pittsburgh-area infants: prevalence and risk factors during the first two years of life. Pediatrics. 1997;99(3):318–33.

107. Tos M. Epidemiology and natural history of secretory otitis media. Am J Otol. 1984;5(6):459–62.

108. Miura MS, Mascaro M, Rosenfeld RM. Association between otitis media and gastroesophageal reflux: a systematic review. Otolaryngol Head Neck Surg. 2012;146(3):345–52.

109. Lo PS, Tong MC, Wong EM, van Hasselt CA. Parental suspicion of hearing loss in children with otitis media with effusion. Eur J Pediatr. 2006;165(12):851–7.

110. Gouma P, Mallis A, Daniilidis V, Gouveris H, Armenakis N, Naxakis S. Behavioral trends in young children with conductive hearing loss: a case-control study. Eur Arch Otorhinolaryngol. 2011;268(1):63–6.

111. Young DE, Ten Cate WJ, Ahmad Z, Morton RP. The accuracy of otomicroscopy for the diagnosis of paediatric middle ear effusions. Int J Pediatr Otorhinolaryngol. 2009;73(6):825–8.

112. Khanna R, Lakhanpaul M, Bull PD, Guideline Development Group. Surgical management of otitis media with effusion in children: summary of NICE guidance. Clin Otolaryngol. 2008;33(6):600–5.

113. Lack G, Caulfield H, Penagos M. The link between otitis media with effusion and allergy: a potential role for intranasal corticosteroids. Pediatr Allergy Immunol. 2011;22(3):258–66.

114. Simpson SA, Lewis R, van der Voort J, Butler CC. Oral or topical nasal steroids for hearing loss associated with otitis media with effusion in children. Cochrane Database Syst Rev. 2011(5):CD001935.

115. Simon F, Haggard M, Rosenfeld RM, et al. International consensus (ICON) on management of otitis media with effusion in children. Eur Ann Otorhinolaryngol Head Neck Dis. 2018; 135(1S):S33–S9.

116. Rosenfeld RM, Shin JJ, Schwartz SR, et al. Clinical practice guideline: otitis media with effusion (update). Otolaryngol Head Neck Surg. 2016;154(1 Suppl):S1–S41.

117. Rosenfeld RM, Schwartz SR, Pynnonen MA, et al. Clinical practice guideline: tympanostomy tubes in children: executive summary. Otolaryngol Head Neck Surg. 2013;149(1):8–16.

118. Monasta L, Ronfani L, Marchetti F, et al. Burden of disease caused by otitis media: systematic review and global estimates. PLoS One. 2012;7(4):e36226.

119. Wiet RJ. Patterns of ear disease in the southwestern American Indian. Arch Otolaryngol. 1979;105(7): 381–5.

120. Jassar P, Murray P, Wabnitz D, Heldreich C. The posterior attic: an observational study of aboriginal Australians with chronic otitis media (COM) and a theory relating to the low incidence of cholesteatomatous otitis media versus the high rate of mucosal otitis media. Int J Pediatr Otorhinolaryngol. 2006;70(7):1165–7.

121. Lehmann D, Tennant MT, Silva DT, et al. Benefits of swimming pools in two remote Aboriginal communities in Western Australia: intervention study. BMJ. 2003;327(7412):415–9.

122. Ovesen T, Blegvad-Andersen O. Alterations in tympanic membrane appearance and middle ear function in 11-year-old children with complete unilateral cleft lip and palate compared with healthy age-matched subjects. Clin Otolaryngol Allied Sci. 1992;17(3):203–7.

123. Sheahan P, Blayney AW, Sheahan JN, Earley MJ. Sequelae of otitis media with effusion among children with cleft lip and/or cleft palate. Clin Otolaryngol Allied Sci. 2002;27(6):494–500.

124. Lee MR, Pawlowski KS, Luong A, Furze AD, Roland PS. Biofilm presence in humans with chronic suppurative otitis media. Otolaryngol Head Neck Surg. 2009;141(5):567–71.

125. Browning GG, Picozzi G, Sweeney G, Calder IT. Role of anaerobes in chronic otitis media. Clin Otolaryngol Allied Sci. 1983;8(1):47–51.

126. Austin DF. Sound conduction of the diseased ear. J Laryngol Otol. 1978;92(5):367–93.

127. Esposito S, D'Errico G, Montanaro C. Topical and oral treatment of chronic otitis media with ciprofloxacin: a preliminary study. Arch Otolaryngol Head Neck Surg. 1990;116(5):557–9.

128. Browning GG, Picozzi GL, Calder IT, Sweeney G. Controlled trial of medical treatment of active chronic otitis media. Br Med J (Clin Res Ed). 1983;287(6398):1024.

129. Esposito S, Noviello S, D'Errico G, Montanaro C. Topical ciprofloxacin vs intramuscular gentamicin for chronic otitis media. Arch Otolaryngol Head Neck Surg. 1992;118(8):842–4.

130. Macfadyen CA, Acuin JM, Gamble C. Systemic antibiotics versus topical treatments for chronically discharging ears with underlying eardrum perforations. Cochrane Database Syst Rev. 2006(1):CD005608.

131. Palva T, Ramsay H. Myringoplasty and tympanoplasty: results related to training and experience. Clin Otolaryngol Allied Sci. 1995;20(4):329–35.

132. Halik JJ, Smyth GD. Long-term results of tympanic membrane repair. Otolaryngol Head Neck Surg. 1988;98(2):162–9.

133. Scally CM, Allen L, Kerr AG. The anterior hitch method of tympanic membrane repair. Ear Nose Throat J. 1996;75(4):244–7.

134. Iurato S, Marioni G, Onofri M. Hearing results of ossiculoplasty in Austin-Kartush group A patients. Otol Neurotol. 2001;22(2):140–4.

135. Austin DF. Ossicular reconstruction. Otolaryngol Clin North Am. 1972;5(1):145–60.

136. Austin DF. Reporting results in tympanoplasty. Am J Otol. 1985;6(1):85–8.

137. Bellucci RJ. Selection of cases and classification of tympanoplasty. Otolaryngol Clin North Am. 1989;22(5):911–26.

138. Kartush JM. Ossicular chain reconstruction: capitulum to malleus. Otolaryngol Clin North Am. 1994;27(4):689–715.

139. Becvarovski Z, Kartush JM. Smoking and tympanoplasty: implications for prognosis and the Middle Ear Risk Index (MERI). Laryngoscope. 2001;111(10):1806–11.

140. Olszewska E, Rutkowska J, Ozgirgin N. Consensus-based recommendations on the definition and classification of cholesteatoma. J Int Adv Otol. 2015;11(1):81–7.

141. Michaels L. An epidermoid formation in the developing middle ear: possible source of cholesteatoma. J Otolaryngol. 1986;15(3):169–74.

142. Potsic WP, Samadi DS, Marsh RR, Wetmore RF. A staging system for congenital cholesteatoma. Arch Otolaryngol Head Neck Surg. 2002;128(9): 1009–12.

143. Sade J, Berco E. Atelectasis and secretory otitis media. Ann Otol Rhinol Laryngol. 1976;85(2 Suppl 25 Pt 2):66–72.

144. Tos M, Stangerup SE, Larsen P. Dynamics of eardrum changes following secretory otitis: a prospective study. Arch Otolaryngol Head Neck Surg. 1987; 113(4):380–5.

145. Dornhoffer JL, Friedman AB, Gluth MB. Management of acquired cholesteatoma in the pediatric population. Curr Opin Otolaryngol Head Neck Surg. 2013; 21(5):440–5.

146. Stankovic M. Follow-up of cholesteatoma surgery: open versus closed tympanoplasty. ORL J Otorhinolaryngol Relat Spec. 2007;69(5):299–305.

147. Luntz M, Avraham S, Sade J. The surgical treatment of atelectatic ears and retraction pockets in children and adults. Eur Arch Otorhinolaryngol. 1991; 248(7): 400–1.

148. Koch U. [Long-term results following tympanoplasty in complete atelectasis of the tympanum]. Laryngol Rhinol Otol (Stuttg). 1986;65(9):502–5.

149. Schilder AG. Assessment of complications of the condition and of the treatment of otitis media with effusion. Int J Pediatr Otorhinolaryngol. 1999; 49(Suppl 1): S247–51.

150. Tay HL, Mills RP. Tympanic membrane atelectasis in childhood otitis media with effusion. J Laryngol Otol. 1995;109(6):495–8.

151. Dodson EE, Hashisaki GT, Hobgood TC, Lambert PR. Intact canal wall mastoidectomy with tympanoplasty for cholesteatoma in children. Laryngoscope. 1998; 108(7):977–83.

152. Osborn AJ, Papsin BC, James AL. Clinical indications for canal wall-down mastoidectomy in a pediatric population. Otolaryngol Head Neck Surg. 2012; 147(2):316–22.

153. Sarcu D, Isaacson G. Long-term results of endoscopically assisted pediatric cholesteatoma surgery. Otolaryngol Head Neck Surg. 2016; 154(3):535–9.

154. Bennett M, Wanna G, Francis D, Murfee J, O'Connell B, Haynes D. Clinical and cost utility of an intraoperative endoscopic second look in cholesteatoma surgery. Laryngoscope. 2018;128(12):2867–71.

155. Han SY, Lee DY, Chung J, Kim YH. Comparison of endoscopic and microscopic ear surgery in pediatric patients: a meta-analysis. Laryngoscope. 2019;129(6):1444–52.

156. Ghadersohi S, Carter JM, Hoff SR. Endoscopic transcanal approach to the middle ear for management of pediatric cholesteatoma. Laryngoscope. 2017;127(11):2653–8.

157. Singh B, Maharaj TJ. Radical mastoidectomy: Its place in otitic intracranial complications. J Laryngol Otol. 1993;107(12):1113–8.

158. Feinmesser M, Tell L, Levi H. Decline in the prevalence of childhood deafness in the Jewish population of Jerusalem: ethnic and genetic aspects. J Laryngol Otol. 1990;104(9):675–7.

159. Torroni A, Cruciani F, Rengo C, et al. The A1555G mutation in the 12S rRNA gene of human mtDNA: recurrent origins and founder events in families affected by sensorineural deafness. Am J Hum Genet. 1999;65(5):1349–58.

160. Yoshinaga-Itano C, Sedey AL, Coulter DK, Mehl AL. Language of early- and later-identified children with hearing loss. Pediatrics. 1998;102(5):1161–71.

161. Chadha S, Moussy F, Friede MH. Understanding history, philanthropy and the role of WHO in provision of assistive technologies for hearing loss. Disabil Rehabil Assist Technol. 2014;9(5):365–7.

162. Anne S, Lieu JEC, Cohen MS. Speech and language consequences of unilateral hearing loss: a systematic review. Otolaryngol Head Neck Surg. 2017;157(4):572–9.

163. Appachi S, Specht JL, Raol N, et al. Auditory outcomes with hearing rehabilitation in children with unilateral hearing loss: a systematic review. Otolaryngol Head Neck Surg. 2017;157(4):565–71.

164. Peters JP, Ramakers GG, Smit AL, Grolman W. Cochlear implantation in children with unilateral hearing loss: a systematic review. Laryngoscope. 2016;126(3):713–21.

165. Tavora-Vieira D, Rajan GP. Cochlear implantation in children with congenital and noncongenital unilateral deafness. Otol Neurotol. 2015;36(8):1457–8.

166. Rahne T, Plontke SK. Functional result after cochlear implantation in children and adults with single-sided deafness. Otol Neurotol. 2016;37(9):e332–40.

167. Stachler RJ, Chandrasekhar SS, Archer SM, et al. Clinical practice guideline: sudden hearing loss. Otolaryngol Head Neck Surg. 2012;146(3 Suppl):S1–35.

168. Wilson WR, Byl FM, Laird N. The efficacy of steroids in the treatment of idiopathic sudden hearing loss: a double-blind clinical study. Arch Otolaryngol. 1980;106(12):772–6.

169. Sloan-Heggen CM, Bierer AO, Shearer AE, et al. Comprehensive genetic testing in the clinical evaluation of 1119 patients with hearing loss. Hum Genet. 2016;135(4):441–50.

170. Shearer AE, Black-Ziegelbein EA, Hildebrand MS, et al. Advancing genetic testing for deafness with genomic technology. J Med Genet. 2013;50(9):627–34.

171. Kiringoda R, Kozin ED, Lee DJ. Outcomes in endoscopic ear surgery. Otolaryngol Clin North Am. 2016; 49(5):1271–90.

172. Isaacson G. Endoscopic anatomy of the pediatric middle ear. Otolaryngol Head Neck Surg. 2014; 150(1):6–15.

173. Landegger LD, Cohen MS. Use of the flexible fiber $CO_2$ laser in pediatric transcanal endoscopic middle ear surgery. Int J Pediatr Otorhinolaryngol. 2016; 85:154–7.

174. Kakehata S, Watanabe T, Ito T, Kubota T, Furukawa T. Extension of indications for transcanal endoscopic ear surgery using an ultrasonic bone curette for cholesteatomas. Otol Neurotol. 2014;35(1):101–7.

175. Rivera T, Sanz L, Camarero G, Varela-Nieto I. Drug delivery to the inner ear: strategies and their therapeutic implications for sensorineural hearing loss. Curr Drug Deliv. 2012;9(3):231–42.

176. Hannon GJ. RNA interference. Nature. 2002; 418(6894):244–51.

177. Chen W, Johnson SL, Marcotti W, Andrews PW, Moore HD, Rivolta MN. Human fetal auditory stem cells can be expanded in vitro and differentiate into functional auditory neurons and hair cell-like cells. Stem Cells. 2009;27(5):1196–204.

178. Venekamp RV, Sanders S, Glasizou PP, et al. Antibiotics for acute otitis media in children. Cochrane Database Syst Rev 2013;1: CD000219.

# 2 Hearing Loss in Adults

*Amit Sood*

## CONTENTS

## INTRODUCTION

Hearing loss is one of the commonest symptoms for which patients report to the ENT clinics. Causes of hearing loss are varied and are different across the spectrum of age; the ENT surgeon as such should be aware of various causes of hearing loss and should be able to deduce the underlying causes using history, clinical examination, audiological findings and other investigations like imaging (1).

Various estimates place hearing loss as the fifth commonest disability affecting world population and it ranks fourth when number of years lived with disability is considered (2). The burden of disease in terms of numbers is staggering, with WHO estimates showing about 466 million people in the world with disabling hearing loss (thresholds worse than 40 dB in better hearing ear). Out of these, 432 million people are adults, 56% being males and 44% females (Figure 2.1) (3). Adults in lower socio-economic status are more commonly effected (4).

Presentation of hearing loss is variable according to the type of loss and underlying aetiology. Due to the large numbers of patients affected, hearing loss has a huge economic effect in terms of man hours lost due to disability and also as litigation/compensation for occupational hearing loss. The disease also has a tremendous psychological burden as it leads to social isolation and depression, especially in older individuals. As the disease has multiple aspects, the otolaryngologist should be prepared to tackle each of them to achieve a high resolution rate in patients.

## SEVERITY OF HEARING LOSS
### Assessment of Hearing Loss

Hearing loss is a symptom and identification of the location of lesion is the first step towards management of these cases. The basic physics of sound and the physiology of conduction of sound is important for this understanding, but these topics will not be discussed here.

Assessment of hearing loss can be done both subjectively and objectively. For subjective assessment, the method used is psycho-acoustic audiometry. In this method an acoustic stimulus presented to the ear is tested, which requires a conscious patient who can understand the instructions and cooperate with the assessor, hence the "psych" part of psycho-acoustic audiometry. Objective methods for assessment of hearing include otoacoustic emissions (OAE), short latency responses like brainstem-evoked response audiometry (BERA), mid-latency response like auditory steady-state response (ASSR) and long-latency response like cerebral auditory evoked potential (CAEP).

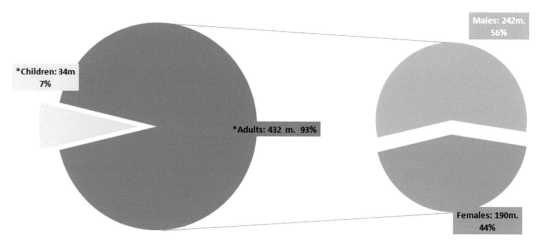

**Figure 2.1**  Prevalence of hearing loss (3).

Of all these methods, Pure Tone Audiometry (PTA) is the most widely used and the thresholds achieved in PTA are used to assess the type and severity of hearing loss. PTA provides information that can be plotted in a graphical form where Air Conduction (AC) and Bone Conduction (BC) thresholds of the patient are assessed by providing stimuli in the form of pure tones. There are standards for pure tone audiometers (IEC 60645-1:2017 & BSEN 60645-1:2017), the type of room and the procedure to be followed (ISO 8253-1:2010). It is crucial to adhere to these conventions in order to obtain valid and comparable results across sessions and clinicians.

The local professional societies publish their own guidelines in line with current international standards, which are then followed in their respective regions (5). The audiometer has to be calibrated yearly in order for it to provide valid and reliable results. In addition, certain daily checks are also recommended to maintain accuracy of results (ISO 8253-1:2010) (6).

The AC threshold assessment is the basic test to assess the degree of hearing loss being faced by the patient. BC thresholds are needed to differentiate between conductive and Sensorineural Hearing Loss (SNHL). On subtracting the BC thresholds from AC thresholds, we get the Air-Bone (AB) gap, which signifies the degree of conductive hearing loss; a minimum of 15 dB AB gap is required for conductive hearing loss to be considered clinically significant. In case there is an asymmetry between the two ears, then the better ear is tested first, and while testing the second ear the better ear has to be masked so that it does not interfere in the testing of the worse ear. The interaural attenuation for AC is 40 dB using over the ear headphones and 55 dB using insert-type headphones. Adequate level of masking is arrived at by using Hood's plateau seeking method (7) (Figure 2.2).

Depending on the type of audiogram obtained, hearing loss can be divided into the following types:

1. *SNHL* (Figure 2.3):

    a. Increased thresholds both in AC and BC curves.

    b. No significant AB gap.

    c. Pathology of the sensory organ (cochlea) or in the neural connections between the inner hair cells (IHC) and the cochlear nerve.

    d. Usually permanent.

2. *Conductive hearing loss* (Figure 2.4):

    a. Normal BC thresholds, i.e. <20 dB.

    b. AB gap (>15 dB).

    c. Pathology in conduction of sound from the external ear to the inner ear.

    d. Reduced hearing sensitivity, but most of the other aspects of sound perception remain intact.

    e. Respond well to hearing augmentation.

3. *Mixed hearing loss* (Figure 2.5):

    a. Increased thresholds both in AC and BC curves.

    b. Significant (>15 dB) AB gap.

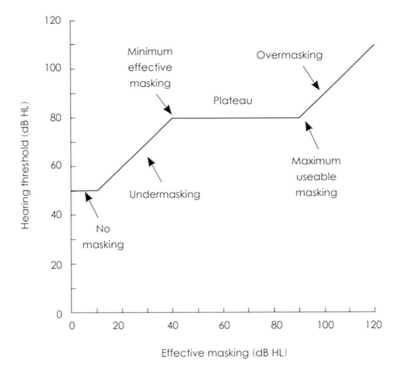

**Figure 2.2** Hood's plateau method for masking.

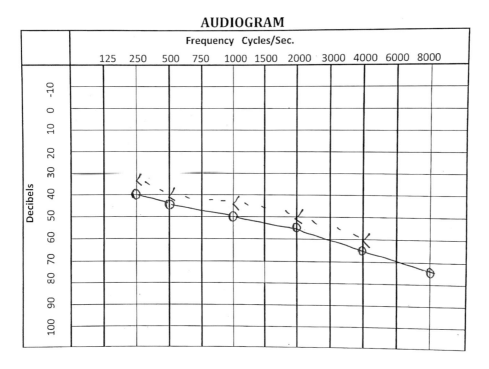

**Figure 2.3** Sensorineural hearing loss (R) ear.

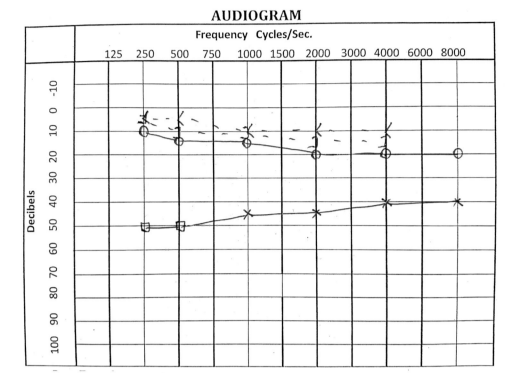

**Figure 2.4** Conductive hearing loss (L) ear.

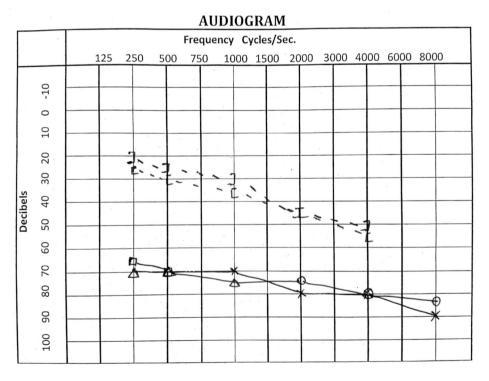

**Figure 2.5** Mixed hearing loss.

4. *Auditory Neuropathy Spectrum Disorder* (ANSD):

a. Patient is able to hear the sound, but there is difficulty in processing these sounds into meaningful speech.

b. Good PTA scores with poor speech recognition.

c. Lesion may affect the cochlear nerve or the auditory pathway or even the auditory cortex.

d. Various reasons like diminished neural firing or asynchronous neural firing.

### Severity of Hearing Loss

Various classifications have been given for severity of hearing loss, of which the Goodman (Clark) classification (8) and the WHO classification (9) are most commonly used (Tables 2.1 and 2.2).

While these classifications are useful in categorization of patients, these are only broad categories and actual disability being faced by the patient is not reflected by them. For calculation of disability, government departments dealing with disabilities provide lists of percentage of disability in consultation with the professional bodies. In India, the Ministry of Social Justice and Empowerment has provided a list containing percentage of disability according to the severity of hearing loss depicted by PTA thresholds (Figure 2.6).

### Table 2.1: Goodman (Clark) Classification for Severity of Hearing Loss (8)

| S. No. | PTA Thresholds | Hearing Loss Classification |
|---|---|---|
| 1 | <25 dB | Normal |
| 2 | 26–40 dB | Mild |
| 3 | 41–55 dB | Moderate |
| 4 | 56–70 dB | Moderately severe |
| 5 | 71–90 dB | Severe |
| 6 | >90 dB | Profound |

### Table 2.2: WHO Classification for Severity of Hearing Loss (9)

| S. No. | PTA Thresholds | Hearing Loss Classification |
|---|---|---|
| 1 | <25 dB | Normal |
| 2 | 26–40 dB | Mild |
| 3 | 41–60 dB | Moderate |
| 4 | 61–80 dB | Severe |
| 5 | >80 dB | Profound |

The disability is calculated for each ear separately and then composite disability is calculated using the following formula: %disability in worse ear + (% disability in better ear × 5)/6 (10).

Another important aspect of severity of hearing loss is the level defined as "hard of hearing" and "deaf"; these terms have medico-legal implications as well as financial implications and hence these terms should be used cautiously. In India, a person is "deaf" if hearing thresholds are worse than 70 dB in both ears and "hard of hearing" if hearing thresholds are worse than 60 dB in both ears (11).

### DIFFERENTIAL DIAGNOSIS
### Sensorineural Hearing Loss
#### Presbycusis

The word presbycusis is derived from the Greek words "Presbys", meaning elder, and "acusis", meaning hearing. It is a term used synonymously with age-related hearing loss, which is the commonest cause of hearing loss in general population (12). The prevalence of hearing loss increases with an increase in the age of the subjects: the prevalence below 15 years is 1.7%, which increases to 7.6% in subjects above 15 years of age and almost 30% in people above the age of 65 years (13).

Humans have best hearing in late teens and early 20s from where the hearing thresholds start declining (14, 15), this worsening is more prominent in males and in manual workers probably due to added effects of occupational noise exposure (16). There is no consensus on the age at which presbycusis sets in, but maximum cases present at the age of 40–60 years (17). It has been noted that patients with age-related hearing loss have higher incidence of falls and subsequent trauma (18). It is also associated with dementia, social isolation, loss of confidence and depression (19, 20).

Age-related changes occur in outer, middle and inner ear but only the changes in inner ear contribute significantly to hearing loss. Age-related hearing loss was divided into six distinct types according to their histopathological findings by Schuknecht et al. (21–23) (Table 2.3). In addition to the cochlear changes, there are following changes in the Central Nervous System (CNS):

- Reduced neural plasticity (24)
- Decline in central auditory processing
- Reduced word recognition
- Reduced speech discrimination (25)

Various risk factors have been identified for presbycusis (Table 2.4).

| Monaural PTA in dB | % of Disability | | Monaural PTA in dB | % of Disability |
|---|---|---|---|---|
| 0 to 25 | 0 | | 61 | 41.71 |
| 26 | 1 | | 62 | 43.42 |
| 27 | 1 | | 63 | 45.13 |
| 28 | 1 | | 64 | 46.84 |
| 29 | 1 | | 65 | 48.55 |
| 30 | 1 | | 66 | 50.26 |
| 31 | 1 | | 67 | 51.97 |
| 32 | 1 | | 68 | 53.68 |
| 33 | 1 | | 69 | 55.39 |
| 34 | 2 | | 70 | 57.1 |
| 35 | 3 | | 71 | 58.81 |
| 36 | 4 | | 72 | 60.52 |
| 37 | 5 | | 73 | 62.23 |
| 38 | 6 | | 74 | 63.94 |
| 39 | 7 | | 75 | 65.65 |
| 40 | 8 | | 76 | 67.36 |
| 41 | 9 | | 77 | 69.07 |
| 42 | 10 | | 78 | 70.78 |
| 43 | 11 | | 79 | 72.49 |
| 44 | 12 | | 80 | 74.2 |
| 45 | 13 | | 81 | 75.91 |
| 46 | 14 | | 82 | 77.62 |
| 47 | 15 | | 83 | 79.33 |
| 48 | 16 | | 84 | 81.04 |
| 49 | 17 | | 85 | 82.75 |
| 50 | 18 | | 86 | 84.46 |
| 51 | 19 | | 87 | 86.17 |
| 52 | 20 | | 88 | 87.88 |
| 53 | 21 | | 89 | 89.59 |
| 54 | 22 | | 90 | 91.3 |
| 55 | 23 | | 91 | 93.01 |
| 56 | 24 | | 92 | 94.72 |
| 57 | 25 | | 93 | 96.43 |
| 58 | 26 | | 94 | 98.14 |
| 59 | 27 | | 95 | 100 |
| 60 | 40 | | | |

**Figure 2.6**  Calculation of disability (10).

## Table 2.3: Types of Hearing Loss According to Histopathological Findings

| S. No. | Type | Features |
|---|---|---|
| 1 | Sensory | Loss of hair cells<br>Loss of sustentacular cells<br>Basal turn involvement |
| 2 | Neural | Degeneration of cochlear nerve neurons<br>Loss of spiral ganglion cells |
| 3 | Vascular/ metabolic | Atrophy of stria vascularis<br>Involvement of apical and middle turns |
| 4 | Mechanical/ cochlear conductive | Stiffening of basement membrane |
| 5 | Intermediate | Changes in cochlear duct<br>Changes in cell metabolism<br>Changes in endolymph composition |
| 6 | Mixed | Combination of the five types mentioned above |

## Table 2.4: Risk Factors for Presbyacusis

| Non-modifiable Factors | Modifiable Factors | Comorbid Conditions |
|---|---|---|
| • Age<br>• Sex<br>• Genetics | • Environmental<br>• Noise exposure<br>• Smoking<br>• Alcohol consumption | • Hypertension<br>• Cardiovascular disease<br>• CNS stroke |

To make a diagnosis of age-related hearing loss, usually the only investigation required is a PTA which will show a SNHL that is worse at higher frequencies in early stages; as the disease progresses, middle and low frequencies are also involved (Figure 2.7). The hearing loss is usually symmetrical; if asymmetrical, it warrants further investigation with a contrast-enhanced MRI of the brain to evaluate the Cerebello-Pontine (CP) angle and the posterior cranial fossa (Figure 2.8).

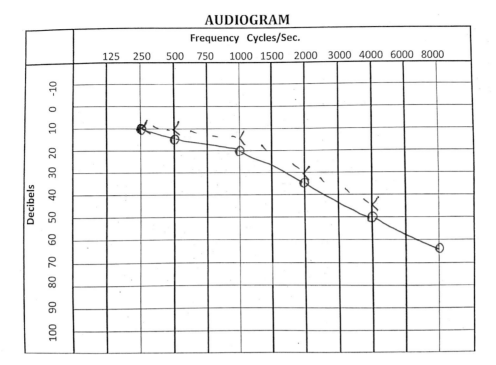

**Figure 2.7** Early presbyacusis (R) ear.

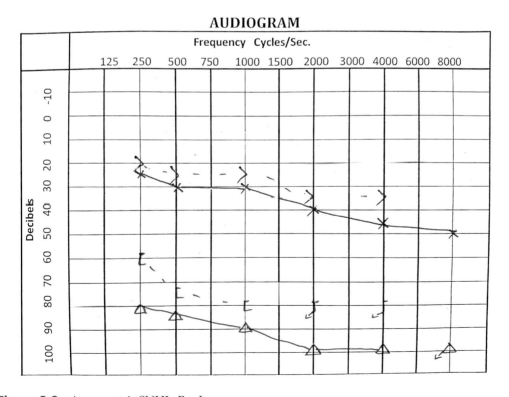

**Figure 2.8** Asymmetric SNHL: R > L.

The treatment of age-related hearing loss is multipronged; it includes certain practical measures to be taken by the patient like reducing background noise, face-to-face conversation, focusing on non-verbal cues, lip reading, use of volume-controlled telephones, use of louder doorbells and alternative alerting mechanism like pets/vibrating alerts. Another major aspect for treatment of presbycusis is accepting the disease and overcoming its psychological effects which may range from isolation to depression. As the hearing loss is irreversible, the mainstay for management is use of amplification, most commonly hearing aids. Hearing aids can be of various types like behind the ear, in the canal and completely in canal type, which can be chosen on the basis of age of the patient and their choice. A bilateral hearing aid fitting gives a better hearing outcome as compared to unilateral fitting.

*Occupational/Noise-Induced*
*Hearing Loss (NIHL)*

NIHL is defined as reduced hearing sensitivity consequent to excessive noise exposure. Thomas Barr in 1886 described the "boiler-maker's deafness" related to ship-building, then the histological features of NIHL in the organ of Corti of the inner ear were demonstrated by Haberman in 1890. Fowler described the characteristic noise-induced 4 kHz notch on PTA and later in 1939, Bunch explained broadly the audiometric findings of NIHL (26). NIHL can be broadly classified into the following types:

a. Temporary Threshold Shift (TTS)

b. Permanent Threshold Shift (PTS)

c. Acoustic trauma

TTS is a short-term reversible effect on the hearing threshold, which may follow an exposure to noise. Above a certain frequency and intensity, the outer hair cells show signs of metabolic exhaustion with drooping of stereocilia. This correlates with the phenomenon of TTS, which recovers within a few hours (27). This also highlights the fact that it is the outer cells rather than the inner cells that get damaged in TTS, and eventually in NIHL. If in any particular person the level of exposure compatible with recovery is exceeded, recovery from threshold shift will not be complete and the residue is known as PTS. Most episodes of TTS recover within 16 hours; however, no formal timeline has been laid out to differentiate TTS from PTS (28–30).

Acoustic trauma is characterized by a sudden change in hearing as a result of a single exposure to a sudden burst of sound, such as an explosive blast (31). An impulse noise may damage the middle ear as well as the inner ear. It may result in conductive hearing loss as well as SNHL due to damage to inner ear. The human Tympanic Membrane (TM) is known to rupture at an intensity of 180 dB. Other changes in middle ear due to acoustic trauma include fracture or dislocation of ossicles, hemotympanum and tearing of round window membrane (32).

A large number of occupations/activities expose people to harmful levels of noise, e.g. gunfire, heavy industry, aviation industry, clubs/concerts etc. (33). Various estimates place the prevalence of NIHL as high as 25% in the male population, making it the second commonest cause of SNHL after presbycusis (34). The effects of noise on hearing are variable and unpredictable but one thing is clear that the damage increases with an increase in exposure to noise. Sounds below 80 dB in intensity usually cause no damage while those above 130 dB can cause NIHL even after a short-term exposure (35). Noise level in various occupational activities and the physiological response to those noise levels are illustrated in Table 2.5 (36).

## Table 2.5: Effects of Various Levels of Noise

| Noise Level (dB) | Response | Example |
|---|---|---|
| 150 | Instantaneous damage | Heavy calibre weapon firing |
| 140 | Damage over a small period of time | Rifle firing |
| 130 | Threshold of pain | Jet craft taking off |
| 115 | Some hearing damage after approximately 30 s | Power saw |
| 100 | Some hearing damage after approximately 15 minutes | Grinding metal, lawn mower |
| 85 | Some hearing damage after approximately 8 hours | Noise in a very busy street |
| 70 | Damage to hearing unlikely to occur | Assembly work without noisy tools |
| 60 | Difficulty in hearing a conversation over telephone | Busy office |
| 50 | Hearing with comfort | Urban noise level away from roads |
| 30 | Undisturbed sleep | Average bedroom |
| 0 | Hearing threshold | Anechoic chamber |

The middle ear may be affected in NIHL, but the predominant site for pathological manifestation is the cochlea. Various mechanisms have been described for pathological changes in cochlea following noise exposure, the most commonly accepted are the metabolic and the structural mechanisms leading to NIHL.

Various metabolic mechanisms have been postulated:

- Excessive stimulation of cochlea due to noise causes excessive neurotransmitter release, the excess glutamate accumulates at the synapse and the glutamate receptors auto-regulate leading to reduced hearing, which manifests itself as TTS (37, 38).

- Changes in blood flow associated with noise exposure also lead to NIHL. It has been seen in animal studies that moderate sound levels cause increased cochlear blood flow while stimulation by loud noise leads to reduced blood flow (39, 40).

- Cochlear hair cell damage by Reactive Oxygen Species (ROS) after noise exposure. The cochlea is a metabolically active organ, several ROS are generated under normal metabolic circumstances which can cause damage to DNA, proteins and membranes. Normally, antioxidant systems are present to neutralize ROS (41, 42), but if the ear is not given a chance to rest and recover, the ROS acts to damage hair cell nuclei and cell wall membranes, resulting in cell death and resultant NIHL (43).

The following structural changes are caused by noise:

- Depolymerization of actin filaments of stereocilia following exposure to loud noise lead to structural changes in stereocilia leading to NIHL.

- Swelling of the stria vascularis, afferent nerve endings and supporting cells of organ of Corti (44).

Outer Hair Cells (OHCs) are more vulnerable to noise as compared to Inner Hair Cells (IHCs). Caspase 10 has been implicated in apoptosis of OHCs following noise exposure (45). Another mechanism for causation of NIHL is synaptopathy; the synapses between the IHCs and spiral ganglion are highly vulnerable to noise and are damaged on exposure to loud noise. This type of NIHL presents as a "hidden hearing loss", i.e. the patient has difficulty in hearing especially in noise, but the PTA thresholds remain unchanged (46).

Many factors determine the vulnerability of individuals to NIHL, the most commonly accepted factor being genetic (47, 48). It is generally accepted that certain individuals are more prone to develop NIHL and have been termed as "Green ears". In addition, factors like age, smoking, presence of diseases like diabetes mellitus, cardiovascular diseases or history of cerebrovascular accident also decide an individual's susceptibility to develop NIHL (49–51). NIHL has been known to damage hearing synergistically along with ototoxic medications/environmental toxin exposure (52).

A classic case of NIHL is a middle-aged male who has a long-term history of noise exposure and presents with hearing loss. Initial complaints include difficulty in hearing in noise and a loss of clarity rather than volume (53). Other features may include tinnitus, hyperacusis and social withdrawal/depression. Otoscopy is usually normal; however, presence of chronic otitis media (COM) does not preclude the diagnosis.

As with other causes of hearing loss, the investigation of choice for quantifying the hearing loss is PTA. PTA characteristically shows a bilateral symmetrical high-frequency hearing loss with an audiometric notch at higher frequencies 3–6 kHz with a recovery at 8 kHz (54), the lower frequencies are usually spared (55) (Figure 2.9). However, in later stages all the frequencies may be involved. If PTA shows asymmetry, then imaging has to considered to rule out a CP angle or posterior cranial fossa lesion. In cases of exposure to fire arms, asymmetry on PTA may be attributed to the "head shadow effect" where hearing loss is worse on the side where the weapon is carried/fired; this is however true only for recreational firearms where the breech does not open automatically to eject the spent case. This is not seen with military firearms as the noise escapes from both the muzzle and the chamber/breech (56, 57).

The patient of NIHL reports to ENT clinic in one of two conditions: (a) deterioration of hearing, i.e. clinical, and (b) demand for compensation/disability, i.e. medico-legal. There are various confounding factors which make the diagnosis more difficult, like individual susceptibility, long-term exposure to noise and contribution from presbycusis. Age-wise hearing thresholds are available for normative population and these can be subtracted from actual thresholds to arrive at contribution of NIHL towards entire hearing loss. There are guidelines to ascertain the contribution of NIHL in the entire hearing loss and these are taken into consideration while awarding disability (58, 59).

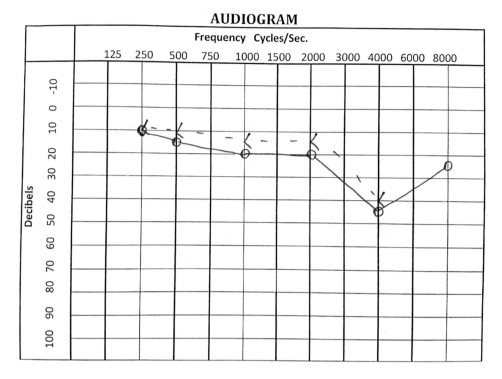

**Figure 2.9** Noise-induced hearing loss (R) ear.

The management of NIHL is primarily prevention as it is preventable with use of appropriate protective equipment. Preventive measures include reducing exposure to loud noise, use of protective equipment and change of workplace/sheltered appointment for known cases of NIHL (60). It is the responsibility of employers to identify all areas where harmful noise exposure is present and mark these areas appropriately with warning signs. The employers are required to identify two peak sound levels – at the first sound peak level, the use of hearing protection devices is advisable but is on the discretion of the employee; on the second peak, however, the use of hearing protection devices is mandatory (60, 61). In addition, regular hearing tests have to be performed on employees working in areas with loud noise.

Various types of hearing protection devices are available. These include the ear plugs (insert type), earmuffs (over the ear) and active noise cancellation devices. The ear plugs are difficult to fit properly and hence offer poor protection from noise. The earmuffs are more reliable and offer an attenuation of 10–15 dB, which is similar to properly fitted ear plugs (62, 63). Active noise cancellation devices are highly effective; they act by producing sound inside the earmuffs, which is 180° out of phase with the ambient noise. However, these devices are very expensive and are presently used only in the military and aviation industry (64). All hearing protection devices are given noise reduction ratings (NRR) in decibels, which depict their efficacy in reducing the sound exposure in a given work environment.

Recovery of thresholds is unlikely once NIHL has occurred and its management is similar to that of presbycusis. In addition, many methods have been tried for treatment of NIHL, including intra-tympanic steroid injections, hyperbaric oxygen therapy, antioxidants, carbogen inhalation etc., but all these treatment modalities are presently in experimental stage.

*Ototoxicity*

Ototoxicity is the process by which drugs, environmental agents and toxins cause damage to the peripheral end organs of hearing and balance. The definition does not include agents that act on neural pathways or respective centres in the brain. For a drug to cause ototoxicity, it has to enter the perilymph or the endolymph; therefore, only the drugs that can cross the

## Table 2.6: **Mechanisms of Ototoxicity**

| Drugs Causing Acute Effect on the Stria Vascularis (68, 69) | Drugs Causing Temporary Impairment of Hair Cell Function (70, 71) | Drugs Causing Death of Hair Cells (72) |
|---|---|---|
| • Target the $Na^+/K^+/Cl^-$ co-transporter (loop diuretics) or $Na^+/K^+$-ATPase (macrolides)<br>• Reduce the endocochlear potential from its normal value of +80 mV to up to −40 mV<br>• Hearing loss is usually reversible<br>  • Loop diuretics like frusemide<br>  • Macrolide antibiotics like erythromycin | • Target are the OHCs<br>• OHC damage leads to loss of cochlear amplification<br>• Hearing loss is usually reversible<br>• Associated symptoms like tinnitus<br>  • Quinine<br>  • Salicylates | • Cause hair cell death on repeated administration<br>• Permanent threshold shift<br>• Associated with vestibular dysfunction<br>  • Aminoglycosides<br>  • Platinum agents |

blood-perilymph barrier are able to cause ototoxicity (65, 66). The primary effect of ototoxic agents is on the OHCs, while the IHCs are usually spared (67).

Various mechanisms have been described by which drugs cause ototoxicity; the most commonly accepted ones are listed in Table 2.6 (68–72).

In the vestibular system, the type I hair cells are more susceptible to damage from ototoxic drugs. The cristae are affected more severely followed by utricle and then the saccule (73). Various types of drugs which cause ototoxicity are listed in Table 2.7.

Aminoglycosides are the clinically most important group of drugs that cause ototoxicity. All aminoglycosides are ototoxic; however, they can be classified into groups according to severity of ototoxicity and organ preference within the inner ear. Neomycin is the most ototoxic, followed by gentamicin, kanamycin and tobramycin. Amikacin is the least ototoxic. Streptomycin and gentamicin are more vestibulotoxic, while amikacin and neomycin are primarily cochleotoxic (74). The effect of these drugs become apparent only after prolonged treatment. A single

### Table 2.7: **Common Drugs Implicated in Causing Ototoxicity**

| Category of Drugs | Compounds |
|---|---|
| Aminoglycosides antibiotics | Amikacin, gentamicin, kanamycin, streptomycin, tobramycin, framycetin |
| Macrolide antibiotics | Erythromycin, azithromycin, clarithromycin |
| Antitumour agents | Cis-platin, carboplatin, bleomycin |
| Anti-inflammatory agents | Salicylate, ibuprofen, indomethacin |
| Antimalarials | Quinine, chloroquine |
| Loop diuretics | Frusemide, ethacrynic acid |
| Iron chelators | Desferrioxamine |
| Industrial chemicals | Trimethyltin, toluene, xylene |

parenteral dose does not usually cause inner ear damage; however, idiosyncratic ototoxicity has been reported. Topical application of even a single dose can initiate ototoxicity. This property has led to use of intra-tympanic gentamicin in intractable vertigo of Ménière's disease (75).

The classical finding in case of ototoxicity is a high-frequency SNHL which is symmetrical and occurs after exposure to a drug/toxin. To be considered significant, the ototoxic changes must meet the following criteria (76):

■ >20 dB change at any one test frequency.

■ >10 dB change at two consecutive test frequencies.

■ Loss of response at three consecutive frequencies where responses were earlier present.

It is important to note that these changes are always calculated in relation to baseline audiometry done before starting the ototoxic agent and have to be confirmed by repeat testing. If any changes develop in the audiometry, then it needs to be recorded and drug or dose may be modified if possible. However, there are many confounding factors which make it difficult to assess the ototoxicity caused by these agents like age, status of renal system, dosage regime, concurrent use of other drugs, presence of infection, nutritional status and genetic predisposition (77).

There is no treatment for hearing loss caused by ototoxicity as the recovery of hearing thresholds is unlikely once PTS has occurred; however, the PTA thresholds may recover after stopping the offending drug if they cause ototoxicity by the reversible mechanisms. Hearing aids may be offered to patients who develop significant permanent hearing loss.

### *Genetic Hearing Loss*

Hearing loss is known to occur in familial patterns; however, no single gene has been identified for causing genetic hearing loss (78). Out of all cases of genetic hearing loss, about 70% are non-syndromic. Of the non-syndromic SNHL, about 80% are transmitted in an autosomal recessive pattern, 15% in autosomal dominant pattern and the rest in X-linked or mitochondrial inheritance. These are represented as DFNA, DFNB and DFNX where DFN stands for deafness, A for autosomal dominant, B for autosomal recessive and no alphabet for X-linked/mitochondrial inheritance (79).

In clinical presentation the autosomal dominant SNHL is usually post-lingual and progressive in contrast to syndromic or autosomal recessive types of SNHL, which are usually pre-lingual and non-progressive (80).

The field of molecular genetics in hearing loss is currently under research and more developments are likely to improve the understanding of genetic hearing loss with improving ability to predict the likely course of disease, genetic counselling, early intervention and also potential development of molecular treatments (81).

### Autoimmune Hearing Loss

Autoimmune SNHL is a rare disorder in which the patient has progressive bilateral hearing loss which may be fluctuating and even asymmetric developing over a period of 5–90 days and shows benefit with steroids/immune-suppressive therapy. The patient may also have symptoms like tinnitus, hyperacusis and vestibular symptoms in up to 30% of cases. Incidence of this disorder is <5/1,00,000 population per year in the United States, it accounts for less than 1% of all cases of SNHL and is more common in females between third and sixth decades of life (82). At present there are no standardized diagnostic criteria or tests for autoimmune SNHL and it remains a diagnosis of exclusion (83).

Various mechanisms have been postulated for damage to ear caused in autoimmune SNHL:

- Deposition of immune complex (type III immune reaction)

- Antibodies against cochlea-vestibular antigens (type II immune reaction)

- Vasculitis

- Microthrombosis

- Electrochemical alterations in cochlea

- Part of systemic autoimmune disorder

As this is a diagnosis of exclusion, a detailed history must be taken to rule out all other causes of SNHL. Laboratory testing for autoimmune diseases should be carried out along with a contrast-enhanced MRI of the brain to rule out a retro-cochlear pathology.

Treatment of choice is administration of systemic steroids, which may help in reduction of symptoms, but data shows variable efficacy (14–70%). Use of immune-suppressive agents may be considered if steroids are contraindicated or poorly tolerated. Various drugs have been tried like methotrexate, cyclosporine and azathioprine, but the evidence regarding their efficacy is limited. Use of hearing aids can be advised in case hearing loss is affecting communication and in case of profound hearing loss, use of cochlear implants can also be considered.

### Non-Organic Hearing Loss (NOHL)

NOHL refers to a condition in which a patient reports hearing loss despite having normal hearing. It can be of two types:

- *Psychogenic:* There is an underlying psychological disorder in which the patient presents with hearing loss.

- *Malingering:* In these cases, the patient has normal hearing but feigns deafness for personal gain like claiming disability.

The tests for NOHL include the following (84, 85):

**Observation:** A patient with NOHL tries to aggravate his hearing loss with repeated requests of repeating and trying to bring the better ear forward, these patients will also avoid eye contact.

**Speech tests:** Various tests have been described like the Erhard's test, Lombard's test, delayed auditory feedback test and swinging story test.

**Tuning fork tests:** Many tuning fork tests have been described of which the most important is the Stenger's test. Other tuning fork tests include the Chimani-Moos test.

**PTA**: There are many features on PTA that can indicate a case of NOHL:

- Inconsistent PTA on repeat testing

- Flat PTA curve

- Absence of a shadow curve

- Positive Stenger's test

**Objective tests**: Objective tests like OAE, BERA and ASSR can confirm the hearing status of the individual.

The management for psychogenic NOHL includes psychological counselling and treatment of underlying disorder. In case of malingering, the patient needs to be made aware about the findings of NOHL.

## Conductive Hearing Loss
### External Ear Conditions

**Wax:** Presence of wax is normal in the EAC; it rarely causes any symptoms and does not warrant removal unless it is hindering the visualization of the TM. In some cases, the wax causes occlusion of the EAC and results in hearing loss; this condition is more frequent in elderly due to factors like laxity of canal skin, collapse of EAC and presence of hair in the EAC (86, 87).

**Otitis externa:** Otitis externa can be divided into two types – the localized type known as furunculosis/folliculitis, which involves infection of a hair follicle in the EAC, and a generalized form, where the entire EAC is involved. Predisposing factors are swimming and use of ear buds. The presenting symptom is usually otalgia, which is severe and aggravated by movement of the pinna (88). These patients may have hearing loss due to oedema and occlusion of the EAC. Treatment involves aural toilet along with the use of topical steroids and antibiotic ointments, systemic antibiotics providing Gram-positive cover and supportive therapy like pain relief (89). Hearing loss resolves on resolution of otitis externa.

**Keratosis obturans:** It is the accumulation of a large plug of desquamated keratin in the external auditory canal. A geometrically patterned keratin plug is seen within an expanded/ballooned out EAC. It mostly occurs in young patients who present with otalgia and conductive hearing loss (90). Treatment is removal of the keratin plug, which may have to be done under anaesthesia; in cases of recurrent disease, canalplasty may be considered (91).

**Myringitis:** It is an inflammation of the TM which can be acute/bullous myringitis or chronic/granular myringitis. Studies indicate that in almost all cases of bullous myringitis, concurrent otitis media is seen. Patients present with otalgia and conductive hearing loss due to presence of fluid in the middle ear; some patients may also have SNHL which usually resolves. Treatment is similar to that of AOM, which includes symptomatic therapy with or without incision of bullae. Role of antibiotics is controversial and so is the role of steroids in treatment of associated SNHL (92). Granular myringitis is a chronic inflammatory process in which there is de-epithelialization of outer layer of TM and its replacement with granulation tissue. It is thought to be caused due to injury to lamina propria of the TM, e.g. in infections or during surgery. Patients present with painless otorrhoea and mild conductive hearing loss. Treatment includes meticulous aural toilet followed by application of antibiotic and anti-inflammatory ointment. Debulking the granulation tissue with cold steel instruments/cryosurgery or use of nitrous oxide cautery can also be considered (93).

### Middle Ear Conditions

**Acute otitis media:** It is an acute inflammation of the middle ear cleft. It is predominantly a disease of children with greatest incidence in first two years of life (94); however, the disease is not as uncommon in adults as was previously considered. Majority of cases reporting to ENT centres with AOM are bacterial infections with the commonest causative organisms being *Haemophilus influenzae*, *Streptococcus pneumoniae* and *Moraxella catarrhalis* (95). All these infections are preventable with use of vaccination. Patients present with severe otalgia, which may reduce following onset of mucopurulent otorrhoea and associated with hearing loss. Examination may reveal a bulging red TM or a perforated TM with mucopurulent discharge in the EAC (96). Treatment consists of symptomatic therapy with pain relief. Antibiotics are commonly used and may help in pain reduction in addition to preventing TM perforation, but there is mixed quality of evidence for their use (97).

**Otitis media with effusion:** OME is a collection of fluid in the middle ear, it is also predominantly a disease of childhood (98). It may occur secondary to an episode of URTI, it may also precede AOM or occur during resolving phase of AOM. Other causes of OME in adults include nasal allergy, barotrauma and eustachian tube dysfunction (99). Patients present with sensation of ear blockage, hearing loss, tinnitus or sensation of popping of ears. Examination may reveal fluid behind an intact TM. PTA reveals a conductive hearing loss and tympanometry reveals a "B"-type curve. In case of a unilateral OME in adults, a diagnostic nasal endoscopy is mandatory to rule out any lesion in nasopharynx (100). Most of the cases of OME in adults resolve spontaneously. Management may include non-medical treatment in the form of Toynbee manoeuvre and Valsalva manoeuvre or use of Otovent® balloon. Medical management may include use of topical decongestants for a short duration, but evidence for their efficacy is limited as also evidence for use of topical steroid sprays. Non-resolving cases can be offered surgery in the form of myringotomy with/without placement of grommet/ventilation tubes (99, 101). Hearing aids may be offered to patients who are unwilling for surgical intervention (102).

**Chronic Otitis Media:** COM is long-standing infection of a part or whole of the middle ear cleft

## Table 2.8: **Causes of Hearing Loss in COM**

| Conductive Hearing Loss | SNHL |
|---|---|
| • *TM perforation:* Loss of areal ratio, CHL is generally proportional to size of the perforation.<br>• *Ossicular destruction:* Loss of lever ratio. The destruction follows in decreasing order: long process of incus, stapes crura, body of incus and manubrium (105).<br>• *Tympanosclerosis:* Stiffening of TM or ossicular fixation.<br>• Presence of discharge which may also increase the conductive hearing loss.<br>• Iatrogenic<br>  • Due to requirement of removing Incus to achieve disease clearance (107)<br>  • In cholesteatoma, hearers (sound being conducted through cholesteatoma) postoperative hearing will be worse than preoperative status. | • Diffusion of toxins through the round window membrane can cause labyrinthitis and hence SNHL (106)<br>• SNHL due to damage caused by moving drill touching the intact ossicular chain (108) |

characterized by a permanent abnormality of TM (pars flacida or pars tensa) (103). There are various factors that are involved in aetiology of COM: history of AOM or OME which may cause degenerative changes making TM more vulnerable to chronic perforation, genetics, low socio-economic status, eustachian tube function, cranio-facial anomalies, GERD and recurrent respiratory tract infections. The present system of classification divides COM into mucosal and squamous types, as discussed in the previous section.

WHO estimates that about 65–330 million people are affected by COM worldwide and of these almost 50% have hearing loss (104). Various ways in which hearing loss occurs in COM are listed in Table 2.8.

There are some important considerations in treatment of hearing loss due to COM:

■ The worse hearing ear is taken up for surgery first in bilateral disease; in case both are equally affected, the patient's choice decides which ear to be operated first.

■ Belfast rule of thumb: It states that in order for the patient to perceive a benefit in hearing postoperatively the hearing thresholds should be brought up to 30 dB or better or within 15 dB of the better hearing ear (109).

■ Glasgow benefit plot: The preoperative and postoperative hearing thresholds of both ears are represented in a graphical to assess the benefit in hearing perceived by the patient after surgery (110).

■ In case of a mixed hearing loss, the poorer prognosis of hearing has to be explained to the patient and consent has to be taken for the same.

■ A conductive hearing loss of more than 35 dB should alert the surgeon for a possible ossicular discontinuity and hence an ossiculoplasty should be performed to improve

hearing outcomes. Most of ossicular defects are covered by the Austin-Kartush classification, which has been discussed in the previous section (111, 112). Broadly speaking, two types of ossiculoplasty procedures are done – the short columella, where the stapes superstructure is present and the prosthesis/refashioned incus is placed over it, and the long columella, where the prosthesis/refashioned incus is placed directly over the stapes footplate (113).

■ In some cases of COM squamous, the patient may have good hearing despite ossicular damage due to conduction of sound through cholesteatoma (cholesteatoma hearers) and in them hearing will worsen following surgery and this has to be explained to the patient.

■ In case a canal wall down procedure is planned, the patient has to counselled regarding possible permanent residual conductive hearing loss following surgery (114).

■ Hearing aids have an important role in rehabilitation of patients with COM:

  – In cases of healed COM with conductive hearing loss.

  – In cases of inactive COM where hearing loss is disabling, and patient is unfit/unwilling for surgery.

  – Postoperatively in case hearing loss persists after surgery, especially in cases of pre-existing SNHL.

  – However, hearing aids have to be avoided in cases of COM active as they will increase chances of infection due to stasis of secretions.

  – In cases of canal wall down mastoidectomy, open-fit hearing aids may be required.

*Post-traumatic*

**Ossicular discontinuity:** Ossicular discontinuity is commonly caused by head injury causing temporal bone trauma and in up to 60% cases, concomitant temporal bone fractures are present (115); other causes include surgery like tympanoplasty and stapes surgery and intra-tympanic injections. Ossicular fractures are relatively rare, mostly involving the long process of incus (116). The patient has a conductive hearing loss which may have components due to TM perforation or hemotympanum (117), rarely SNHL may also be present. Ossicular discontinuity with an intact TM gives a severe conductive hearing loss. Tympanometry may reveal an "Ad" type of curve. Majority of the ossicular injuries are identifiable on HRCT of temporal bones and this should be the investigation of choice when ossicular discontinuity is suspected (118).

Ossicular discontinuity may heal by fibrosis with good hearing results; therefore, up to 3 months of conservative management should be given following trauma before considering surgical intervention (119). Ossiculoplasty can be performed according to the site of discontinuity (111, 112) Option of hearing aids may be offered to patient and an informed decision should be taken.

**Hemotympanum:** Presence of blood in the middle ear cavity is a relatively common finding in cases of head injury/barotrauma. Detailed clinical examination is required to look for associated injuries like temporal bone fracture, head injury etc. Imaging should be done to rule out skull base fracture leading to CSF in the middle ear. Treatment of hemotympanum is conservative and most of the cases resolve within a period of 3 months (120, 121).

**Ruptured tympanic membrane:** Traumatic TM rupture can occur following blast injury, head injury, due to foreign body or due to iatrogenic trauma like syringing. A careful history and detailed clinical examination is required to look for other injuries like fracture of EAC, fracture of mandible, fracture of temporal bone, head injury etc. (122). The patient will present with pain and bleeding from the ear associated with conductive hearing loss (123). Treatment of traumatic TM perforation is conservative and consists of aural toilet to remove any foreign body/debris from the EAC and instillation of topical antibiotic drops to treat any infection. Most of the traumatic perforations (up to 95%) heal spontaneously in a time period of up to 3 months in the absence of a pre-existing pathology and this time should be allowed to pass before considering formal repair by surgery. The prognosis is poorer for larger perforations,

for patients with advanced age and for caustic injuries. Presence of infection in the middle ear slows the recovery; however, the location of TM perforation does not impact the rate of healing (124). Use of treatments like application of cigarette paper, absorbable gel foam or epidermal growth factor may help to speed up the recovery process but do not significantly improve the prognosis (125).

**Otosclerosis:** Otosclerosis is a hereditary disorder affecting endochondral bone of the otic capsule. It is characterized by disordered resorption and deposition of bone (126).The most common site of otosclerosis is the area anterior to oval window (80–95% of cases), called the fissula ante fenestram (127). Other sites of involvement include the round window niche (about 30%), the apical medial wall of the cochlear labyrinth (about 15%), the stapes footplate (about 12%) and posterior to the oval window (5–10%) (128).

The disease usually begins early in third decade of life, it is twice as common in females and is aggravated during pregnancy. The disease is often familial but sporadic cases of otosclerosis represent 40–50% of all clinical cases (129). Symptoms include slowly progressive hearing loss, which is bilateral in 75% of cases (130). Tinnitus may be present. Otoscopic examination reveals a normal TM. Tuning-Fork tests reveal signs of conductive hearing loss. The British National Study of Otosclerosis has defined presumptive clinical otosclerosis as an ear where the TM is normal, the tympanogram is peaked with normal pressure range and associated with an air-bone gap of 15 dB or greater over 0.5, 1 and 2 kHz (130).The gold reference standard of diagnosis is exploratory tympanotomy.

PTA usually demonstrates conductive hearing loss with air-bone gap greater at low frequencies. If cochlear involvement is present, a mixed hearing loss is present, with high frequencies more affected.

Carhart's notch is named after the well-known audiologist who first described it in detail as a depression in the BC audiogram of patients with clinical otosclerosis. It is characterized by elevation of BC thresholds of 5 dB at 500 Hz, 10 dB at 1000 Hz, 15 dB at 2000 Hz and 5 dB at 4000 Hz (131, 132) (Figure 2.10). In most of the otosclerosis cases, the BC depression is usually observed at the frequency level 2 kHz region, but it can also be seen in any middle frequencies from 0.5 to 2 kHz, which correspond to the resonance frequency of the middle ear, and can be substantially improved following successful stapes surgery.

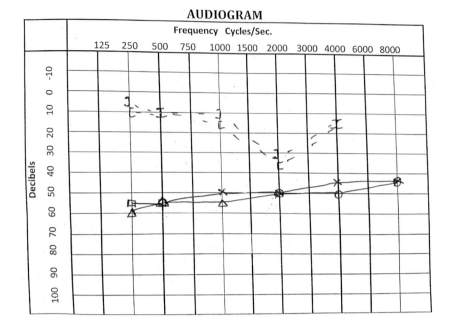

**Figure 2.10**  Carhart's notch.

**BC Over-closure:** Most cases of otosclerosis show an improvement of up to 15 dB from their preoperative BC thresholds in affected frequencies after successful stapes surgery. This phenomenon is known as BC over-closure and leads to "flat-pattern audiogram" postoperatively (133).

Tympanometry usually reveals a type "As" or type "A" curve with reduced compliance at normal pressure. HRCT of temporal bone is used to visualize hypodense foci around otic capsule, measure the stapes footplate thickness and rule out other causes of conductive hearing loss such as ossicular chain discontinuity (134).

Treatment of otosclerosis can be surgical or non-surgical and an informed decision has to be taken by the patient. It is generally agreed that a minimum AB gap of 20 dB is required for the patient to appreciate improvement in hearing postoperatively, but experienced surgeons can choose to operate on ears with lesser AB gap (135). The surgical management of otosclerosis has evolved over a period of time from mobilization to fenestration surgery to stapedectomy to the current standard of treatment, that is stapedotomy with use of piston (136). Stapedotomy can be performed using perforators or drill or LASER. Various types of pistons are in use like fluoroplastic, titanium and thermoplastic pistons, all of which have their own advantages and disadvantages. The point against surgery is that it does nothing to stop

disease progression and eventually the hearing loss recurs, another disadvantage of surgery is the risk of causing permanent SNHL which has to be explained to the patient. In far advanced otosclerosis, use of cochlear implants can be considered but it has disadvantages like obliteration of round window due to disease process and incomplete electrode array insertion (137).

Non-surgical treatment involves medical management like use of sodium fluoride, which has been shown to delay the worsening of conductive hearing loss (138). Another mainstay of treatment is use of hearing aids; as the hearing loss is predominantly conductive, these patients hear well using hearing aids and this option can be considered in patients who are unfit/unwilling for surgery or in cases of recurrence of hearing loss after surgery in otosclerosis.

### Mixed Hearing Loss

**Trauma:** Trauma can cause conductive hearing loss, as discussed earlier. It can also cause SNHL due to mechanisms listed in Table 2.9. These conditions may coexist and present as mixed hearing loss.

**Coexisting COM with SNHL:** Presence of chronic ear disease does not preclude the effect of ageing/noise or ototoxic drugs. Therefore, the conductive component of hearing loss due to middle ear pathology may be superimposed on the SNHL caused by said causes leading to mixed hearing loss (139). Although the SNHL

## Table 2.9: **Causes of SNHL in Trauma**

- Temporal bone fracture otic involving
- Labyrinthine concussion
- Labyrinthine haemorrhage
- Perilymphatic fistula, e.g. round window tear
- Direct trauma to cochlea due to noise (acoustic trauma)
- Iatrogenic, e.g. excessive handling of ossicles or touching the drill to an intact ossicular chain or avulsion of stapes footplate.

component is irreversible, the conductive component of hearing loss can be managed with surgical intervention (140). The patient should be informed and counselled regarding poorer prognosis of hearing in such cases.

**Complication of COM:** Toxins produced in the middle ear due to infection can cross the round window membrane and lead to labyrinthitis causing SNHL, which is superimposed on the existing conductive hearing loss due to COM, causing mixed hearing loss. If only toxins have entered the labyrinth, it is called serous labyrinthitis which is reversible, but an infection of the labyrinth causes purulent labyrinthitis which causes permanent SNHL. COM is managed with surgical intervention which can resolve the conductive part of the mixed hearing loss.

### Auditory Neuropathy Spectrum Disorder

The term auditory neuropathy was coined by Starr et al. in 1996 to describe patients whose hearing loss was supposed to be due to neuropathy of the auditory nerve (141). These patients had absent BERA in presence of OAE and cochlear microphonics. However, research has shown that the disease is multifaceted and the site of origin of this disorder can be many levels, and hence the term auditory neuropathy spectrum disorder was adopted in 2008 (142, 143). The various sites where disease can occur are (144) as follows:

- Inner hair cells

- Tectorial membrane

- Synaptic junctions

- Auditory neurons in spiral ganglion

- Auditory nerve fibres

ANSD is a type of hearing disorder where the patient is able to hear the sound but has difficulty in understanding speech. ANSD is usually diagnosed in paediatric population and is most commonly caused by genetic conditions, but certain genetic conditions manifest with hearing loss only during adult life. There are certain disorders which may cause ANSD as a

part of their spectrum like multiple sclerosis, peripheral neuropathies, hereditary spastic paresis, hereditary motor-sensory neuropathy etc. In a study conducted by Starr et al., it was found that 42% of ANSD cases were associated with hereditary neurological disorders, 10% due to toxic/immunologic/infective/metabolic causes and remaining 48% were idiopathic (141).

Examination reveals normal otoscopy, PTA thresholds are variable and can range from normal to profound hearing loss. Tympanometry is normal but speech audiometry reveals poor thresholds and discrimination scores. OAE is present with absence of contralateral suppression of OAE, cochlear microphonics are present with an absent BERA response. Cortical auditory evoked potential is a measure of cortical maturation and its absence indicates auditory dys-synchrony and poor auditory prognosis.

The patients should undergo an MRI of brain as up to 35–40% cases will have abnormalities on MRI like cochlear/vestibular anomalies, CN VIII anomalies and abnormalities of brain like multiple sclerosis (145). The patients should also undergo evaluation by ophthalmologist, neurophysician and geneticist for associated disorders.

Management of these cases is complex, use of hearing aids has been tried but evidence of benefit is limited (146). Theoretically, cochlear implantation should not be helpful as disease is beyond the cochlea, but some studies have shown that cochlear implantation may help in auditory outcomes (147). Total communication may be offered in cases not responding to treatment. Associated immunologic/metabolic/infective/toxic disorders can be treated according to aetiology.

### CONCLUSION

A wide variety of disorders lead to hearing loss, so when a patient presents with complaints of hearing loss, a history has to be taken for associated ear symptoms like otalgia, otorrhoea, tinnitus, vertigo and facial palsy. In addition, history regarding onset of symptoms, duration, progression of disease, severity of hearing loss, exposure to loud noise, head injury, meningitis and any other history of serious illness for which ototoxic medications like aminoglycosides may have been given also needs to be elicited. After this the patient should undergo physical examination including otoscopy. Otoscopy may reveal the underlying pathology in cases of conductive hearing loss where the disease may be evident on inspection. However, otoscopy may be normal in most cases of SNHL and in some cases of conductive hearing loss like otosclerosis and the clinician should always keep this in mind while evaluating a patient with hearing loss. With use of appropriate audiological and radiological investigations, the clinician should be able to reach a diagnosis.

## REFERENCES

1. Issacson JE, Vora NM, Milton S. Differential diagnosis and treatment of hearing loss. Am Fam Physician. 2003; 68(6):1125–32.

2. Cunningham LL, Tucci DL. Hearing loss in adults. N Engl J Med. 2017;377(25):2465–7.

3. WHO. Addressing the Rising Prevalence of Hearing Loss. Geneva: World Health Organization, 2018.

4. Scholes S, Biddulph J, Davis A, et al. Socioeconomic differences in hearing among middle-aged and older adults: cross-sectional analyses using the Health Survey for England. BMJ Open. 2018;8:e019615.

5. Guidelines Standard Audiometric Procedures. Indian Speech-Language and Hearing Association. Available at Ishaindia.org.in. Accessed in Dec 2019.

6. American Speech-Language-Hearing Association. 2005. Guidelines for manual pure tone threshold audiometry. Available at: www.Asha.org/policy.

7. de Souza Fernandes, KC, Pacheco Russo IC. Clinical masking: applicability of plateau and optimized methods in hearing thresholds testing. Pro Fono. 2009; 21(4):333–8.

8. Clark JG. Uses and abuses of hearing loss classification. ASHA. 1981;230:495–500.

9. WHO Report of the Informal Working Group on Prevention of Deafness and Hearing Impairment Programme Planning, Geneva, 1991.

10. Ministry of Social Justice and Empowerment, Department of Empowerment of Persons with Disabilities (Divyangjan), Notification New Delhi, 4th January 2018.

11. The Rehabilitation Council of India Act, 1992, Ministry of Law, Justice and Company Affairs, No. 34 of 1992, New Delhi, 1992. Available at: http://www.rehabcouncil.nic.in/engweb/rciact.pdf

12. Jennings CR, Jones NS. Presbyacusis. J Laryngol Otol. 2001;115(3):171–8.

13. Davis A. Hearing in Adults. London: Whurr Publishers, 1995.

14. Brandt LJ, Fozard JL. Age changes in pure tone hearing thresholds in a longitudinal study of normal human ageing. J Acoust Soc Am. 1990;88(2):813–20.

15. Glorig A, Nixon J. Hearing loss as a function of age. Laryngoscope. 1962;72:1596–610.

16. Lutman ME, Spencer HS. Occupational noise and demographic factors in hearing. Acta Otolaryngol. 1991;(Suppl 476):74–84.

17. Gates GA, Cooper JC. Incidence of hearing decline in the elderly. Acta Otolaryngol. 1991;111:240–8.

18. Agmon M, Lavie L, Doumas M. The association between hearing loss, postural control and mobility in older adults: a systematic review. J Am Acad Audiol. 2017;28(6):575–88.

19. Thomson RS, Auduong P, Miller AT, Gurgel RK. Hearing loss as a risk factor for dementia: a systematic review. Laryngoscope Investig Otolaryngol. 2017; 2(2):69–79.

20. Rutherford BR, Brewster K, Golub JS, et al. Sensation and psychiatry: linking age related hearing loss to late-life depression and cognitive decline. Am J Psychiatry. 2018;175(3):215–24.

21. Schuknecht H. Presbycusis. Laryngoscope. 1955; 65:402–19

22. Schuknecht HF, Gaecek MR. Cochlear pathology in presbycusis. Ann Otol Rhinol Laryngol. 1993;102:1–16.

23. Schuknecht H. Patholgy of the Ear, 2nd ed. Pennsylvania: Lea & Febiger, 1993.

24. Palmer CV, Nelson CT, Lindley GA. The functionally and physiologically plastic adult auditory system. J Acoust Soc Am. 1998;103:1705–21.

25. Hopkins K, Moore BC. The effects of age and cochlear hearing loss on temporal fine structure sensitivity, frequency selectivity, and speech recognition in noise. J Acoust Soc Am. 2011;130(1):334–49.

26. Azizi MH. Occupational noise induced hearing loss. Int J Occup Environ Med. 2010;1(3):116–23.

27. Prevention of NIHL. WHO report (WHO-PDH), 1997:11. Available at: www.who.int/pbd/deafness/en/noise (accessed 12 Nov 2013).

28. Patuzzi R. Exponential onset and recovery of temporary threshold shift after loud sound: evidence for long-term inactivation of mechano-electrical transduction channels. Hear Res. 1998;125:17–38.

29. Ward WD. General auditory effects of noise. Otolaryngol Clin North Am. 1979;12 (3).

30. Alberti PW. Noise and ear. In: Kerr AG, editor. Scott-Brown's Otolaryngology, 6th ed. Oxford: Butterworth Heinnman, 1996, p. 1–28.

31. Kirchner BD, Evenson Col. Eric, Dobie RA, Rabinowitz P, Crawford J, Kopke R, Hudson TW. Occupational noise-induced hearing loss. ACOEM Task Force on Occupational Hearing Loss. J Occup Environ Med. 2012;54 (1):106–8.

32. Jahrsdoerfer R. The effects of impulse noise on the ear drum and middle ear. Otolaryngol Clin North Am. 1979;12 (3):515–20.

33. Levey S, Fligor BJ, Kagimbi CGL. The effects of noise-induced hearing loss on children and young adults. Contemp Issues Commun Sci. 2012;39:76–83.

34. Robinowitz PM, Rees TS. Occupational hearing loss. In: Rosenstock L, et al., editor. Textbook of Clinical Occupational and Environmental Medicine, 2nd ed. St. Louis, Mo: Elsevier, 2005.

35. Alberti PW. Noise induced hearing loss. BMJ. 1992; 304:522.

36. Noise Induced Hearing Loss of Occupational Origin: A Guide for Medical Practitioners, 1st ed. New Zealand: Occupational Safety and Health Service, Department of Labour, 1994.

37. Puel JL, Ruel J, d'Aldin CG, Pujol R. Excite-toxicity and repair of cochlear synapses after noise trauma induced hearing loss. Neuroreport. 1998;9:2109–14.

38. Chen GD, Kong J, Reinhard K, Fetcher LD. NMDA receptor blockage protects against permanent noise induced hearing loss but not its potentiation by carbon monoxide. Hear Res. 2001;154:108–15.

39. Thorne PR, Nuttall AL. Laser Doppler measurements of cochlear blood flow during loud sound exposure in the Guniea pig. Hearing Research. 1987;27 (1):1–10.

40. Quirk WS, Seidman MD. Cochlear vascular changes in response to loud noise. Am J Otol. 1995;16:322–5.

41. Cheng AG, Cunningham LL, Rubel EW. Mechanisms of hair cell death and protection. Curr Opin Otolaryngol Head Neck Surg. 2005;13:343–8.

42. Wong ACY, Froud KE, Hsieh Y-SY. Noise induced hearing loss in the 21st century: a research and translational update. World J Otorhinolaryngol. 2013;3(3):58–70.

43. Poirrier AL, Pincemail J, Van Den Ackerveken P, Lefebvre PP, Malgrange B. Oxidative stress in the cochlea: an update. Curr Med Chem. 2010;17 (31): 1–14

44. Lim DJ, Dunn DE. Anatomic correlates of noise induced hearing loss. Otolaryngol Clin North Am. 1979;12(3):493–513.

45. Yang WP, Henderson D, Hu BH, Nicotera TM. Quantitative analysis of apoptotic and necrotic outer hair cells after exposure to different levels of continuous noise. Hear Res. 2004;196:69–76.

46. Kobel M, Le Prell CG, Liu J, et al. Noise induced cochlear synaptopathy: past findings and future studies. Hear Res. 2017;349:148–54.

47. Konings A, Laer LV, Camp GV. Genetic studies on noise-induced hearing loss: a review. Ear Hear. 2009;30(2):151–59.

48. David RR, Newlander JK, Ling XB, et al. Genetic basis for susceptibility to noise induced hearing loss in mice. Hear Res. 2001;155:85–90.

49. Kujawa SG, Liberman MC. Acceleration of age related hearing loss by early noise exposure: evidence of a misspent youth. J Neurosci. 2006;26:2115–23.

50. Ohermiller KK. Contribution of mouse models to understanding of age and noise related hearing loss. Brain Res. 2006;1091:89–102.

51. Sung JH, Sim CS, Lee C et al. Relationship of cigarette smoking and hearing loss in workers exposed to occupational noise. Annals Occup Environ Med. 2013;25:8–17.

52. Henderson D, Hu B, Mc Fadden S, Zheng X. Evidence of common pathway in noise induced hearing loss and carboplatin ototoxicity. Noise Health. 1999; 2:53–70.

53. Baguley DM, McCombe A. Noise induced hearing loss. In: Gleeson M, editor. Scott-Brown's Otorhinolaryngology, Head & Neck Surgery, 7th ed. London: Hodder Arnold, 2008:3548–57.

54. Osei-Lah V, Yeoh L. High frequency audiometric notch: an outpatient survey. Int J Audiol. 2010. 49;85–8.

55. Nair S, Kashyap RC. Significance of 6 kHz in noise induced hearing loss in IAF personnel. Ind J Aerospace Med. 2008;52(2):15–20.

56. Cain PA. Update: noise induced hearing loss and the military environment. J R Army Med Corps. 1998; 144:97–101.

57. Ylikoski ME, Ylikoski JS. Hearing loss and handicap of professional soldiers exposed to gunfire noise. Scand J Work Environ Health. 1994;20(2):93–100.

58. Lutman ME, Robinson DW. Quantification of hearing loss for medicolegal purposes based on self-rating. Br J Audiol. 1992 Oct; 26 (5): 297–306.

59. Hall AJ, Lutman ME. Methods for early identification of noise induced hearing loss. Audiology. 1999; 38:277–80.

60. Health and Safety Executive. Noise at Work: Noise Assessment and Control, Noise Guides 3–8. London: HMSO, 1990.

61. Tikka C, Verbeek JH, Kateman E, et al. Interventions to prevent occupational noise induced hearing loss. Cochrane Database Syst Rev. 2017;7: CD006396.

62. Kraaijenga VJ, Ramakers GG, Grolman W. The effect of ear plugs in preventing hearing loss from recreational noise exposure: a systematic review. JAMA Otolaryngol Head Neck Surg. 2016;142 (4): 389–94.

63. Alberti PW, Abel SM, Rico K. Practical aspects of hearing protector use. In: Hamernik RP, Henderson D, Salvi R, editors. New Perspectives on Noise Induced Hearing Loss. New York: Raven Press, 1982.

64. Owen JP. Noise induced hearing loss in military helicopter aircrew: a review of the evidence. J R Army Med Corps. 1995;141:98–101.

65. Hahn H, Salt AN, Schumacher U, Plontke SK. Gentamycin concentration gradients in scala tympani perilymph following systemic applications. Audiol Neurotol. 2013;18 (6):383–91.

66. Salt AN, Hartsock JJ, Gill RM, et al. Perilymph pharmacokinetics of locally applied gentamycin in the guinea pig. Hear Res. 2016;342:101–11.

67. Taylor RR, Neville G, Forge A. Rapid hair cell loss: a mouse model for cochlear lesions. J Assoc Res Otolaryngol. 2008;9(1):44–64.

68. Pike DA, Bosher SK. The time course of the strial changes produced by intra-venous frusemide. Hear Res. 1980;3(1):79–89.

69. Brummet RE. Ototoxic liability of erythromycin and analogues. Otolaryngol Clin North Am. 1993;26(5):811–9.

70. Jastreboff PJ, Hansen R, Sasaki PG, Sasaki CT. Differential uptake of salicylate in serum, cerebrospinal fluid and perilymph. Arch Otolaryngol Head Neck Surg. 1986;112 (10):1050–3.

71. Tange RA, Dreschler WE, Claessen FA, Perenboom RM. Ototoxic reactions of quinine in healthy persons and patients with *Plasmodium falciparum* infection. Auris Nasus Larynx. 1997;24 (2):131–6.

72. Schacht J, Talaska AE, Rybak LP. Cisplatin and aminoglycoside antibiotics: hearing loss and its prevention. Anat Rec. 2012;295(11):1837–50.

73. Lindeman HH. Regional differences in sensitivity of vestibular sensory epithelia to ototoxic antibiotics. Acta Otolaryngol. 1969;67 (2):177–89.

74. Forge A, Schacht J. Aminoglycoside antibiotics. Audiol Neurotol. 2000;5(1):3–22.

75. Blakeley BW. Clinical forum: a review of intra-tympanic therapy. Am J Otol. 1997;18 (4):520–6.

76. Konrad-Martin D, Helt WJ, Reavis KM, et al. Ototoxicity: early detection and monitoring. ASHA Leader. 2005;10(7):1–14.

77. Durrant JD, Campbell K, Fausti S, et al. American Academy of Audiology Position Statement and Clinical Practice Guidelines: Ototoxicity Monitoring, American Academy of Audiology, October 2009.

78. Hereditary Hearing Loss. Available at: http://hereditaryhearingloss.org.

79. Hildebrand MS, DeLuca AP, Taylor KR, et al. A contemporary review of AudioGene profiling: a machine based candidate gene prediction tool for autosomal dominant nonsyndromic hearing loss. Laryngoscope. 2009;119:2211–5.

80. Peterson MB. Non-syndromic autosomal dominant deafness. Clin Genet. 2002;62:1–13.

81. Pan B, Askew C, Galvin A, et al. Gene therapy restores auditory and vestibular function in a mouse model of Usher syndrome type 1c. Nat Biotechnol. 2017;35 (3):264–72.

82. Ciorba A, Corazzi V, et al. Autoimmune inner ear disease: a diagnostic challenge. Int J Immunopathol Pharmacol. 2018;32:1–5.

83. Mijovic T, Zeitouni A, Colmegna I. Autoimmune sensorineural hearing loss: the otology rheumatology interface. Rheumatology. 2013;52:780–9.

84. Mehat AK, Singh VK. Screening tests for nonorganic hearing loss. Med J Armed Forces India. 2000 Jan; 56(1):79–81.

85. Biswas A. Clinical audio-vestibulometry for otologist and neurologist. 2009;4:48–176.

86. Adobamen PR, Ogisi FO. Hearing loss due to wax impaction. Nig Q J Hosp Med. 2012;22(2):117–20.

87. Clegg AJ, Loveman E, Gospodarevskya E, et al. The safety and effectiveness of different methods of ear wax removal: a systematic review and economic evaluation. Health Technol Assess. 2010;14(28):1–192.

88. Hirsch BE. Infections of the external ear. Am J Otolaryngol. 1992;13:145–55.

89. Kaushik V, Malik T, Saeed SR. Interventions for acute otitis externa. Cochrane Database Syst Rev. 2010;20: CD004740.

90. Morrison AW. Keratosis obturans. J Laryngol. 1956;70:317–21.

91. Paparella MM, Goycoolea MV. Canalplasty for chronic intractable external otitis and keratosis obturans. Otolaryngol Head Neck Surg. 1981;89:440–3.

92. Marais J, Dale BA. Bullous myringitis: a review. Clin Otolaryngol Allied Sci. 1997;22(6):497–9.

93. Neilson LJ, Hussain SS. Management of granular myringitis: a systematic review. J Laryngol Otol. 2008;122(1):3–10.

94. Pukander J, Luotonen J, Sipila M, et al. Incidence of acute otitis media. Acta Otolaryngol. 1982;93 (5–6):447–53.

95. Greenberg DP. Update on the development and use of viral and bacterial vaccines for the prevention of acute otitis media. Allergy Asthma Proc. 2001; 22(6):353–7.

96. Shaikh N, Hoberman A, Kaleida PH, et al. Otoscopic signs of otitis media. Paed Infect Dis J. 2011;30 (10):822–6.

97. Venekamp RV, Sanders S, Glasizou PP, et al. Antibiotics for acute otitis media in children. Cochrane Database Syst Rev. 2013;1: CD000219.

98. Robinson PM. Secretory otitis media in the adult. Clin Otolaryngol Allied Sci. 1987;12:297–302.

99. Finkelstein Y, Ophir D, Talmi YP, et al. Adult onset otitis media with effusion. Arch Otolaryngol Head Neck Surg. 1994;120:517–27.

100. Morton RP, Woollons AC, McIvor NP. Nasopharyngeal carcinoma and middle ear effusion: natural history and effect of ventilation tubes. Clin Otolaryngol Allied Sci. 1994;19 (6):529–31.

101. Rosenfeld, RM, Shin JJ, Schwartz SR, et al. Clinical Practice Guideline: Otitis Media with Effusion (Update). Otolaryngol Head Neck Surg. 2016;154(1 Suppl) :S1–41.

102. Otitis Media with effusion in under 12s: surgery. National Institute for Health and Care Excellence Clinical Guidelines, 27 February 2008.

103. Browning GG, Merchant SN, Kelly G, et al. Chronic otitis media. In: Gleeson M, editor. Scott-Brown's Otorhinolaryngology, Head & Neck Surgery, 7th edition, Vol. 3. London: Hodder Arnold.

104. Acuin J, World Health Organization. Chronic suppurative otitis media: burden of illness and management. Geneva : World Health Organization, 2012.

105. Browning GG, Weir J, Kelly G, Swan IRC. Chronic otitis media. In: Watkinson JC, editor. Scott-Brown's Otorhinolaryngology, Head & Neck Surgery. 8th ed. UK: Taylor & Francis Group, 2018, p. 977–1014.

106. Cureoglu S, Schachern PA, Rinaldo A, Tsuprun V, Ferlito A, Paparella MM. Round window membrane and labyrinthine pathological changes: an overview. Acta Otolaryngol. 2005;125(1):9–15.

107. Patil A, Khairnar P. A cross sectional study to assess effects of mastoid drill on hearing levels in chronic suppurative otitis media cases in a tertiary care hospital in northern Maharashtra. Int J Otorhinolaryngol Head Neck Surg. 2017;3(2):264.

108. Domenech J, Carulla M, Traserra J. Sensorineural high-frequency hearing loss after drill-generated acoustic trauma in tympanoplasty. Arch Otorhinolaryngol. 1989;246(5):280–2.

109. Smythh GD, Patterson CC. Results of middle ear reconstruction: do patients and surgeons agree. Am J Otol. 1985,6.276–9.

110. Browning GG, Gatehouse S, Swan IRC. The Glasgow benefit plot: a new method for reporting benefits from middle ear surgery. Laryngoscope. 1991;101:180–5.

111. Austin DF. Ossicular reconstruction. Arch Otolaryngol. 1971;94:525–35.

112. Kartush J. Ossicular chain reconstruction: capitulum to malleus. Otolaryngol Clin North Am. 1994;27(4):689–715.

113. Mudhol RS, Naragund AI, Shruthi VS. Ossiculoplasty revisited. Indian J Otolaryngol Head Neck Surg. 2013; 65(Suppl 3):451–4.

114. Azevedo AF, Soares ABC, et al. Tympanomastoidectomy: comparison between canal wall-down and canal wall-up techniques in surgery for chronic otitis media. Int. Arch. Otorhinolaryngol. 2013;17 (3):242–5.

115. Kim JP, Kim SC, Yoon HV, et al. Clinical study of traumatic ossicular disruption without tympanic membrane perforation. Korean J Otorhinolaryngol Head Neck Surg. 2001;44(7):696–9.

116. Spector GJ, Pratt LL, Randall G. A clinical study of delayed reconstruction in ossicular fractures. Laryngoscope. 1973;83:837–51.

117. Podoshin L, Fradis M. Hearing loss after head injury. Arch Otolaryngol Head Neck Surg. 1975;101:15–8.

118. Meriot P, Veillon F, Garcia JF, et al. CT appearances of ossicular injuries. Radiographics. 1997;17:1445–54.

119. Holzapfel AR, Chang CYJ, Pereira KD. Ossicular chain disruption with normal hearing. Ear Nose Throat J. 2005;84:351–3.

120. Kim, C, Shin, JE. Hemorrhage within the tympanic membrane without perforation. J Otolaryngol Head Neck Surg. 2018 47, 66:1–7.

121. Pulec JL, DeGuine C. Hemotympanum from trauma. Ear Nose Throat J. 2001;80(8):486.

122. Lou ZC, Lou ZH, Zhang QP. Traumatic tympanic membrane perforations: a study of etiology and factors affecting outcomes. Am J Otolaryngol. 2012;33(5):549–55.

123. Hempel JM, Becker Muller JA, et al. Traumatic tympanic membrane perforations: clinical and audiometric findings in 198 patients. Otol Neurotol. 2012;33:1357–62.

124. Orji FT, Agu CC. Determinants of spontaneous healing in traumatic perforations of the tympanic membrane. Clin Otolaryngol. 2008;33:420–6.

125. Orji FT, Agu CC. Patterns of hearing loss in tympanic membrane perforation resulting from physical blow to the ear: a prospective controlled cohort study. Clin Otolaryngol. 2009;34(6):526–32.

126. Chole RA, McKenna M. Pathophysiology of otosclerosis. Otol Neurotol. 2001;22(2):249–57.

127. Schuknecht HF, Barber W. Histologic variants in otosclerosis. Laryngoscope. 1985;95(11):1307–17.

128. Merchant SN, Mckenna MJ, Browning GG, Rea PA, Tange RA. Otosclerosis. In: Gleeson M, Browning GG, Burton MJ, et al., editors. Scott-Brown's Otorhinolaryngology, Head & Neck Surgery, 7th ed. London: Hodder Arnold; 2008:3453–85.

129. Menger D, Tange R. The aetiology of otosclerosis: a review of the literature. Clin Otolaryngol Allied Sci. 2003;28(2):112–20.

130. Browning GG, Gatehouse S. The prevalence of middle ear disease in the adult British population. Clin Otolaryngol Allied Sci. 1992;17(4):317–21.

131. Carhart R. Clinical application of bone conduction audiometry. Arch Otolaryngol. 1950;51(6):798–808.

132. Kashio A, Ito K, Kakigi A, et al. Carhart notch 2-kHz bone conduction threshold dip: a nondefinitive predictor of stapes fixation in conductive hearing loss with normal tympanic membrane. Arch Otolaryngol Head Neck Surg. 2011;137(3):236–40.

133. Vijayendra H, Parikh B. Bone conduction improvement after surgery for conductive hearing loss. IJOHNS. 2011;63(3):201–4.

134. Lagleyre S, Sorrentino T, Calmels M-N, et al. Reliability of high-resolution CT scan in diagnosis of otosclerosis. Otol Neurotol. 2009;30(8):1152–9.

135. Lippy WH, Burkey JM, Schurung AG, Rizer FM. Stapedectomy in patients with small AB gaps. Laryngoscope. 1997;107:919–22.

136. Tange RA. The history of otosclerosis treatment. Amsterdam; Kugler Publications, 2014.

137. Rea P, Abrahams Y, Sanli H, Gibson W. Severe Otosclerosis: The Pitfalls and Outcomes of Cochlear Implantation. Paper presented at British Cochlear Implant Conference, Manchester UK, 2002.

138. Colletti V, Florino FG. Effect of sodium fluoride early otosclerosis. Am J Otol. 1991;12:195–8.

139. Amali A, Hosseinzadeh N, Samadi S, Nasiri S, Zebardast J. Sensorineural hearing loss in patients with chronic suppurative otitis media: is there a significant correlation? Electron Phys. 2017;9(2):3823–7.

140. Sharma R, Sharma VK. Analysis of sensorineural hearing loss in chronic suppurative otitis media with and without cholesteatoma. Indian J Otol. 2012;18(2):65–8.

141. Starr A, Picton TW, Sinninger Y, et al. Auditory neuropathy. Brain. 1996;119:741-53.

142. Kaga K. Auditory nerve disease and auditory neuropathy spectrum disorders. Auris Nasus Larynx. 2016;43(1):10–20.

143. Ruosch P. Auditory neuropathy spectrum disorder: evaluation and management. Hear J. 2008;61 (11):1–5.

144. Berlin CI, Hood LJ, et al. Multi-site diagnosis and management of 260 patients with auditory neuropathy/dys-synchrony (auditory neuropathy spectrum disorder). Int J Audiol. 2010;49:30–43.

145. De Seze J, Assouad R, Stojkovik T, et al. Hearing loss in multiple sclerosis: clinical, electro-physiological and radiological study. Rev Neurol. 2001;157:1403–9.

146. Hassan DM. Auditory neuropathy spectrum disorder: a new approach to hearing aid fitting. Egypt J Otolaryngol. 2017;33:67–77.

147. Teagle HFB, Roush PA, Woodard, JS, et al. Cochlear implantation in children with auditory neuropathy spectrum disorder. Ear Hear. 2010;31(3):325–35.

# 3 Sudden Sensorineural Hearing Loss

*Atul Gupta*

## CONTENTS

## INTRODUCTION

Sudden Sensorineural Hearing Loss (SSNHL) is an alarming symptom that often prompts an urgent or emergent visit to a physician. First described by De Klevn in 1944, it is a familiar entity which is easier to recognize than to define. It is commonly defined as a rapid onset of hearing impairment in one or both ears occurring over a period of 72 hours. The most frequently used audiometric criteria include a worsening in hearing of ≥30 dB, affecting at least three consecutive frequencies. Since pre-morbid audiometry is generally unavailable and most commonly the loss is unilateral, hearing loss is defined in relation to the opposite ear's thresholds, assuming both ears were normal before the event. Early recognition and commencement of treatment of SSNHL improve the chances of hearing recovery and favourably impact the patient's quality of life.

## REVIEW OF LITERATURE

**Epidemiology**: SSNHL affects 5–20 cases per 100,000 population/year (1). It can affect any age, more often at 43–53 years, with equal male-to-female ratio. It is bilateral in <1% cases. Vestibular symptoms are reported to be associated with 28–57% of cases.

**Aetiology**: The aetiology of SSNHL is diverse and is summarized in Table 3.1. Of the total cases of SSNHL, 80–90% are idiopathic and almost exclusively unilateral. Retrocochlear disorders (vestibular schwannoma, stroke) constitute 1% of the total cases. Other identifiable causes (Ménière's disease, trauma, autoimmune disease, syphilis, Lyme disease or perilymphatic fistula) are seen in 10–15% of the cases of SSNHL.

**Pathogenesis:** Most common findings reported in temporal bone histopathological studies include atrophy of the organ of Corti, loss of cochlear neurons, labyrinthine fibrosis, labyrinthine haemorrhage, formation of a new bone and degeneration of the spiral ligament, stria vascularis, hair cells, dendrites and apical spiral ganglion cells (2).

SSNHL is not a disease but represents a common symptom of a number of different pathologies (Table 3.2; 3). The following are some of the mechanisms by which SSNHL can be caused:

■ *Vascular theory:* Proposed by Rasmussen in 1949, the theory suggests vascular occlusion or ischaemia as a cause of SSNHL. Rasmussen postulated that the labyrinthine artery being an end artery (Figure 3.1) is highly prone to occlusion in conditions such as Buerger's disease, hypercholesterolemia, leukaemia and sickle cell anaemia, and this interruption of blood flow can cause tissue injury within 60 seconds. This leads to damage to hair cells, ganglion cells, spiral ligament, neuronal loss and alteration of the tectorial membrane. Treatment regimes based on this theory include fibrinogen apheresis, dextran infusion, hyperbaric oxygen and pentoxifylline

■ *Immunological theory:* Based upon clinical data and pathological findings in autoimmune diseases, McCabe, in 1979, gave the immunological theory for causation of SSNHL. It is based on the findings of immune complexes found in stria vascularis, endolymphatic sac and ducts, supporting cells and spiral ligament. Glucocorticoid receptors in the stria vascularis and supporting cells suggest their role as immune targets. The rationale behind treatment with corticosteroids was a result of this theory. This theory supports the increased occurrence of SSNHL in diseases like Cogan's syndrome, Wegener's granulomatosis and systemic lupus erythematosus.

## Table 3.1: Aetiology of Sudden Sensorineural Hearing Loss

| Infectious | Immunological | Neoplastic |
|---|---|---|
| • Meningitis (streptococcal, meningococcal, cryptococcal)<br>• Mumps<br>• Rubeola<br>• Rubella<br>• Syphilis<br>• Herpes virus (simplex, zoster, varicella)<br>• Lassa fever<br>• HIV<br>• Mononucleosis<br>• Mycoplasma<br>• Toxoplasmosis<br>• Cytomegalovirus | • Wegener's granulomatosis<br>• Cogan's syndrome<br>• Primary immune inner ear disease<br>• Temporal arteritis<br>• Systemic lupus erythematosus | • Acoustic neuroma<br>• Meningioma<br>• Lymphoma<br>• Leukaemia<br>• Myeloma<br>• Meningeal carcinomatosis |
| Circulatory | Traumatic | Metabolic |
| • Cerebrovascular accident<br>• Sickle cell disease<br>• Cardiopulmonary bypass<br>• Vertebrobasilar insufficiency | • Temporal bone fracture<br>• Acoustic trauma<br>• Barotrauma<br>• Perilymph fistula<br>• Otological surgery<br>• Lightening | • Renal failure<br>• Diabetes mellitus<br>• Hyperlipidaemia<br>• Hypothyroidism |
| Neurological | Toxic | Other Causes |
| • Multiple sclerosis<br>• Neurosarcoidosis | • Snake bite<br>• Ototoxic agents | • Idiopathic<br>• Ménière's disease<br>• Ulcerative colitis<br>• Scleroderma |

## Table 3.2: Categories of Sudden Sensorineural Hearing Loss

| Category | Description |
|---|---|
| SSNHL of specific cause | Clearly identifiable cause from history, examination, investigation |
| Possible idiopathic SSNHL | Cause not clearly identified |
| Definite idiopathic SSNHL | No obvious cause detected |

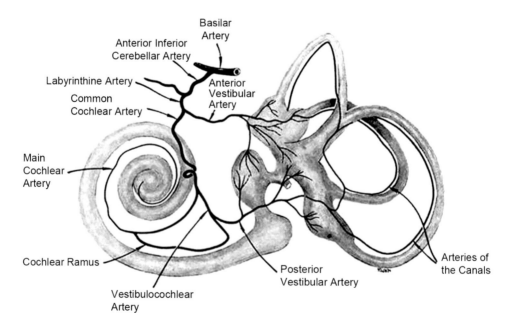

**Figure 3.1**  Blood supply of cochlea.

- *Infectious theory:* Hunt first reported Herpes zoster as a cause of SSNHL in 1907. Acute viral infections or reactivation of a latent viral infection with Herpes virus have been postulated to cause SSNHL (4). SSNHL is also seen in other infectious diseases such as syphilis, mumps, cytomegalovirus infection and rubella. The pathological changes include damage to organ of Corti, ganglion cells, nerve fibres, tectorial membrane and stria vascularis. Antiviral drugs, such as acyclovir and valacyclovir, are used to treat SSNHL as a result of this theory.

- *Genetic theory:* In 1853, Wilde first reported the genetic cause of congenital deafness. Gackler et al. (2010) found that majority of individuals with SSNHL had a family history of SSNHL.

About 32–65% of cases of SSNHL recover spontaneously (5). Clinical experience however indicates that this recovery rate may be an overestimation. The specific definition of what constitutes "improvement" or "recovery" after sudden hearing loss is not uniform among studies and reports. Vague subcategories of recovery, such as partial recovery or minimal recovery, are presented in literature without universally accepted definitions. Perhaps the most lenient and possibly the most commonly encountered definition of improvement is an improvement of 10 dB in pure tone average (PTA) or an improvement of 10% or 15% in Speech Discrimination Score (SDS). An alternative, stricter interpretation is improvement of 20 dB in PTA or 20% in SDS (6).

Using absolute values of improvement has the advantage of being relatively simple and being able to be performed without knowledge of prior hearing function or a normally hearing contralateral ear. The disadvantage is that absolute values can be misleading in certain patients. For example, a patient who has a 90 dB PTA and a 10% SDS could be considered improved at an 80 dB PTA and a 10% SDS, even though the patient may not notice any subjective improvement. Furthermore, patients who experience improvement in PTA but a worsening SDS (or vice versa) may be classified as improved. Presenting recovery as a percentage is more complex but provides consideration for a varying spectrum of severity of sudden loss. A major drawback of presenting recovery as a percentage is the need to know or assume the functional status of the ear before the SSNHL has occurred. In most cases, an audiogram before the SSNHL event is not available and must be assumed. Typically, the ear is assumed to be normal or similar to the contralateral ear. The validity of these assumptions has an impact on the calculation of a recovery percentage. Most importantly, the lack of a uniform definition of recovery limits the ability to compare or combine data across studies. It seems reasonable to speculate that perhaps the applied definition of recovery is the single most important factor in determining what percentage of patients with SSNHL recover.

Treatment in cases of idiopathic sudden sensorineural hearing loss (ISSNHL) is a controversial topic and various treatment agents and regimens are mentioned in literature (7). Use of more than one agent is common for successful treatment in case of ISSNHL. To date, no treatment agent or scheme is universally accepted and no single agent has been determined to improve patient outcomes beyond the natural history of the disease. The American Academy of Otolaryngology Head and Neck Surgery has given recommendations for treatment of SSNHL which are summarized in Table 3.3 (8).

## DIFFERENTIAL DIAGNOSIS
## ISSNHL

When there is no obvious cause detected for SSNHL, it may be referred to as ISSNHL. Fortunately, ISSNHL is almost always unilateral. Tinnitus is usually present along with SSNHL in idiopathic cases. Vertigo is frequent, either spontaneous (as in vestibular neuritis) or as isolated positional vertigo.

*Diagnostic criteria:* Pure tone audiometry confirms ≥30 dB hearing loss at three consecutive frequencies occurring in less than 3-day period and an underlying condition cannot be identified by history, physical examination and investigations (9).

*Incidence:* ISSNHL affects about 1 person per 10,000 per year.

*Causation theories:* Since ISSNHL is by definition idiopathic, the cause is not known. Nevertheless, there has been considerable speculation about viral, vascular and multiple other causes, with more evidence for the former than the latter. Many otologists believe that viral infection (or reactivation of latent viruses) is the most important cause of ISSNHL. In 1983, Wilson and colleagues in their study found out that viral seroconversion rates were greater in patients with ISSNHL (63%) compared to control (40%) (10). Current belief supports that viral cochleitis causes the majority of cases of ISSNHL.

## Table 3.3: American Academy of Otolaryngology-Head and Neck Surgery Recommendations for Sudden Sensorineural Hearing Loss

| | |
|---|---|
| Strong recommendations | • Distinguish sensorineural from conductive hearing loss<br>• Educate patients with ISSNHL, about the natural history of the condition, the benefits and risks of medical interventions and the limitations of existing evidence regarding efficacy<br>• Counsel patients with incomplete recovery of hearing and about the possible benefits of amplification |
| Recommendations | • Assess patients with presumptive SSNHL for bilateral SHL, recurrent episodes of SHL or focal neurological findings<br>• Diagnose presumptive ISSNHL if audiometry confirms a 30-dB hearing loss at three consecutive frequencies over 72 hours and an underlying condition cannot be identified by history and physical examination<br>• Evaluate for retrocochlear pathology by obtaining MRI, ABR or audiometric follow-up<br>• Offer intratympanic steroid perfusion when patients have incomplete recovery from ISSNHL after failure of initial management<br>• Obtain follow-up audiometric evaluation within 6 months of diagnosis for patients with ISSNHL |
| Recommendation against | • Routinely prescribing antivirals, thrombolytics, vasodilators, vasoactive substances or antioxidants to patients with ISSNHL |
| Strong recommendation against | • Ordering CT scan of the head in the initial evaluation of a patient with presumptive SSNHL<br>• Obtaining routine laboratory tests |

The circumstantial evidence for viral aetiology can be summarized as follows:

■ Many viral diseases (e.g. mumps, rubella, Varicella-zoster virus [VZV], influenza B) can cause congenital or sudden SNHL.

■ Cochlear histopathology after these viral diseases resembles that seen after ISSNHL.

■ Patients with ISSNHL often demonstrate immunological evidence for viral infection. Rates of seroconversion for herpes virus family are significantly higher in sudden hearing loss population (11).

■ Viruses such as herpes simplex may lie dormant in neural tissue for years and have also been identified in human spiral ganglia.

■ High prevalence of recent viral-type illness.

Although viral cause is implicated as the most common cause of ISSNHL, causation has not been definitely proved in any study till now. Another theory which can be postulated to be a causative factor in ISSNHL is the "Vascular Compromise" theory in which there is obstruction/blockade in the labyrinthine artery (end artery with no collaterals). Since cochlear function is sensitive to changes in blood supply and in case of blockage, there is reduced oxygen supply to the stria vascularis which may lead to SSNHL.

SSNHL can also be caused by leak of perilymph fluid into middle ear via round window or oval window like in cases of barotraumas. Intracochlear membrane breaks lead to mixing of endolymph and perilymph which alters endocochlear potential and there is possibility of causation of SSNHL.

*Evaluation:* The goal of the evaluation should be to detect the following:

■ Is there a loss?

■ How severe is the loss?

■ How quickly did the loss occur?

■ Is there an identifiable cause?

Cause of sudden SNHL should be ascertained based on history, onset, duration, progression or fluctuation of the hearing loss. Enquiry should be made to know about associated symptoms such as vestibular symptoms (Ménière's' disease), tinnitus and ear pain (infectious causes). Any history related to trauma to the ear (noise, direct, barotrauma) and exposure to ototoxic agents should be elicited. Enquiry related to autoimmune diseases in the patient or family members, sexually transmitted disease exposure, other neurological deficits and comorbid conditions like hypertension and diabetes should be sought.

Physical examination should include standard ear, nose and throat (ENT) examination with specific attention to known causes of SSNHL. Otoscopic evaluation should be done carefully to rule out effusion, infection or trauma. Complete neurotological examination, including examination of all cranial nerves and cerebellar function, should be done.

Pure tone audiogram (PTA) and SDS should be done to assess the severity of initial loss and the degree of recovery by serial PTA at 2, 6 and 12 months. Impedance audiometry should be done to assess the status of middle ear and to rule out conductive causes of sudden hearing loss. Other tests which can be done include oto-acoustic emissions (OAEs), electrocochleography (ECochG) and auditory brainstem response audiometry (ABR).

Imaging studies include gadolinium-enhanced contrast MRI, which should be routinely done in every case of SSNHL. Contrast-enhanced MRI (CEMRI) of brain helps to diagnose lesions like acoustic neuroma and cerebrovascular accidents leading to SSNHL. It can also identify changes in the inner ear, VII, VIII nerves in cases of an infective process, especially in viral infections. Cadoni et al. noted that CEMRI could identify some abnormalities in 57% of patients presenting with SSNHL, and in 6 out of 54 cases the abnormality was directly corroborated with the clinical picture (labyrinthine haemorrhage, cochlear inflammation, acoustic neuroma and white matter lesions consistent with demyelinating pathology like multiple sclerosis) (12).

Lab investigations are not done routinely, but may vary from case to case as per suspected cause. In case of suspicion of an infectious or a haematological cause, complete blood count, erythrocyte sedimentation rate, plasma viscosity and sickle cell tests can be done. Cerebrospinal fluid for serology, viral titres and fluorescent treponemal antibody testing can be done. To ascertain any metabolic cause, blood glucose, thyroid function test, electrolyte levels, lipid profile and renal function test results are prescribed. Rheumatologic workup is necessary when the history is suggestive of an autoimmune cause.

*Management:* About 50–60% of patients recover completely with or without treatment, most within 2 weeks (13). Individuals with low-frequency hearing losses have a better prognosis than those with high-frequency losses (14). Prognosis for recovery is dependent on a number of factors, as listed in Table 3.4 (15). Drug therapy and alternative regimen options for the treatment of ISSNHL are listed in Table 3.5.

Steroids are the mainstay of treatment for SSNHL (6). Golden period is 72 hours, i.e. the time after the onset of SSNHL when steroids should ideally be started; however, steroid therapy can be started up to 6 weeks after the onset of symptoms. The specific action of steroids on

## Table 3.4: Prognostic Factors in Idiopathic Sudden Sensorineural Hearing Loss

| Prognostic Factor | Favourable Prognosis |
| --- | --- |
| Age | Young |
| Vertigo at onset | Absent |
| Degree of hearing loss | Mild |
| Audiometric configuration | Upward sloping |
| Time between onset of hearing loss and treatment | Minimal |

the cochlea is still unclear. Steroids decrease inflammation and oedema by increasing anti-oxidants like glutathione at the spiral ganglion by scavenging reactive oxygen species which are produced by noise, ischaemic and ototoxic trauma. Two forms of steroids used most commonly are the systemic steroids (oral and intravenous) and intratympanic steroids; the dosage schedules and differences between the two modalities have been enumerated in Table 3.6. Better outcomes are achieved with combination therapy (16, 17).

## Table 3.5: Treatment Option in Idiopathic Sudden Sensorineural Hearing Loss

| | |
| --- | --- |
| Steroids | • Oral<br>• Transtympanic<br>• Intravenous |
| Agents to improve cochlear blood flow | • Pentoxifylline<br>• Dextran<br>• Diuretics<br>• Plasma expanders<br>• Calcium channel blockers<br>• Betahistine |
| Vitamins and antioxidant | • B1, B3, B6, B12, E |
| Dietary/lifestyle modifications | • Restriction of caffeine<br>• Cessation of smoking<br>• Antibiotics |
| Others | • *Antiviral:* aciclovir, valacyclovir<br>• Gingko extract<br>• Prostacycline<br>• Heparin infusion (anticoagulant)<br>• Hyperbaric oxygen<br>• Carbogen<br>• Hypaque (TM)<br>• Diazepam<br>• Plasmapheresis<br>• Stellate ganglion block<br>• Dorsal sympathectomy<br>• Interferon-α<br>• Lipoprostaglandin E1<br>• Intravenous lidocaine |

## Table 3.6: **Steroids in Idiopathic Sudden Sensorineural Hearing Loss**

| | Systemic Steroids | Intratympanic Steroids |
|---|---|---|
| Timing of treatment | Immediate, ideally within first 14 days. Up to 6 weeks | Immediate Salvage therapy after systemic treatment fails |
| Dose | Oral Prednisolone 1 mg/kg/day or methylprednisolone 48 mg/day or dexamethasone 10 mg/day or *intravenous steroids:* 1000 mg methylprednisolone intravenously for 3 days combined with an oral prednisone taper starting at 60 mg daily | Dexamethasone 24 mg/mL or 16 mg/mL (9) or methylprednisolone 40 mg/mL or 30 mg/mL |
| Duration/frequency | Full dose for 7–14 days, then taper over similar time period | Inject 0.4–0.8 mL into middle ear space every 3–7 days for a total of 3–4 sessions |
| Technique | Single morning dose to prevent hypothalamic–pituitary–adrenal (HPA) axis suppression | Anterosuperior myringotomy: inject solution into the posterior inferior quadrant via narrow-gauge spinal needle to fill middle ear space. Keep head in otological position for 15–30 minutes |
| Monitoring | Audiogram at completion of treatment course and at delayed intervals: 6, 12 months | Audiogram before each subsequent, at completion of treatment course and at delayed intervals. Inspect tympanic membrane (TM) to ensure healing |
| Modifications | Medically treat adverse drug reactions, such as insomnia. Monitor for hyperglycaemia and hypertension | May insert pressure-equalizing tube if planning multiple injections |

As per current belief, since majority of ISSNHL is caused by viral cochleitis, antiviral agents such as Acyclovir (800 mg five times a day for 7 days) or valacyclovir (1 g three times a day [TDS] for 7 days) can be added to steroid therapy for enhanced outcomes in terms of hearing recovery (10, 18).

Therapeutic administration of 100% oxygen at environmental pressures >1 atm (Hyperbaric Oxygen Therapy [HBOT]) in ISSNHL acts by reversing hypoxic event in the cochlear apparatus (19). Patient is placed in an airtight vessel with increased pressure within the vessel and 100% oxygen is administered for respiration. It is shown that there is 25% improvement in hearing in 25% of the cases treated with HBOT. Younger patients respond better to HBOT than older patients (the age cutoffs vary from 50 to 60 years). As with other therapies, HBOT administered within 72 hours gives better results. Contrary to other treatment modalities, HBOT has more benefit in recovery of moderate to severe hearing loss than mild hearing loss. HBOT is time-consuming and patient has to be physically present in the hyperbaric chamber for 90 minutes per cycle for a minimum of ten cycles. Adverse effects are rare, but may include middle ear barotrauma, claustrophobia and rarely pulmonary barotrauma or seizures (20).

Pentoxifylline is a phosphodiesterase inhibitor which increases the oxygen delivery to ischaemic tissues. It acts by decreasing the blood viscosity by increasing the flexibility of the RBC membrane, thus allowing the RBCs to traverse the capillaries more easily to supply oxygen to the ischaemic tissue and is helpful in cases of ISSNHL as adjuvant therapy (21).

Calcium channel blockers increase the cerebral blood flow and prevent vascular smooth muscle contraction induced by neurotransmitters and vasoactive substances. Nimodipine 40 mg TDS for 4 weeks has shown good results in vertebrobasilar insufficiency, but promising results in treatment of ISSNHL are still awaited (22).

Betahistine is a cochlear vasodilator and has histamine-like action on H1 receptors in the cochlea where it increases cochlear blood flow. It is frequently given in cases of ISSNHL in doses of 16–32 mg TDS for a period of 1–3 months (23). Carbogen (combination of 5% $CO_2$ and 95% $O_2$) causes cerebral vasodilatation by increasing $PCO_2$. It is given by inhalation for 30 minutes, eight times per day (24). Ginkgo biloba extract contains flavones and terpenes. It prevents the development of free radicals in cases of ischaemic-related metabolic disturbances and thus counteracts secondary vasoconstriction. Audiological rehabilitation with hearing aids is recommended in refractory cases.

## Table 3.7: Outcomes in Idiopathic Sudden Sensorineural Hearing Loss

| | |
|---|---|
| Complete recovery | • Within 10 dB of normal ear/pre-morbid level<br>• 50% cases |
| Partial recovery | • 50% or more of the prehearing loss<br>• 25–30% of cases |
| No recovery | • <50% recovery of hearing<br>• 10–15% of cases |

One typical treatment regimen where every potential cause is covered includes a "shotgun" regimen of low-molecular-weight dextran, histamine, Hypaque™ (Diatrizoate Meglumine injection), diuretics, steroids, vasodilators and carbogen inhalation (25).

*Outcomes:* Outcomes can be broadly divided as per Table 3.7.

### Barotrauma

It may sometimes result in SSNHL and may occur due to lifting heavy weights, straining, scuba diving, flying in an unpressurized aircraft or blunt trauma. It is also seen in patients undergoing HBOT. Barotrauma is more likely to occur in those with an acute upper respiratory infection. The cause of SSNHL in case of barotrauma is invariably due to the occurrence of a perilymphatic fistula at the oval window, round window or some other site (26). Other possibilities include inner ear membrane breaks and pneumo-labyrinth (usually from rapid ascent during diving). Dizziness and tinnitus often accompany the SNHL. A fistula test in case of a perilymphatic fistula with pneumatic otoscopy may be suggestive of this diagnosis, but there is no definitive diagnostic examination available, except for surgical exploration. Treatment for this condition includes strict bed rest, head elevation and avoidance of straining/lifting heavy weights. If no improvement is seen after 5 days of this conservative regime, patching of the fistula can be done via the middle ear (27).

### Iatrogenic

Iatrogenic inner ear injury leading to SSNHL can result from ear surgeries like stapedectomy or excessive ossicular handling in tympanoplasty. Iatrogenic injury can also result from non-otological surgeries like posterior and middle fossa craniotomies.

### Central causes of SSNHL

An acute infarction of the region supplied by the anteroinferior cerebellar artery may result in a sudden and profound SNHL. This will nearly always be associated with vertigo as well as other significant findings of central nervous system dysfunction. In cases of a transient ischaemic attack, the loss may be temporary. In other cases of a cerebrovascular accident involving the central auditory pathways or centres, auditory perception or speech discrimination may be impaired in the setting of intact threshold detection.

Thirteen per cent of patients with vestibular schwannomas present with SSNHL (28), and MRI of the brain may show a vestibular schwannoma in up to 1–2% of SSNHL cases (29). These cases are identified by CEMRI of the internal auditory meatus and brain and further treated with stereotactic radiotherapy or surgical excision.

### CONCLUSION

SSNHL is an otological emergency. Though there are minor differences between authors in defining SSNHL, but commonly it is defined as the sudden onset of decrease in hearing of at least 30 dB at three consecutive frequencies within 3 days. In the majority of cases, the aetiology remains unknown and there are no fixed treatment protocols. Corticosteroids are the most widely used form of therapy. The use of HBOT is optional. Antiviral agents can be added when there is high suspicion of viral infection. The other treatment options such as volume expanders and vasodilators have not shown statistically significant benefit and are not recommended for routine use. Routine lab tests are not recommended. A suggested algorithm for management of SSNHL is as depicted in Figure 3.2.

### TAKE HOME POINTS/KEY LEARNING POINTS

- SSNHL is considered an otological emergency.

- Most common cause is idiopathic.

- Diagnosis is by pure tone audiometry.

- Imaging (MRI brain) is recommended to rule out CP Angle pathologies.

- Treatment includes oral/intratympanic steroids, antivirals and supportive therapy.

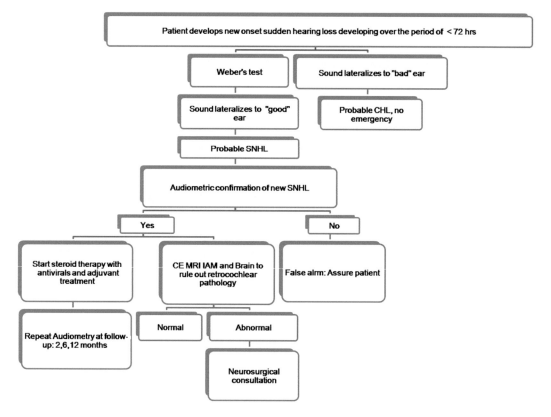

**Figure 3.2** Algorithm for management of sudden sensorineural hearing loss.

## REFERENCES

1. Schreiber BE, Agrup C, Haskard DO, Luxon LM. Sudden sensorineural hearing loss. Lancet. 2010; 375(Issue 9721):1203–11.

2. Schuknecht HF, Donovan ED. The pathology of idiopathic sudden sensorineural hearing loss. Arch Otorhinolaryngol. 1986;243:1–15.

3. O'Malley MR, Haynes DS. Sudden hearing loss. Otolaryngol Clin North Am. 2008;(41):633–49.

4. Pitkaranta A, Vasama JP, Julkunen I. Sudden deafness and viral infections. Otorhinolaryngol Nova. 1999; 9:190–7.

5. Yeo SW, Lee DH, Jun BC, Park SY, Park YS. Hearing outcome of sudden sensorineural hearing loss: long term follow up. Otolaryngol Head Neck Surg. 2007;136(2):221–4.

6. Wilson WR, Byl FM, Laird N. The efficacy of steroids in idiopathic sudden hearing loss. Arch Otolaryngol. 1980;106:772–6.

7. Rauch SD. Idiopathic sudden sensorineural hearing loss. N Engl J Med. 2008;359:833–40.

8. Stachler RJ, Chandrasekhar SS, Tsai BS, et al. Clinical practice guideline: sudden hearing loss. Otolaryngol Head Neck Surg. 2012;146:S1–35.

9. National Institute of Deafness and Communication Disorders. Sudden deafness. 2000. Available from http://www.nidcd.nih.gov/health/hearing/sudden.htm. Accessed 18 May 2011.

10. Wilson WR, Veltri RW, Laird N, et al. Viral and epidemiologic studies of idiopathic sudden hearing loss. Otolaryngol Head Neck Surg. 1983;91(6):653–8.

11. Koide J, Yanagita N, Hondo R, Kurata T. Serological and clinical study of herpes simplex virus infection in patients with sudden deafness. Acta Otolaryngol Suppl. 1988;456:21–6.

12. Cadoni G, Clanfoni A, Agostino S, et al. Magnetic resonance imaging findings in sudden sensorineural hearing loss. J Otolaryngol. 2006;35(5):310–6.

13. Fetterman BL, Saunders JE, Luxford WM. Prognosis and treatment of sudden sensorineural hearing loss. Am J Otol. 1996;17(4):529–36.

14. Mattox DE, Simmons FB. Natural history of sudden sensorineural hearing loss. Ann Otol Rhinol Laryngol. 1977;86(4, Pt 1):463–80.

15. Conlin AE, Parnes LS. Treatment of sudden sensorineural hearing loss, I: a systematic review. Arch Otolaryngol Head Neck Surg. 2007;133(6): 573–81.

16. Conlin AE, Parnes LS. Treatment of sudden sensorineural hearing loss, II: a meta-analysis. Arch Otolaryngol Head Neck Surg. 2007;133(6):582–6.

17. Haynes DS, O'Malley M, Cohen S, Watford K, Labadie RF. Intratympanic dexamethasone for sudden sensorineural hearing loss after failure of systemic therapy. Laryngoscope. 2007;117:3–15.

18. Stokroos RJ, Albers FW, Tenvergert EM. Antiviral treatment of idiopathic sudden sensorineural hearing loss: a prospective, randomized, double-blind clinical trial. Acta Otolaryngol. 1998;118:488–95.

19. Bennett MH, Kertesz T, Yeung P. Hyperbaric oxygen for idiopathic sudden sensorineural hearing loss and tinnitus. Cochrane Database Syst Rev. 2006;(1):CD004739.

20. Bayoumi AB, De-Ru JA. Use of hyperbaric oxygen therapy in acute hearing loss: a narrative review. Eur Arch Oto Rhino Laryngol. 2019;276:1859–80.

21. Reisser CH, Weidauer H. Ginkgo biloba extract EGb 761 or pentoxifylline for the treatment of sudden deafness: a randomized, reference-controlled, double-blind study. Acta Otolaryngol. 2001;121(5): 579–84.

22. Mann W, Beck C. Calcium antagonists in the treatment of sudden deafness. Arch Otorhinolaryngol. 1986;243:170–3.

23. Toroslu T, Erdogan H. Comparison of different treatment methods for idiopathic sudden sensorineural hearing loss. Turk Arch Otorhinolaryngol. 2018;56(4):226–32.

24. Fisch U, Nagahara K, Pollak A. Sudden hearing loss: circulatory. Am J Otol. 1984;5(6):488–91.

25. Wilkins SA, Mattox DE, Lyles A. Evaluation of "Shotgun" regimen for sudden hearing loss. Otolaryngol Head Neck Surg. 1987;97(5):474–80.

26. Jaffe BF. Clinical studies in sudden deafness. Adv Otorhinolaryngol. 1973;20:221–8.

27. Maitland CG. Perilymphatic fistula. Curr Neurol Neurosci Rep. 2001;1(5):486–1.

28. Berg HM, Cohen NL, Hammerschlag PE, Waltzman SB. Acoustic neuroma presenting as sudden hearing loss with recovery. Otolaryngol Head Neck Surg. 1986;94(1):15–22.

29. Aarnisalo AA, Suoranta H, Ylikoski J. Magnetic resonance imaging findings in the auditory pathway of patients with sudden deafness. Otol Neurotol. 2004;25(3):245–9.

# 4 Single-Sided Deafness: A Long-Neglected Entity in Otology

*Garima Upreti and Uma Patnaik*

## CONTENTS

## INTRODUCTION

The term "single-sided deafness" (SSD) dawned with the advent of bone-anchored hearing devices being offered for the condition per se. SSD is a condition in which an individual has non-functional hearing in one ear (without benefit from acoustic amplification) and normal contralateral hearing (1).

A person with SSD has distinct disabilities that transcend the degree of auditory disadvantage. The binaural cues of interaural latency, intensity and head shadow effect that predicate sound localization are absent or distorted. Lack of binaural summation and binaural squelch beget difficulty in understanding speech in noise and overall increased listening effort.

In congenital/paediatric SSD, binaural hearing is traded for a stronger cerebral representation of the hearing ear, impacting higher auditory processing. This restricts the options available to restore hearing in the deaf ear and deliver binaural localization, later in life. Such children show relatively poor verbal cognition, speech and language impairment and poor academic performance.

These factors coupled with late detection of SSD and lack of objectivity in quantifying the associated disability highlight the need for early identification of hearing asymmetry and early rehabilitation.

## REVIEW OF LITERATURE
### Definitions

Unilateral hearing loss (UHL) refers to any degree of permanent hearing impairment in one ear with normal hearing in the opposite ear, irrespective of type and aetiology of hearing loss (1).

Various audiological criteria have been described for SSD. While it may simply be referred to as severe-profound UHL, Van de Heyning et al. suggest that SSD should meet all of the following criteria: in the poorer ear, the pure tone average (PTA) is 70 dB hearing level (HL) or more, in the better ear PTA is 30 dB HL or less and the interaural threshold gap is ≥40 dB. Similar definitions have been given by other authors (2–4). According to Macias et al., the main criterion for defining SSD is that the worse ear does not receive benefit with traditional acoustic amplification, and the "good" ear has a pure tone threshold of 20 dB HL or better (5).

According to the American Academy of Audiology, a person with SSD has normal hearing in one ear and unaidable hearing in the opposite ear with poor word recognition scores

## AUDIOLOGICAL CLASSIFICATION CRITERIA

| | |
|---|---|
| **Unilateral hearing loss (UHL)** | Any degree of permanent hearing loss in one ear, regardless of aetiology, with normal hearing* in the opposite ear |

| | | | |
|---|---|---|---|
| **Single-sided deafness (SSD)** | Severe-to-profound UHL | | |
| | Poorer ear | PTA $\geq$ 70dB HL | |
| | Better ear | PTA $\leq$ 20 dB HL[#] | OR |
| | | $\leq$ 30 dB HL[@] | |

| | | |
|---|---|---|
| **Asymmetric hearing loss** | Poorer ear | PTA $\geq$ 70dB HL |
| | Better ear | PTA > 30 dB HL $\leq$ 55 dB HL[@] |
| | Interaural threshold gap $\geq$ 15 dB HL | |

PTA = pure tone average threshold measured at 0.5, 1, 2, and 3 kHz
*Normal hearing is defined as a pure tone average air-conduction hearing threshold of better than or equal to 20 dB HL.
# American Academy of Audiology Clinical Practice Guidelines [1]
@ Van de Heyning et al [2], Vincent C et al [3], Usami et al [4]

**Figure 4.1**  Relevant definitions.

or an inability to tolerate amplified sound. On the other hand, the "good" ear must have hearing thresholds no poorer than 20 dB HL for PTA of 0.5, 1, 2 and 3 kHz (1). Relevant definitions have been presented in Figure 4.1.

### Problem Statement

SSD is estimated to affect 12–27 individuals every 100,000 people, with the majority of hearing loss being sudden and idiopathic. The overall prevalence of UHL in adult Americans is 7.2%, with 1.5% (0.1–2.1%) experiencing moderate or worse UHL (6). As per the American Association of Audiology, about 60,000 new cases of SSD are detected annually in the United States (1). Data for India is not available.

At least one-third of all children born with hearing loss have UHL. Prevalence of UHL amongst newborns is reported to be approximately 0.6–0.7 per 1000 births in the Unites States. Despite the introduction of universal newborn hearing screening, UHL is recognized late. Moreover, UHL progresses to bilateral hearing loss in 7.5–11% of cases. The number of children with UHL increases considerably after the newborn period. It is reported that approximately 2.5–3% of school-age children have UHL (7).

The common misconception amongst many clinicians as well as the general population that monaural listeners have less disability and that normal hearing in one ear is sufficient for most everyday communication further impedes the detection and seeking rehabilitation for SSD.

### Problems Associated with Single-Sided Deafness

Individuals with SSD lose access to critical cues provided through binaural hearing regarding the timing and intensity of sound signal, which prevents them from performing complex tasks of auditory function. Consequently, monaural listeners have reduced sound awareness, poor speech perception in noise and inability to localize sounds. Figure 4.2 summarizes the auditory problems associated with SSD.

*Binaural Summation:* The sensitivity to sound increases when input is received through both ears simultaneously rather than just one ear, due to central auditory summation. This summation gives advantage of 2–3 dB at threshold level, when sound is just detectable, and increases up to 10 dB at 90 dB sensation level. Speech discrimination scores are known to improve at a rate of

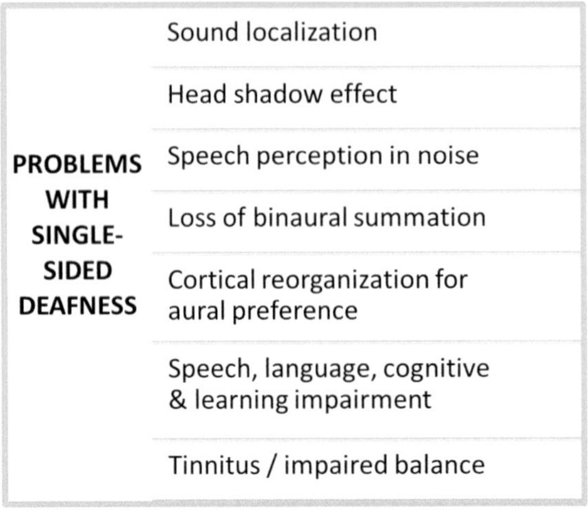

| | |
|---|---|
| **PROBLEMS WITH SINGLE-SIDED DEAFNESS** | Sound localization |
| | Head shadow effect |
| | Speech perception in noise |
| | Loss of binaural summation |
| | Cortical reorganization for aural preference |
| | Speech, language, cognitive & learning impairment |
| | Tinnitus / impaired balance |

**Figure 4.2** Problems associated with single-sided deafness.

6% per decibel, 2–3 dB can result in improved speech discrimination score of 12–18% (8).

*Head Shadow Effect:* It refers to attenuation of sound signal by the mere presence of head between the two ears. Tillman et al. described a 6.4-dB reduction of signal intensity from one side of the head to the other. For pure tones, the head shadow effect is greatest at high frequencies, 20 dB for 5000–6000 Hz, hence it impacts speech recognition.

As a binaural benefit, the head shadow effect leads to different signal-to-noise ratio (SNR) in the two ears and hence aids in sound localization. In SSD, the head shadow effect results in a bad ear side and good ear side, depending on where sound signal originates. Patients need to develop compensatory coping mannerisms, such as positioning the head to receive auditory signal in the "good" ear (1, 8, 9).

*Sound Localization:* As the sound arrives earlier in the ear nearer to the sound source, the resultant interaural time difference (ITD) relates to the angular direction of the source in the horizontal plane. In humans, ITD ranges from 0 to 700 µs, and ITD in the order of 10 µs can be discerned. The accuracy of localization achieved with the analysis of ITD is a few degrees, depending on whether the sound source is in front of the subject or sideways.

While the ITD cues cannot be used at high frequencies, the head shadow effect increases with frequency (as mentioned above). It leads to different sound intensities reaching the two ears, depending on the location of sound source, called the interaural level difference (ILD). Below 200 Hz, ILD hardly reaches a few decibels and shows little dependence on source direction, while for 1000 Hz, ILD varies between 5 and 10 dB as a function of source direction. Above 1000 Hz, ILD and its directional dependency continues to increase with frequency. ITD processing occurs in the medial superior olive, while ILD processing occurs in the lateral superior olive, being excited by ipsilateral inputs and inhibited by contralateral ones. Thus, ITD and ILD help in source localization in the horizontal plane.

For source localization in the vertical plane, cues are provided by diffraction patterns produced by the head and pinna, which result in characteristic spectral dips. The frequency at which a spectral dip occurs relates to the angular vertical position of the source, so the changes in spectrum of a broadband source inform about vertical displacements (9).

*Squelch Effect or Binaural Release of Masking:* Squelch effect or 'cocktail party effect' refers to the ability to pick a desired signal from background noise. When competing auditory signals (speech and background noise) are presented to one ear, the target signal (speech) might get masked by the background noise, depending on their respective incident intensities.

However, when presented to a person with binaural hearing, the competing signals get spatially separated by virtue of spatial separation of the two ears. The central auditory system takes cues from interaural differences in time, sound level, phase and spectrum of incident signals to identify the target signal (speech) in noise. This binaural release of masking/binaural squelch leads to improved signal identification and speech intelligibility.

The binaural squelch effect is strongest for low-frequency sounds (up to 15 dB below 2500 Hz) and decreases to 2–3 dB for frequencies above 2500 Hz. Improvement in SNR of 3 dB improves word recognition scores by about 18% (8, 9).

*Cortical Reorganization for Aural Preference:* In early-onset SSD (congenital/pre-lingual), monoaural deprivation of hearing induces compensatory adaptations in central auditory pathways, such that the hearing ear is more extensively represented in the brain. This aural reorganization is more pronounced if its onset is during development, when the brain is highly plastic, with modifiable cortical connections (10, 11). This leaves the deaf ear at a significant disadvantage in the competition for cortical resources.

Sacrificing the binaural localization for strengthening monaural hearing is an optimal adaptation for SSD, but it compromises possibilities to restore hearing in the deaf ear and binaural auditory function later in life. This reiterates the need for early identification and early intervention to rehabilitate the deaf ear in a child (preferably less than 3.5 years of age). For adults, monoaural auditory deprivation is not as detrimental (10, 11).

*Cognitive Speech and Language and Academic Impact of SSD:* UHL negatively impacts early auditory behaviour and preverbal vocalization, speech and language development, academic attainment and cognition (12–15). Young children with UHL have a ten times higher rate of repeating grades compared to those without hearing loss. In addition, 12–41% of children with UHL receive additional educational assistance or have association with educational or behavioural problems. Children with UHL have more academic problems in comparison to not only normal-hearing controls but also to those with moderate to severe bilateral hearing loss. This may be due to frequent lack of acknowledgement of disability in case of UHL, whereas those with bilateral hearing loss receive extra services (8).

Lieu et al., in their controlled studies on schoolchildren, documented a strong negative effect of UHL on speech-language scores (significantly poorer scores on the Oral and Written Language Scales, 2.6 times greater odds of receiving speech therapy, 4.4 times greater odds of receiving extra help in school and lower verbal intelligence quotient scores) (13–15). Fischer and Lieu reported that the gap in language scores between those with UHL and normal-hearing siblings did not diminish with time but perhaps even widened (16). A study on working memory and phonological processing depicted deficits in executive function in children with UHL compared with their normal-hearing siblings (8).

Functional neuroimaging studies too have corroborated that UHL affects not only the regions of the brain involved with auditory perception and processing but also non-auditory cortical regions. This information is relevant when considering the educational and behavioural difficulties faced by children with UHL (17).

## AETIOLOGY OF SINGLE-SIDED DEAFNESS

Usami et al. evaluated the causes of SSD/asymmetrical hearing loss in a cohort of 527 cases. Amongst congenital/early-onset SSD, most common cause was cochlear nerve deficiency (40%), followed by cytomegalovirus (CMV) and mumps infection. Inner ear anomalies accounted for 3.8% congenital/early-onset SSD cases. Incomplete partition type-I (IP-I) was the most frequent anomaly. Auditory neuropathy spectrum disorder (ANSD) was found in 2.4% of these cases. Other studies on children with SSD have found the prevalence of cochlear nerve aplasia or hypoplasia around 50%. Inner ear malformations in SSD children are found in 25–35% of cases by CT or MRI. Commonly reported abnormalities include enlarged vestibular aqueduct (EVA), Mondini's deformity, cochlear and vestibular malformations and common cavity malformations (8).

For post-lingual SSD, idiopathic sudden sensorineural hearing loss (SSNHL; 54.6%) was the most common aetiology, followed by various forms of otitis media. Cerebellopontine angle (CP) tumours, trauma and perilymph fistula were other noted causes of SSD among adults (4).

The frequency of congenital CMV infection in children with unilateral sensorineural hearing loss (SNHL) is reportedly around 25%. Although children with symptomatic congenital CMV infection are more likely to have bilateral hearing loss, children with asymptomatic CMV infection are more likely to have UHL (18). Congenital mumps and measles are frequent causes of hearing loss in the developing world. Mumps is more often associated with UHL than measles.

Genetic causes are usually associated with bilateral hearing loss. Variants of genes associated with bilateral deafness, including Pendred syndrome (SLC26A4) associated with EVA, have been identified in but not found to be major determinants of UHL.

## Table 4.1: Aetiology of Single-sided Deafness

### AETIOLOGY OF SINGLE-SIDED DEAFNESS

**Congenital structural malformations**
- Inner ear malformations
- Cochlear nerve hypoplasia / aplasia

**Neurological**
- Auditory neuropathy Spectrum disorder
- Demyelinating conditions like multiple sclerosis

**Ototoxic drugs**
- Aminoglycosides
- Loop diuretics
- Platinum-based drugs
- Vancomycin
- Salicylates

**Inflammatory**
- Cholesteatoma
- Labyrinthitis
- Meningitis
- Encephalitis
- Viral infections – herpes, CMV, mumps, measles, rubella, HIV
- Syphilis
- Toxoplasmosis
- Lyme disease

**Autoimmune**
- Cogan syndrome
- Wegener's granulomatosis
- Systemic lupus Erythematosus
- Takayasu arteritis
- Systemic sclerosis
- Antiphospholipid antibody syndrome
- Autoimmune inner ear disease

**Traumatic**
- Temporal bone trauma
- Acoustic trauma
- Barotrauma
- Perilymph fistula
- Ear surgery (e.g. stapedectomy, translabyrinthine, transcochlear surgery )

**Vascular**
- Stroke involving AICA / vertebrobasilar insufficiency
- Sickle cell disease
- Waldenstrom macroglobulinemia

**Metabolic**
- Diabetes mellitus
- Hyperlipidemia
- Thyrotoxicosis

**Neoplastic**
- Cerebellopontine angle tumours e.g. vestibular, schwannoma, meningioma

May be caused by tumour or as an outcome of surgical removal

**Endolymphatic hydrops** – Ménière's disease

**Idiopathic sudden sensorineural hearing loss**

Although familial occurrence of UHL has been reported, no specific genetic mutations have been identified (7, 19). Syndromic causes of childhood hearing loss may initially present, or simply be associated with UHL, for example, branchio-oto-renal syndrome and Waardenburg syndrome (8). Possible aetiologies for SSD have been listed in Table 4.1.

### MANAGEMENT OPTIONS

Earlier, patients with SSD met with insouciant advice of "nothing required to be done if the other ear is properly functioning", which unfortunately protracts to this date. Nevertheless, various devices have been developed and approved for auditory rehabilitation in SSD.

### CROS Hearing Aids

Traditionally, the first option offered for SSD is a CROS (Contralateral Routing of Signal) configuration hearing aid, in which a microphone is placed on the deaf ear. The signal picked up by the microphone is routed to an amplifying system fitted on the better side. Thus, the sound incident onto the deaf ear is heard over the good ear.

The early devices were hardwired, spectacle-mounted designs and used ear moulds or open-tube fittings to allow the signal to cross over. Later, Behind The Ear (BTE), In The Canal (ITC) and Completely In Canal (CIC) configurations were manufactured for better cosmesis. These configurations use real-time audio streaming transmission to provide a broadband signal to cross the head.

The *transcranial CROS* uses a CIC hearing device fitted in the dead ear without occlusion of the functional ear. The sound pressure in the residual volume is loud enough to allow osseo-tympanic transmission of sound from the dead ear to the contralateral cochlea.

The poor ear must be able to handle the high level of sound pressure without tolerance or recruitment issues. Hence, it is not a good option for people having residual hearing in the poor ear. Also, it cannot be used in case of ear infection, open mastoid cavity, narrow ear canal or canal atresia. Outcomes are variable compared to conventional CROS devices.

Overall, CROS devices are inexpensive, relatively convenient and non-invasive. They overcome the head shadow effect. Speech understanding in noise is improved when speech is the dominant signal on the side with hearing loss. However, since the head shadow effect for noise too is eliminated, there is reduced speech understanding when noise is

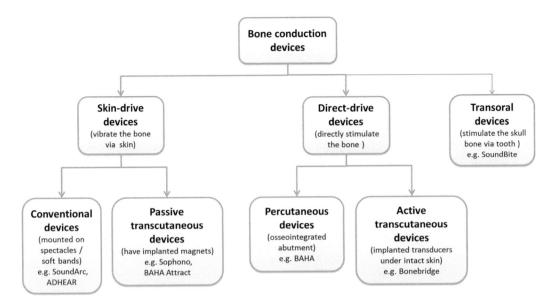

**Figure 4.3** Classification of bone conduction devices.

the dominant signal on deaf side. Since binaural hearing is not restored, they do not help in sound localization.

Demerits include poor cosmesis, occlusion of normal hearing ear canal (conventional devices), poor hearing advantage as compared to other options and acceptance issues, especially with children. Despite these problems, a fair percentage of individuals with SSD do perceive enough benefit to accept and continue using CROS devices (20).

### Bone Conduction Devices (BCDs)

These devices are based on bone conduction (BC) of sound vibrations through the skull to the functional contralateral cochlea. BCDs that vibrate the bone via the overlying skin are called skin-drive devices and are divided into conventional devices (mounted on spectacles or headbands) and passive transcutaneous devices (having implanted magnets). BCDs that directly stimulate the bone are referred to as direct-drive devices and are further divided into percutaneous (BAHA®) and active transcutaneous devices (Bonebridge®) (21). Figure 4.3 illustrates this classification. Figures 4.4 and 4.5 depict BCD mounted on spectacle and soft band, respectively.

*Conventional BCDs*: These skin-drive devices use a sound processor attached to spectacles, steel spring headbands or soft headbands. Examples include SoundArc® and ADHEAR®.

A high static pressure (approximately 2 N) exerted on the skin and soft tissues is required to transmit the sound vibrations effectively to

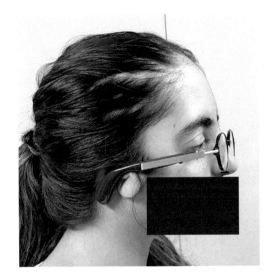

**Figure 4.4** Girl with aural atresia wearing bone conduction device mounted on a spectacle frame.

the underlying bone. This may cause discomfort, skin problems (due to compression in the area of contact) and even tension headaches. Furthermore, the skin attenuates sound vibrations, especially the high frequencies (>1 kHz). This attenuation is more significant in SSD as sound has to cross over to the opposite side and lack of higher frequencies increases the difficulty in discerning speech.

Another issue relates to feedback, where sound is radiated from the transducer back to

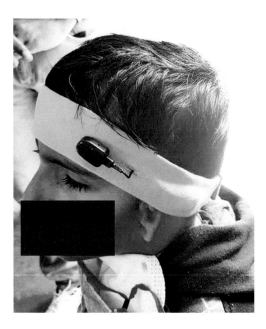

**Figure 4.5**  Child with aural atresia wearing bone conduction device on soft band.

the microphone. In order to reduce feedback, the microphone is placed on the side opposite to the transducer or in a separate casing on the same side of the head (21).

*Percutaneous Device (BAHA):* Percutaneous BCD, also called bone-anchored hearing aid (BAHA) is based on the principle of osseointegration of titanium. Classically, a titanium fixture is implanted into the skull with a skin-penetrating abutment, which in turn facilitates attachment of the sound processor unit. BAHA is FDA approved for management of SSD in candidates aged 5 years and above.

BAHA has several advantages over conventional BCDs. The skin is not compressed, vibrations are transmitted directly to the bone, signal attenuation is less and higher frequencies are preserved. Demerits include invasive procedure for implantation, loss of osseointegration and skin complications.

BAHA processor is sometimes used on a headband, as a conventional skin-drive device. This is valuable for hearing rehabilitation in children who are too young for implantation, and also for preoperative assessment of benefit. The final hearing outcome with implanted BAHA is better than BAHA on a headband. Verstraeten et al. showed that hearing sensitivity through the skin as compared to a skin-penetrating abutment is 8–20 dB lower for the frequency range of 1–4 kHz (21).

For lateralized speech, directed to the worse ear in patients with SSD, a lower (significantly improved) SNR has been reported under BAHA-aided condition as compared to the unaided condition. For lateralized speech directed to the better ear, studies have failed to demonstrate a statistically significant advantage of BAHA (22).

Schroder et al. reported that even though 80% of patients with SSD perceived a subjective handicap, only 24% cases agreed for BAHA implantation after trial on a headband. The short-term compliance amongst the implanted cases was good (95% using the device after 6 months). All cases claimed subjective benefit. However, the sound quality with BAHA was metallic or radio-like in 45% cases. Minor local adverse effects occurred in 40% cases (23). Faber et al. found that 47% of the patients with SSD opted for a BCD after a headband trial (24). The reasons for not opting to use a definitive BCD included the need for surgical intervention, wearing a device behind the ear, cosmetic aspect and "visibility of deafness".

Desmet et al. reported 14% device discontinuation over a period of 50 months (25). Faber et al. reported a 17% discontinuation rate over an average follow-up of 61.7 months, whereas in those with the longest follow-up (average of 10 years) the discontinuation rate was 30% (26). Possible explanations of decreased compliance over long term might be adaptation to the benefits of the new hearing device and progressive deterioration of hearing in the better ear. Nevertheless, on SSD questionnaire, 61% BAHA users reported improved quality of life post-implantation.

*Passive Transcutaneous Skin-Drive BCDs:* Passive transcutaneous skin-drive devices, e.g. Sophono® and BAHA Attract, use retention magnets implanted in the temporal bone. The sound processor is attached on the skin by magnetic attraction force. The vibrations of the transducer are transmitted through soft tissue. In order to avoid skin problems related to high pressure, these devices use a soft pad with a larger surface area over magnetic plate for attachment.

Briggs et al. in their prospective, multicentre study on BAHA Attract users found statistically significant improvement in hearing performance (including speech recognition in noise) compared with unaided hearing and sound processor on a soft band. The device provides significant functional gain at all frequencies, maximum being in the speech frequency range (up to and including 3000 Hz). Above 3000 Hz, the performance drops due to soft tissue attenuation. Minimal soft tissue complications, favourable pain and numbness scores together with a high mean daily use (7 hours/day) suggested good wearing comfort (27).

Transcutaneous BCDs have advantage over skin-penetrating devices of improved cosmesis, less cutaneous complications and eliminates the daily cleaning of implantation site. This provides a significant advantage for patients with disabilities or reduced dexterity.

*Active Transcutaneous Direct-Drive BCD:* In an active transcutaneous device (Bonebridge), the transducer is implanted under intact skin. Hence, vibrations are transmitted from the transducer directly to the skull bone. The sound processor is attached to the skin by retention magnets in the implanted unit and the sound signal is transmitted via an inductive link to the implanted transducer. Bonebridge is FDA approved for patients aged 12 years and above.

Magele et al. performed a systematic review of studies on active transcutaneous BCD users. The functional gain was 28.94 dB in subjects with SSD. Word recognition scores in SSD subjects showed an improvement of 16%. Speech understanding in noise was better, especially when noise was presented from the normal-hearing side and speech input was provided on the deaf side. However, no improvement in sound localization was seen. Subjective measures evaluating the impact of implant on quality of life in subjects with SSD reported definite benefit over unaided condition, and also over conventional hearing aids. Minor complications occurred in 7.7% cases, while major complications (requiring revision surgery or explantation) occurred in 1.7% cases (28). The big size of the FMT can be a challenge in patients with open mastoid cavity and children with small temporal bones. Preoperative imaging is indicated to find the appropriate site for implantation. This site could be retrosigmoid if enough space is not found in the mastoid (29).

*In-the-Mouth BCD (SoundBite®):* SoundBite uses an in-the-mouth transducer anchored to the teeth. A microphone placed behind the ear on the deaf side transmits sound wirelessly to the transducer. The vibrations are generated by piezoelectric effect in the transducer and conducted through the teeth to the skull bone and received by the healthy contralateral cochlea.

Evaluations by Murray et al. (30) show that the SoundBite system is safe and effective, with a substantial benefit with continual daily use. SoundBite has the highest output and gain in the frequency ranges above 2 kHz. This is indeed beneficial in SSD patients who need high-frequency gain for better speech perception. The problems reported with SoundBite include acoustic feedback and less output at lower frequencies. There might be distortion and discomfort using this device while eating, thereby impeding conversation during meals.

## CROS vs. BCDs in SSD

Niparko et al. compared the outcomes of CROS and BAHA in subjects with SSD. Subjects were fitted with CROS devices for 1 month before implantation of BAHA in the deaf ear. There was poor acceptance of CROS amplification, while consistent satisfaction with BAHA was reported. Both CROS and BAHA produced significantly better speech recognition in noise, compared to unaided condition, BAHA being significantly better than CROS (31).No difference in sound localization was observed between the three conditions (32, 33). Peters et al. in their systematic review reported no significant advantage of BCD or CROS regarding speech perception in noise and sound localization (34).

CROS and BAHA have shown differential benefit on the subscales of APHAB (Abbreviated Profile of Hearing Aid Benefit) questionnaire. Significant benefit was identified from BAHA over CROS in the domains of aversiveness of sound, reverberation and hearing in background noise (32).

## Cochlear Implant (CI)

A CI is the only modality which provides auditory stimulation in the ear with impaired hearing and thereby offers opportunity for restoring true binaural hearing. In 2019, CI was accorded FDA approval for the indication of SSD and asymmetric hearing loss in candidates aged 5 years or older.

Binaural hearing benefit of CI usage in these patients has been shown as an improvement in speech recognition in noise and in sound localization performance (35–39). From the localization findings as well as from tests of binaural summation (36), it can be concluded that there is binaural processing and representation of acoustically and electrically transmitted stimuli, particularly ILD in the auditory brainstem in case of dichotic stimulus presentation. Wesarg et al. showed that CI users with SSD are able to process sentence segments presented to either the normal hearing or the implanted ear, even though the respective speech recognition performance was worse for the implanted ear compared to the normal ear. Under dichotic listening conditions, speech recognition was considerably improved, which indicates the ability to integrate bilaterally presented, electrically and acoustically transmitted information via

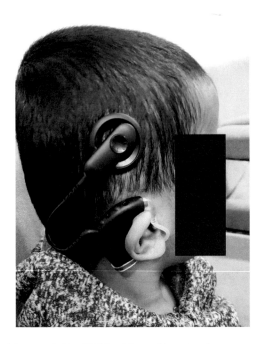

**Figure 4.6** Child with cochlear implant.

This supports emphasis on screening for deafness and continued vigilance during childhood. The Joint Committee on Infant Hearing recommends hearing screening by 1 month of age, definitive diagnosis of hearing loss by 3 months of age and early intervention by 6 months of age (19).

High-risk infants include those with TORCH infection, birth weight <1500 g, hyperbilirubinemia, ototoxic medication, bacterial meningitis, mechanical ventilation/NICU stay >5 days, head trauma, neurodegenerative disorders and family history of hearing loss. These should be screened with both otoacoustic emission (OAE) and automated brainstem evoked response audiometry (BERA). Others can be screened with OAE alone, with automated BERA for absent or diminished OAE responses. A child who fails screening protocols should undergo a confirmatory BERA.

Speech, language and developmental milestones should be monitored in children. The American Academy of Pediatrics recommends developmental and behavioural screening at 9, 18 and 24/30 months of age.

binaural processing in the central auditory system (40).

CI additionally benefits patients with tinnitus. Tinnitus suppression primarily occurs during active CI use and is stable over time (38, 41). Some CI recipients experience residual inhibition of tinnitus even when the implant is switched off, and these periods can extend overnight such that the recipient experiences a complete relief from tinnitus (42). Figure 4.6 shows a child using CI. The key features of these auditory devices have been noted in Table 4.2.

## APPROACH TO A PATIENT WITH SINGLE-SIDED DEAFNESS
### Diagnosis of SSD

An adult, who has experienced binaural hearing, can easily perceive UHL when it occurs. The diagnosis of SSD is straightforward with clinical history and audiometry. SSD in a child is more challenging to diagnose. These children are often missed in the home environment where there is one-on-one interaction and less ambient noise. Their condition usually gets unmasked in the school setting, where they attend classes and participate in group interactions. The common complaints are selective hearing, inability to hear from a distance, speech/language impairment, not paying attention in class, lack of participation in group activities and poor academic performance.

### Identification of the Underlying Aetiology

*History and Examination:* Comprehensive history taking and otological examination is essential. Onset of hearing loss should be enquired about, whether congenital or acquired, pre-lingual or post-lingual. Pre-lingual/congenital SSD requires more vigilant monitoring and prompt rehabilitative measures.

Sudden onset acquired SSD could be due to idiopathic SSNHL, and it requires search for aetiology and prompt treatment with steroids (oral/intratympanic) or hyperbaric oxygen therapy which may salvage the deaf ear. History of trauma might indicate temporal bone fracture. Antecedent history of air travel or underwater diving could imply barotrauma or perilymph fistula.

Accompanying vestibular complaints should be considered. Association with recurrent episodes of rotatory vertigo lasting >20 minutes, aural fullness and tinnitus could suggest Ménière's disease. Internal auditory meatus (IAM)/CP angle tumours may lead to progressive or sudden hearing loss on side of lesion, and maybe associated with vertigo and tinnitus. History of fever, vomiting and headache could indicate meningitis. History of painful parotid swelling with fever indicates mumps. History of systemic disorders in the patient and family should be enquired. Any other focal neurological deficit should be elicited to rule out stroke.

**Table 4.2: Hearing Devices for Single-sided Deafness**

| Hearing Device | Principle | Advantage | Disadvantage | Considerations |
|---|---|---|---|---|
| CROS Devices | Route signals from the impaired to the functioning ear | Non-invasive<br><br>Overcome the head shadow effect<br><br>Improved detection of speech on the side of hearing loss, in quiet<br><br>Improved speech understanding in noise when speech is the dominant signal on the side with hearing loss | Reduced speech understanding when noise is the dominant signal on the side with hearing loss.<br><br>Do not help in sound localization<br><br>Conventional CROS occludes the normal hearing ear | Acceptance issues<br><br>Requires ability to manage the device and environment<br><br>Transcranial CROS requires a customized ear-mould that snugly fits in the bony ear canal, may cause discomfort or may not be feasible in some.<br><br>Cannot be used in case of narrow ear canal, aural atresia or discharging ear |
| Bone Conduction Devices | Transcranial bone conduction of sound vibrations to the contralateral cochlea | Overcome the head shadow effect<br><br>No occlusion of "better" ear<br><br>Most direct path of bone conduction<br><br>Suitable for microtia, aural atresia, discharging ear<br><br>Outcomes better than CROS devices<br><br>No risk of osseointegration failure or cutaneous complications and better cosmesis with transcutaneous devices | Invasive<br><br>Do not help in sound localization<br><br>Sound quality inferior to that of CROS (mechanical quality)<br><br>Percutaneous devices (BAHA) have risk of failure of osseointegration, cutaneous complications, trauma to abutment, especially in children<br><br>Limited wearing comfort<br><br>Transcutaneous devices cause soft tissue attenuation of sound vibrations, especially in high frequencies | Acceptance issues<br><br>Not approved for children under 5 years of age (BAHA) and 12 years of age (Bonebridge)<br><br>MRI compatibility/produces artifact<br><br>Identifying site for implantation (anatomic considerations) |
| Cochlear Implant | Electrical stimulation of cochlear the nerve in the poor ear | Only modality to restore binaural auditory function<br><br>Provides distinct binaural processing for advanced auditory processing abilities.<br><br>Improved speech recognition in noise, improved localization, improved health related quality of life<br><br>Only modality which benefits cases with tinnitus | Might prevent candidacy from future advancements in hearing restoration<br><br>Performance might depend on period of auditory deprivation and amount of aural rehabilitation.<br><br>Contraindicated in certain inner ear malformations, cochlear nerve deficiency.<br><br>Offer with caution in retro cochlear pathologies. | Candidacy issues (approved for 5 years of age and above for SSD or asymmetrical hearing loss)<br><br>Must have compelling audiological evidence that the ear to be implanted will not benefit from other non-surgical forms of technology<br><br>Length of auditory deprivation has a negative impact on performance<br><br>Imaging for inner ear malformations, identify absolute and relative contraindications<br><br>Cost factors |

History of ototoxic drug intake should be elicited. Any antecedent ear surgery should be ruled out. While SSD might be a complication of certain otological surgeries (such as stapedectomy), it is a consequence of certain lateral skull base approaches like trans-labyrinthine, trans-cochlear approaches.

*Audiology:* Complete audiological workup should include pure tone audiometry with air and BC thresholds, speech recognition threshold (SRT) and word recognition score (WRS), tympanometry, acoustic reflex thresholds and reflex decay, OAE and BERA. The diagnosis of ANSD is given when otoacoustic emissions and/or cochlear microphonics are present in the setting of absent or abnormal BERA. BERA also rules out functional hearing loss. Assessment of speech in noise, formal assessment of localization and evaluation of speech and language development are required to determine the degree of disability.

*Imaging:* High-resolution computed tomography (HRCT) of temporal bone and MRI of brain with gadolinium contrast are recommended in cases of unilateral/asymmetric hearing loss. In children with SNHL, overall diagnostic yield of MRI is 34% and of CT is 20%. About 52% of children with asymmetric SNHL and 30% with symmetric SNHL have a causative abnormality on imaging. Children with more severe SNHL are more likely to have an abnormality on imaging. In addition, MRI has a significantly higher diagnostic yield, identifying abnormalities in 14% of children who have normal CT findings (43).

While HRCT is preferred for structural abnormalities such as inner ear malformations and temporal bone trauma, MRI is preferable to evaluate the cochlear nerve status and brain (e.g. IAM/CP angle pathology, stroke, meningitis etc.). Both investigations should be considered in the setting of ANSD, wherein MRI may reveal abnormalities in up to two-thirds of patients.

Choice of imaging should include deliberation on the suspected cause, diagnostic yield of each study, exposure to radiation and possible need for sedation.

*Laboratory Investigations:* Hematological, biochemical and serological investigations to rule out identifiable causes should be guided by history and imaging. These include complete blood count, erythrocyte sedimentation rate (ESR), urea and electrolytes, lipid profile, blood glucose levels, thyroid function tests, coagulation profile, serology for syphilis and Lyme's disease and autoantibodies (antinuclear antibodies, anticardiolipin, lupus anticoagulant, antineutrophil cytoplasmic antibodies).

International Pediatric Otolaryngology Group (IPOG) recommends testing for CMV in case of congenital hearing loss with CMV saliva/urine PCR or shell viral culture within 3 weeks of life, and blood spot PCR after 3 weeks (19).

*Genetic Testing:* As per IPOG recommendations, non-syndromic children with UHL need not be subjected to genetic testing as part of initial workup (19).

### Non-auditory Needs Assessment

Non-auditory factors should be assessed to determine the need for cross-speciality referral, selection of hearing device, managing patient expectations and further counselling.

Such factors include symptoms accompanying hearing loss, patient's physical, mental, and psychosocial well-being, personality, manual dexterity, visual acuity etc. Patient factors may be internal (e.g. morbidities, cognition, personality and dexterity) and external (e.g. support system, work and social environment).

For example, a patient with cerebrovascular event causing SSD requires neurology referral. Some patients may perceive tinnitus to be more bothersome than the hearing loss. For a person with Ménière's disease, vestibular complaints are more troublesome than hearing loss. A person who has undergone surgery to remove a vestibular schwannoma may not be willing to undergo another surgery for device implantation. For a patient with poor manual dexterity, and lacking a good support system, BAHA may not be an optimal option.

Patients with SSD might experience emotional distress, such as feelings of depression, embarrassment and anger, for which counselling and possibly psychotherapy are required. For paediatric/pre-lingual onset of SSD, speech and developmental assessment with appropriate therapy is required. Hence, a holistic approach should be adopted to address the patient's needs.

### Management of Tinnitus and Vertigo

The prevalence of tinnitus is reported to be 68–100% in severe hearing loss, and the treatment of tinnitus is difficult in these cases. Tinnitus retraining therapy (TRT) is free of contraindications and side effects and is known to be effective for any type of tinnitus irrespective of aetiology.

TRT in SSD has shown improvement in 83% of subjects based on Tinnitus Handicap Inventory, and visual analogue scale on annoyance at the initial interview and 6 months after TRT (44). CI has been used in severe unilateral tinnitus in patients with SSD, with reported 81–95% improvement in tinnitus (38, 41, 45).

A patient with SSD may have accompanying vestibular complaints, especially if the onset is acute, which does not allow time for central compensation. Vertigo may be the presenting symptom in labyrinthitis, endolymphatic hydrops, perilymph fistula, posterior circulation stroke or CP angle tumours. Evaluation of vestibular symptoms may uncover the aetiology of hearing loss. Short-term management with vestibular sedatives and long-term management with vestibular rehabilitation therapy may be required.

### Auditory Rehabilitation

*Candidacy:* Audiological examination should be used as an initial assessment for candidacy. Best air conduction (AC) responses in the better ear are used for air conduction devices (e.g. conventional CROS), whereas best BC responses in the better ear are used in BC devices (e.g., transcranial CROS, BC aids).

Following a confirmed diagnosis of SSD, transcranial attenuation (TA) should be measured for any patient considering rehabilitation with a BCD. TA varies significantly (as much as 35 dB per frequency) between patients and is a function of the output of the transmitting device. The lower the TA, the better the efficiency for a BC transmitted signal. TA is best measured clinically by calculating the difference between the BC threshold at the good mastoid and the BC threshold at the stimulation site. An average TA of less than 10 dB at 250–4000 Hz is a good predictor of postoperative performance with a device using BC transmission. Speech-in-noise measurements are useful for quantifying the change in performance with hearing devices.

Numerous studies recommend using a pretreatment trial at home with either a CROS hearing device or the BCD worn on a test-band. It should be ensured that the BCD is programmed according to patient's TA, all hearing devices are electromechanically verified and patients adequately trained on device use and placement. Additional considerations include monitoring of hearing in the better ear at least annually, ensuring the SSD is stable prior to rehabilitative intervention.

*Device Selection:* **Age:** BAHA is approved for candidates aged 5 years and above, Bonebridge for those above 12 years of age and CI for candidates 5 years and older in case of SSD.

**Anatomical Considerations:** Most devices rely on distinct anatomical characteristics for determination of candidacy. Narrow ear canal or canal atresia are contraindications for CROS devices which require well-fitted ear moulds. Also, a discharging ear or open mastoid cavity is a contraindication. In these cases, BCD may be better suited.

Osseointegrated devices such as BAHA require adequate skull thickness for stability. The large size of floating mass transducer of Bonebridge may cause dural or sigmoid sinus compression. Retrosigmoid location may be chosen for implantation if the mastoid cavity is not large enough.

Aetiologies related to deafferentation of the cochlea or inner malformations (cochlear aplasia, rudimentary otocyst, complete labyrinthine aplasia) are contraindications for CI.

**Device Features:** Device selection should include consideration for the following factors: cosmesis, willingness to undergo surgery, comfort and ease of use, reluctance to occlusion of better hearing ear, battery life and manipulation, perceived benefit, ability to maintain site and device and cost and insurance benefits.

CROS/BICROS systems have the flexibility to be reprogrammed to accommodate hearing loss in the better hearing ear. Clinicians should consider the presence of hearing loss in the better ear and the potential for further progression, particularly when considering a more permanent solution such as BAHA. Device selection should also consider the presence and severity of tinnitus. Only CI can offer benefit in tinnitus.

*Counselling and Follow-up:* Patients should be trained to use the hearing device or access special programs in the device to improve speech recognition in noise. Patients should follow-up at 2–4 weeks post-fitting to determine comfort of fit, need for fine-tuning, re-counselling on care and maintenance and addressing any queries. They should have regular hearing device checks and annual audiological evaluations.

*Hearing-Assistive Technology (HAT):* HAT can be used to further improve the hearing environment, such as in background noise, hearing speech from a distance, classroom setting, group discussions, watching television etc. HAT includes personal frequency modulation (FM) systems, Bluetooth devices, telephone amplifier, telecoil, telecommunication device for the deaf (TDD), integrated wireless radio or magnetic induction systems, video-calling services etc.

Auditory devices, including air and BC hearing aids, BAHA and CIs are Bluetooth compatible, enabling connectivity with devices such as phone, television etc. FM system picks up the sound from the source and transmits it directly to a sound-generating transducer at the ear of the listener. The sound is presented at a favourable SNR with minimal ambient noise. Such system can be used in a classroom setting.

An algorithm for managing a case of SSD is presented in Figure 4.7.

## DISCUSSION

SSD has been a neglected entity in otology practice for long. The problems are multifold and include late detection, lack of awareness amongst patients as well as clinicians and lack of acknowledgement of the disability it causes.

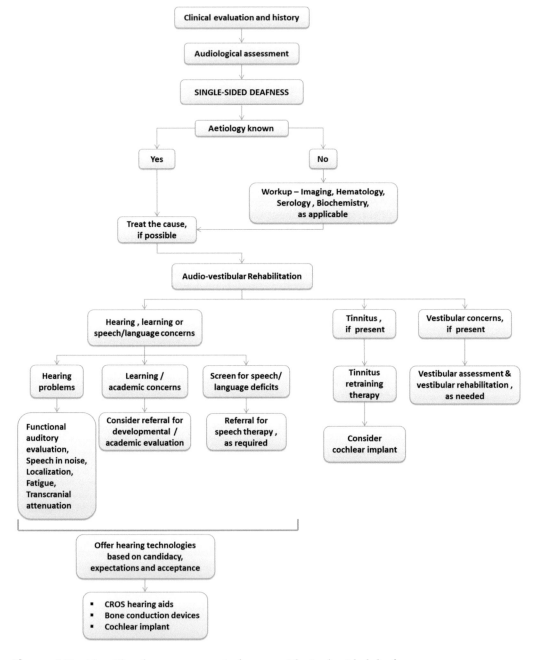

**Figure 4.7** Algorithm for management of a case with single-sided deafness.

Adults with SSD, even after diagnosis, may not want rehabilitation. The causes include lack of awareness, lack of resources, acceptance issues with the available rehabilitation options or reluctance to undergo surgical procedure.

The problem with the paediatric age group is even greater. Lack of universal newborn screening facilities, especially in developing countries, or lack of follow-up during development years may lead to missed diagnosis. As these children have never experienced binaural hearing, they are not able to identify the unilateral deafness, leading to late diagnosis. Also, there is reluctance amongst the parents to subject their child to hearing amplification devices "till absolutely necessary".

In government/institutional policies for provision for disabled, hearing disability percentage is calculated based on the absolute hearing threshold of each ear on PTA. The maximum overall hearing impairment in a case with SSD would therefore be 16.7% (46). Hence, these patients are not eligible for disability benefits such as provision of hearing devices, financial aid, rehabilitation services etc. Criteria for the determination of hearing impairment should be updated to include speech recognition in noise testing with and without the spatial separation of the speech and noise stimuli.

One-third of cases with UHL are never referred to an otolaryngologist by primary care physicians. Many physicians, audiologists and health professionals still hold onto the belief that one ear is enough for hearing. Even if the patients get evaluated for aetiology of SSD, rehabilitation is not offered.

Comprehensive approach should be adopted to identify the underlying aetiology as well as assess the non-auditory needs, such as additional evaluation, cross-speciality referral, management of non-auditory complaints, need for counselling and rehabilitation therapy.

Since SSD in children is often unmasked in the school environment, the onus lies on teachers to identify these cases. They can contribute to management with preferential seating, using hearing-assistive devices, avoiding discrimination and attending to the special needs of these children.

Auditory rehabilitation should be offered based on candidacy, expectations and acceptance of patients. Device selection should be based on age, anatomical considerations, device features, cognition, dexterity, support system and hearing environment.

Studies have depicted varied perception of disability amongst people with SSD. The perceived benefit of hearing device and patient compliance are better if self-selection principle is practised while opting for hearing device. Home-trial of CROS as well as BCD on a headband for 2–3 weeks is recommended before the patient chooses the device.

It is also pragmatic to offer sequential interventional approach based on the degree of invasiveness or risk associated with each intervention. For example, initially CROS or BCD on a headband can be recommended. If that proves unsatisfactory, implantable devices may be offered, failing which CI may be considered (47).

Regular follow-up must be impressed upon for post-fitting counselling, device care, assessment of device usage and benefit derived, concomitant rehabilitation therapy and auditory assessment of the better ear.

## KEY LEARNING POINTS

- SSD leads to distinct disabilities that transcend degree of auditory disadvantage, due to loss of binaural auditory function.

- Early detection of SSD is important, as it may have profound effects on cognitive function, speech and language development, academic performance and quality of life.

- Attempt should be made to identify the aetiology.

- Early hearing rehabilitation, especially in paediatric and pre-lingual deafness, must be done.

- Auditory rehabilitation should be offered based on candidacy, expectations and acceptance of patients.

- Non-auditory aspects – vestibular symptoms, tinnitus, management of systemic conditions and psychological factors must also be addressed.

- Follow up is required for post-fitting counselling, device care, assessment of device usage and benefit derived, concomitant rehabilitation therapy or use of hearing-assistive devices as applicable.

- Regular long-term auditory assessment is required for the functional ear.

## REFERENCES

1. American Academy of Audiology Clinical Practice Guidelines. Adult Patients with Severe-to-Profound Unilateral Sensorineural Hearing Loss American Academy of Audiology Clinical Practice Guidelines. 2015.

2. Van De Heyning P, Távora-Vieira D, Mertens G, et al. Towards a unified testing framework for single-sided deafness studies: a consensus paper. Audiol Neurotol. 2017;21(6):391–8.

3. Vincent C, Arndt S, Firszt JB, et al. Identification and evaluation of cochlear implant candidates with asymmetrical hearing loss. Audiol Neurotol. 2015;20(Suppl 1):87–9.

4. Usami S, Kitoh R, Moteki H, et al. Etiology of single-sided deafness and asymmetrical hearing loss. Acta Otolaryngol. 2017;137(Suppl 565):S2–7.

5. Ramos Macías Á, Borkoski-Barreiro SA, Falcón González JC, de Miguel Martínez I, Ramos de Miguel Á. Single-sided deafness and cochlear implantation in congenital and acquired hearing loss in children. Clin Otolaryngol. 2019;44(2):138–43.

6. Golub JS, Lin FR, Lustig LR, Lalwani AK. Prevalence of Adult Unilateral Hearing Loss and Hearing Aid Use in the United States. Laryngoscope. 2018; 128(7):1681–6.

7. Bagatto M, DesGeorges J, King A, et al. Consensus practice parameter: audiological assessment and management of unilateral hearing loss in children. Int J Audiol. 2019;58(12):805–15.

8. Lieu JEC. Management of children with unilateral hearing loss. Otolaryngol Clin North Am. 2015; 48(6):1011–26.

9. Avan P, Giraudet F, Büki B. Importance of binaural hearing. Audiol Neurootol. 2015;20(Suppl 1):3–6.

10. Kral A, Hubka P, Heid S, Tillein J. Single-sided deafness leads to unilateral aural preference within an early sensitive period. Brain. 2013;136(1):180–93.

11. Kral A, Hubka P, Tillein J. Strengthening of hearing ear representation reduces binaural sensitivity in early single-sided deafness. Audiol Neurotol. 2015; 20(Suppl 1):7–12.

12. Kishon-Rabin L, Kuint J, Hildesheimer M, Ari-Even Roth D. Delay in auditory behaviour and preverbal vocalization in infants with unilateral hearing loss. Dev Med Child Neurol. 2015;57(12):1129–36.

13. Lieu JEC. Unilateral hearing loss in children: speech-language and school performance. B-ENT. 2013; (Suppl. 21):107–15.

14. Lieu JEC, Tye-Murray N, Karzon RK, Piccirillo JF. Unilateral hearing loss is associated with worse speech-language scores in children. Pediatrics. 2010;125(6):e1348–55.

15. Lieu JEC. Speech-language and educational consequences of unilateral hearing loss in children. Arch Otolaryngol Head Neck Surg. 2004;130(5):524–30.

16. Vaish. 基因的改变 NIH Public Access. Bone. 2012;23(1):1–7.

17. Heggdal POL, Brännström J, Aarstad HJ, Vassbotn FS, Specht K. Functional-structural reorganisation of the neuronal network for auditory perception in subjects with unilateral hearing loss: review of neuroimaging studies. Hear Res. 2016;332:73–9.

18. Goderis J, De Leenheer E, Smets K, Van Hoecke H, Keymeulen A, Dhooge I. Hearing loss and congenital CMV infection: a systematic review. Pediatrics. 2014;134(5):972–82.

19. Liming BJ, Carter J, Cheng A, et al. International Pediatric Otolaryngology Group (IPOG) consensus recommendations: hearing loss in the pediatric patient. Int J Pediatr Otorhinolaryngol. 2016; 90:251–8.

20. Hill SL, Marcus A, Digges ENB, Gillman N, Silverstein H, Stevens J. Assessment of patient satisfaction with various configurations of digital CROS and BiCROS hearing aids. Ear Nose Throat J. 2006;85(7):427–30.

21. Reinfeldt S, Håkansson B, Taghavi H, Eeg-Olofsson M. New developments in bone-conduction hearing implants: a review. Med Devices Evid Res. 2015; 8:79–93.

22. Linstrom CJ, Silverman CA, Yu GP. Efficacy of the bone-anchored hearing aid for single-sided deafness. Laryngoscope. 2009;119(4):713–20.

23. Schrøder SA, Ravn T, Bonding P. BAHA in single-sided deafness: patient compliance and subjective benefit. Otol Neurotol. 2010;31(3):404–8.

24. Faber HT, Kievit H, De Wolf MJF, Cremers CWRJ, Snik AFM, Hol MKS. Analysis of factors predicting the success of the bone conduction device headband trial in patients with single-sided deafness. Arch Otolaryngol Head Neck Surg. 2012;138(12):1129–35.

25. Desmet J, Wouters K, De Bodt M, Van De Heyning P. Long-term subjective benefit with a bone conduction implant sound processor in 44 patients with single-sided deafness. Otol Neurotol. 2014;35(6):1017–25.

26. Faber HT, Nelissen RC, Kramer SE, Cremers CWRJ, Snik AFM, Hol MKS. Bone-anchored hearing implants in single-sided deafness patients: long-term use and satisfaction by gender. Laryngoscope. 2015;125(12):2790–5.

27. Briggs R, Van Hasselt A, Luntz M, et al. Clinical performance of a new magnetic bone conduction hearing implant system: results from a prospective, multicenter, clinical investigation. Otol Neurotol. 2015;36(5):834–41.

28. Magele A, Schoerg P, Stanek B, Gradl B, Sprinzl GM. Active transcutaneous bone conduction hearing implants: systematic review and meta-analysis. PLOS ONE. 2019;14(9):1–19.

29. Håkansson B, Eeg-Olofsson M, Reinfeldt S, Stenfelt S, Granström G. Percutaneous versus transcutaneous bone conduction implant system: a feasibility study on a cadaver head. Otol Neurotol. 2008;29(8):1132–9.

30. Murray M, Popelka GR, Miller R. Efficacy and safety of an in-the-mouth bone conduction device for single-sided deafness. Otol Neurotol. 2011;32(3):437–43.

31. Niparko JK, Cox KM, Lustig LR. Comparison of the bone anchored hearing aid implantable hearing device with contralateral routing of offside signal amplification in the rehabilitation of unilateral deafness. Otol Neurotol. 2003;24(1):73–8.

32. Baguley DM, Plydoropulou V, Prevost AT. Bone anchored hearing aids for single-sided deafness. Clin Otolaryngol. 2009;34(2):176–7.

33. Bishop CE, Hamadain E, Galster JA, Johnson MF, Spankovich C, Windmill I. Outcomes of hearing aid use by individuals with unilateral sensorineural hearing loss (USNHL). J Am Acad Audiol. 2017;28(10):941–9.

34. Peters JPM, Smit AL, Stegeman I, Grolman W. Review: bone conduction devices and contralateral routing of sound systems in single-sided deafness. Laryngoscope. 2015;125(1):218–26.

35. Vermeire K, Van De Heyning P. Binaural hearing after cochlear implantation in subjects with unilateral sensorineural deafness and tinnitus. Audiol Neurotol. 2009;14(3):163–71.

36. Arndt S, Aschendorff A, Laszig R, et al. Comparison of pseudobinaural hearing to real binaural hearing rehabilitation after cochlear implantation in patients with unilateral deafness and tinnitus. Otol Neurotol. 2011;32(1):39–47.

37. Wesarg T, Arndt S, Wiebe K, et al. Speech recognition in noise in single-sided deaf cochlear implant recipients using digital remote wireless microphone technology. J Am Acad Audiol. 2019;30(7):607–18.

38. Galvin JJ, Fu QJ, Wilkinson EP, et al. Benefits of cochlear implantation for single-sided deafness: data from the House Clinic-University of Southern California-University of California, Los Angeles Clinical Trial. Ear Hear. 2019;40(4):766–81.

39. Zeitler DM, Dorman MF, Natale SJ, Loiselle L, Yost WA, Gifford RH. Sound source localization and speech understanding in complex listening environments by single-sided deaf listeners after cochlear implantation. Otol Neurotol. 2015;36(9):1467–71.

40. Wesarg T, Richter N, Hessel H, et al. Binaural integration of periodically alternating speech following cochlear implantation in subjects with profound sensorineural unilateral hearing loss. Audiol Neurotol. 2015;20(Suppl 1):73–8.

41. Punte AK, Vermeire K, Hofkens A, De Bodt M, De Ridder D, Van de Heyning P. Cochlear implantation as a durable tinnitus treatment in single-sided deafness. Cochlear Implants Int. 2011;12(Suppl 1): S26–9.

42. Ramos Macías A, Falcón González JC, Manrique M, et al. Cochlear implants as a treatment option for unilateral hearing loss, severe tinnitus and hyperacusis. Audiol Neurotol. 2015;20(Suppl 1):60–6.

43. Liu CC, Anne S, Horn DL. Advances in management of pediatric sensorineural hearing loss. Otolaryngol Clin North Am. 2019;52(5):847–61.

44. Kim SH, Byun JY, Yeo SG, Park MS. Tinnitus retraining therapy in unilateral tinnitus patients with single side deafness. J Int Adv Otol. 2016;12(1):72–6.

45. Mertens G, Kleine Punte A, De Bodt M, Van De Heyning P. Binaural auditory outcomes in patients with postlingual profound unilateral hearing loss: 3 years after cochlear implantation. Audiol Neurotol. 2015;20(Suppl 1):67–72.

46. Vermiglio AJ, Griffin S, Post C, Fang X. An evaluation of the World Health Organization and American Medical Association ratings of hearing impairment and simulated single-sided deafness. J Am Acad Audiol. 2018;29(7):634–47.

47. Heubi C, Choo D. Updated optimal management of single-sided deafness. Laryngoscope. 2017; 127(8):1731–2.

# THE DISCHARGING EAR: DIFFERENTIAL DIAGNOSIS AND MANAGEMENT

# 5 The Discharging Ear: Differential Diagnosis and Management

*Anandita Gupta*

## CONTENTS

## INTRODUCTION

Otorrhea is a common symptom of ear pathology and one of the foremost causes of visits to the ear, nose and throat (ENT) outpatient department. It is a very distressing symptom and may require repeated hospital visits for resolution. All age groups can be affected by a multitude of disorders which can result in otorrhea. It can be associated with otalgia and foul odour and can have a considerable negative impact on the quality of life. A detailed history and clinical examination are essential to establish the source of ear discharge prior to making any attempt to treat it.

## CLINICAL ASSESSMENT

*History:* Patients must be asked about the onset, nature, chronicity, quantum of discharge and presence of any foul odour to infer the nature of ear disease. Other cardinal symptoms of ear disease which must be enquired about are as follows:

- Otalgia
- Vertigo
- Facial paralysis
- Tinnitus
- Hearing loss

Acute onset otorrhea would indicate conditions like Otitis Externa (OE), myringitis, furunculosis or Acute Otitis Media (AOM). A history of recurrent episodes of otorrhea is seen in diseases of chronic nature such as chronic otitis media (COM). The nature of discharge could also indicate its origin. Disorders of the external ear will give rise to purulent otorrhea. As the External Auditory Canal (EAC) is devoid of mucus glands, presence of a mucoid element would indicate involvement of middle ear cleft. Copious discharge may indicate involvement of middle ear cleft due to the glandular secretions from a larger surface area.

Presence of blood intermingled with mucoid or purulent discharge would indicate the presence of granulations associated with chronic infections. Frank blood can be seen in trauma such as fracture of temporal bone, ear bud injury or traumatic rupture of tympanic membrane (TM). Cerebrospinal fluid (CSF) otorrhea can present as clear or blood-tinged watery discharge and should prompt the physician to evaluate for traumatic or spontaneous tegmen defects.

A foul-smelling discharge is indicative of putrefaction associated with cholesteatoma. Ear discomfort or pruritus is associated with OE especially of fungal origin. Hearing loss can occur either due to otitis media or secondary to occlusion of EAC with discharge, debris or oedema. Otalgia is seen in acute conditions such as furunculosis, OE, AOM, osteitis or skull base osteomyelitis (SBO).

Facial paralysis when associated with otorrhea may indicate the presence of Ramsay Hunt syndrome or serious underlying conditions such as complicated otitis media, Malignant Otitis Externa (MOE) or Temporal Bone Malignancy (TBM) malignancy. Vertigo and tinnitus are sinister symptoms and may indicate involvement of inner ear. Entry of the bacteria or their toxins into the inner ear through the round window, oval window or a labyrinthine fistula may cause suppurative or serous labyrinthitis. Compromised function of other cranial nerves such as glossopharyngeal, vagus, spinal accessory and hypoglossal may indicate SBO or skull base tumours with extension into middle or external ears.

*Clinical Examination:* A general examination should precede the ENT evaluation. A good headlight is mandatory for a thorough clinical examination of ear, nose, head and neck region. Any swelling, erythema, scar in the pre- and post-aural region should be noted. Examination of the EAC and TM should be initially done with a headlight to note the conditions involving the outer part of EAC which may be missed if an otoscope is directly introduced into the EAC. Pain elicited on movement of pinna or tragus is diagnostic of OE. Tenderness on palpation of concha, root of zygoma and mastoid tip are pathognomonic of acute mastoiditis. In case the EAC is filled with discharge, a pus swab can be obtained prior to ear toileting. Visualization of the ear and better delivery of topical medications is possible only after meticulous cleaning of EAC. Ear toileting should be done with sterile instruments using a headlight or preferably a microscope. A microsuction or cotton wool tipped sterile probe can be used for removing discharge and debris. A fungal aetiology should be suspected when spores or mass of hyphae is visualized on otoscopy. Curd-like greyish white discharge blocking the EAC is also typically seen in fungal OE.

Water should preferably not be used for clearing EAC as it may exacerbate the inflammation or its inadvertent entry through a perforation in TM may aggravate the infectious process in middle ear. A well-illuminated otoscope should then be used to visualize the TM and middle ear through a perforation if present. Sometimes oedema or granulations in EAC may preclude visualization of TM. Placement of antibiotic or ichthammol glycerine-infused wick in EAC for a few days may reduce the oedema or granulations and allow better visualization.

Any perforation, presence of tympanostomy tube, retraction of TM or part of it and presence of epithelial debris should be noted. Condition of the middle ear mucosa should be noted through the TM perforation. Hearing status can be assessed by performing tuning fork tests. Presence of jerk nystagmus or unilateral vestibular weakness evident on Romberg's test or Unterberger's test can warn the clinician of inner ear involvement.

*Investigations:*

- **Pure tone audiogram:** A baseline audiogram for documentation of type and degree of hearing loss should be obtained when feasible. It must be done once the discharge or oedema in the EAC has reduced.

- **Microbiologic tests:** Sterile cotton wool tipped applicators should be used to obtain the pus or debris from deep part of the meatus. Prior to sampling, the concha should be cleaned with an alcohol-based preparation to avoid contamination with skin flora. The material should then be processed for Gram stain and cultured to identify the causative organisms. A 10% potassium hydroxide mount is an inexpensive and quick test to identify fungal elements. Inoculation of the specimen on Sabouraud dextrose agar with antibiotics allows identification of fungal species and susceptibility testing. AFB staining and culture can be done when mycobacterial infection is clinically suspected.

Both fungi and mycobacteria are slow growing and require specialized culture media and techniques for isolation. Utilization in routine practice is limited due to longer test turnaround time and it should be resorted to in refractory cases only.

- **Radiological investigations**: Highresolution Computed Tomography (HRCT) of the Temporal Bone (TB) or Magnetic Resonance Imaging (MRI) is rarely required in the initial management of a discharging ear. Radiological investigations may be considered early when complicated otitis media, MOE, malignancy or Temporal Bone (TB) fracture is suspected.

### DIFFERENTIAL DIAGNOSIS

Otorrhea as a presenting complaint is seen in benign conditions such as OE to more sinister conditions like Temporal Bone (TB) malignancy. The clinician should consider the following conditions while diagnosing the cause of otorrhea.

### Diseases of the External Ear

#### *Furunculosis*

It is a condition caused by *Staphylococcal* infection of hair follicles present in the outer third of the EAC (1). It generally starts as folliculitis, but later involvement of multiple hair follicles may result in diffuse oedema or formation of an abscess which narrows the calibre of the meatus. The usual inciting event is self-cleansing with finger nails or ear buds. Water entry in an abraded EAC can also initiate the infection.

Intense otalgia is usually the presenting complaint. The hallmark is local tenderness on movement of pinna, tragus or jaw. Headlight examination will show diffuse erythema, oedema, pus filled or a discharging lesion associated with hair follicle in outer one-third of EAC. During otoscopic examination, a smaller size ear speculum can be gently inserted beyond the inflamed area to note the condition of the TM.

### *Otitis Externa*

Swimmer's ear or diffuse OE occurs when the pathogenic organisms flourish in the EAC due to high levels of humidity and alteration of pH. The EAC is colonized with mixed flora such as *Staphylococcus, Streptococcus,* Gram-negative organisms or certain saprophytic fungi which prevent growth of pathogenic organisms. Almost 98% infections are bacterial in origin and the most common pathogens are *Staphylococcus aureus* and *Pseudomonas aeruginosa* (2, 3). Alteration of pH in diabetics or presence of moisture favours growth of pathogenic organisms such as *Pseudomonas*. Loss of protective cerumen due to swimming or self-cleansing, breach of skin integrity due to use of hearing aid ear moulds, fingernail trauma and presence of debris due to various dermatologic disorders also favour growth of pathogenic organisms.

The usual presentation is acute onset of otalgia, pruritus, tragal tenderness, erythema or oedema of EAC with or without the presence of purulent discharge (4) (Figure 5.1). Evaluation of TM using a smaller sized speculum should be attempted to rule out presence of AOM. Often, diffuse OE can be secondary to presence of secretions in acute or COM.

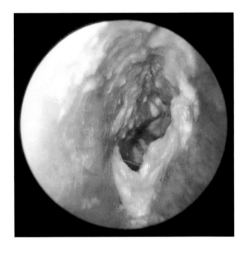

**Figure 5.1** Chronic otitis externa. (From Hawke Library. Dr Michael Hawke, Toronto, Canada.)

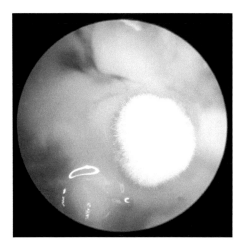

**Figure 5.2** Otomycosis. (From Hawke Library. Dr Michael Hawke, Toronto, Canada.)

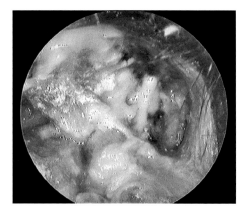

**Figure 5.3** Otomycotic debris blocking the external auditory canal.

### Otomycosis

Primary fungal infection of EAC is commonly seen in geographical areas which are hot and humid and in individuals associated with farming. Personal habits such as use of unsterile sticks, hairpins or instillation of oil in EAC favour deposition of fungal spores. Prolonged use of antibiotic drops in EAC can supress the bacterial organisms and cause overgrowth of fungal elements (Figure 5.2). Discharge and debris in EAC following otitis media or OE can cause maceration of skin which is an excellent medium for growth of fungal spores, especially in immunocompromised hosts.

*Aspergillus* species and *Candida* species are most common causative fungal agents (4). Species from other genera such as *Penicillium*, *Mucoraceae*, *Alternaria* and certain *Dermatophytes* have also been implicated.

Initial presentation may be itching, erythema or scaling in the EAC. Intense otalgia may occur as the infection progresses. Blocked sensation due to desquamated epithelial cells and fungal debris may cause hearing loss. The typical fungal debris has "blotting paper" or "wet newspaper" appearance (5) (Figure 5.3).

### Myringitis

Granular Myringitis (GM) is an inflammatory disorder involving the outer epithelial layer of the TM. It is defined as loss of lateral squamous epithelium of TM without disease in the middle ear cleft. Its pathogenesis is poorly understood, and it is disputable whether the fibrous and the mucosal layers of TM are also primarily involved (6). It is postulated that GM occurs secondary to trauma or infection. It is sometimes encountered

in a postoperative setting as an area of granulation and disturbed epithelialization on the neotympanum. The lesion is seen as focal or diffuse area of de-epithelialization and granulation tissue on the surface of TM.

Makino et al. have suggested that pathological changes in TM such as atrophy, calcification result in impaired epithelial migration. The initiating event is insult to the lamina propria of the TM following which granulations arise. The process of epithelialization over these granulations fails to occur due to suppressed epithelial migration. This process is also perpetuated by infection (6). GM is an important cause of persistent offensive otorrhea, which is usually scanty and purulent in character. It causes only mild ear discomfort and may go unnoticed sometimes as the lesion may be covered with dried crust which can be mistaken for dried wax. Clinically it appears as a well-demarcated denuded area on the TM, or a shallow ulcer or as polypoid granulations on the surface of TM (7). Histologically, the tissue may consist of epithelium alone or associated with chronic inflammatory infiltrate.

Untreated diffuse GM or extensive lesions involving the EAC can result in extensive scarring and secondary stenosis of medial part of EAC. Extensive GM with diffuse involvement of TM and EAC may sometimes be difficult to distinguish from COM.

Bullous myringitis, on the other hand, has a more acute onset and is characterized by severe otalgia. Otorrhea is not a usual complaint. Its occurrence has been usually associated with AOM. Blisters which may be haemorrhagic occasionally appear on the surface of TM and in the EAC. These blisters form between the epithelial layer and the middle fibrous layer of TM. *Streptococcus pneumoniae, Haemophilus influenzae* and *Moraxella catarrhalis* and certain respiratory viruses have been implicated in its causation. Bullous myringitis as an independent disease entity is disputed as some authors consider it as an inflammatory reaction to AOM.

### Malignant Otitis Externa

It is an external otitis with a propensity to spread to the soft tissues, blood vessels, cranial nerves and bones of the skull base resulting in a life-threatening condition. It is almost exclusively seen in individuals who are immunocompromised secondary to diabetes mellitus and haematological malignancies or on chemotherapeutic agents. If unchecked during the initial stage, it can cause severe osteomyelitis of the skull base (8, 9).

The initial presentation is similar to acute OE – erythema, purulent otorrhea, oedema and exuberant granulations in the EAC (Figure 5.4a–c). This condition should be suspected in any immuno-deficient patient with refractory otorrhea and granulations, who complains of severe unrelenting nocturnal otalgia. Also, this diagnosis must be considered when OE is associated with weakness of facial nerve or lower cranial nerves such as cranial nerves IX, X, XI, XII.

Poor phagocytic function of the white blood cells, diabetic microangiopathy and alteration of the pH of cerumen allows the causative organisms to flourish unchecked in the EAC. *P. aeruginosa* is most commonly implicated. Other organisms known to cause it are *S, aureus*, *Candida* sp. and *Streptococcus* sp. The fissures of Santorini in the floor of EAC at the bony cartilaginous junction facilitate the spread of infection to the soft tissues and neurological and vascular structures of the skull base (1).

### Granulomatous Conditions

The skin of EAC can be involved in systemic conditions involving the Temporal Bone (TB).

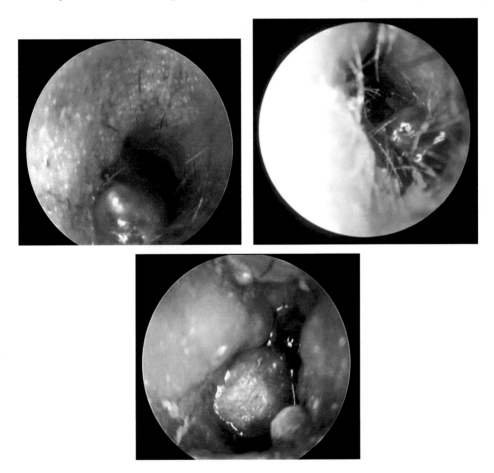

**Figure 5.4** (a) Exuberant granulations arising from the floor of external auditory canal in a case of malignant otitis externa. (b) Malignant otitis externa. (From Hawke Library. Dr Michael Hawke, Toronto, Canada.) (c) Discharge seen behind external auditory canal granulations in a case of malignant otitis externa (right ear).

EAC and middle ear involvement in tuberculous otitis media (TOM), anti-neutrophilic cytoplasmic antibody (ANCA) associated vasculitis, sarcoidosis and invasive fungal disease can cause refractory ear discharge (10). These conditions are not usually suspected at the time of initial presentation. Suitable laboratory investigations should be done in patients who have systemic involvement and who do not respond to routine treatment. Diagnosis can remain elusive when these conditions are solely localized in ear.

### EAC Cholesteatoma

It is an uncommon condition which occurs due to focal epithelial hyperplasia and localized bone erosion in the EAC. It can be either idiopathic or secondary to meatal stenosis, bone loss secondary to trauma or surgery or following exposure to radiation (11). Chronic osteitis associated with it increases the bone erosion and results in ingrowth of epithelium into the mastoid through the EAC. Otorrhea, either intermittent or persistent, is the commonest clinical presentation. An extensive EAC cholesteatoma may rarely be difficult to differentiate from keratosis obturans. Patients usually do not complain of hearing loss as the TM, middle ear and the ossicles are intact. These clinical findings may help to differentiate the two conditions. Clinical picture may also appear similar to EAC malignancy or MOE. In cases of unexplained otorrhea, the bony EAC must be examined microscopically to look for any erosion, sequestered bone and epithelial ingrowth. Probing can be done to note the extent of invasion into the mastoid. Naim et al. have proposed a classification system based on the pathological changes in the skin and the extent of bone erosion (12).

### Keratosis Obturans

It is a condition caused by collection of desquamated keratin plug in the bony part of EAC and its consequent expansion and ballooning. Patients usually present with blocked sensation of ears, otalgia and hearing loss. Ear discharge is not commonly reported unless it is associated with infection (13). Increased desquamation and altered epithelial migration cause the keratin layer to accumulate in an onion peel fashion. This condition needs to be differentiated from EAC cholesteatoma, which is a distinct clinical and pathologic entity (14).

### Meatal Stenosis

This condition may arise consequent to chronic OE. Narrowing of the bony or the cartilaginous part of EAC can also be congenital or acquired, secondary to trauma to the parotid gland, temporo-mandibular joint or EAC (15). Chronic ear discharge and hearing loss are the common presenting complaints. Post-inflammatory medial meatal stenosis has two stages: the initial wet stage is characterized by episodic inflammation and granulations which result in a discharging ear. The second dry phase begins when a fibrous plug develops, which completely occludes the meatus. At this stage, the ear discharge ceases and the patient presents with blocked sensation and conductive hearing loss. Breakdown of the central part of fibrous layer can result in refractory ear discharge (16). Entrapment of squamous epithelium medial to the fibrous plug can result in the formation of a cholesteatoma during this phase.

Post-traumatic stenosis may involve the bony part of EAC due to healing of the misaligned bony fragments. Congenital stenosis has been described by Cole and Jahrsdoerfer as EAC calibre of ≤4 mm (17). Early surgical intervention is necessary to widen the canal to prevent EAC cholesteatoma.

### Herpetic Otitis Externa

Reactivation of Varicella zoster virus in the geniculate ganglion of Facial nerve can result in intense pain, nerve paralysis and erythematous vesicular eruptions in its sensory distribution. These clinical findings may be temporally separated, thus can result in misdiagnosis at the time of initial presentation. The vesicular eruptions in EAC may cause crust formation which can develop secondary bacterial infection and cause otorrhea (18). Due to associated otalgia, the picture may appear similar to acute OE more so when facial nerve paralysis is absent. Associated symptoms such as tinnitus, hearing loss, vertigo, loss of taste sensation or involvement of cranial nerves V, IX, X may help in establishing the diagnosis of Ramsay Hunt syndrome (19).

### Foreign Body in the EAC

Foreign body in the EAC can result in laceration of the canal skin and perforation of the TM. Management by an otolaryngologist is easily accomplished in an OPD set-up using micro ear instruments under direct or microscopic vision and only in rare circumstances is surgical intervention required. Excessive manipulation, incomplete removal or attempted aural syringing in a non-ENT set up may result in OE. A neglected foreign body, especially if vegetative, can cause persistent otorrhea. As vegetative material is hygroscopic, the vegetative foreign body can swell up and occlude the EAC. This predisposes to superimposed bacterial or fungal infection, which can present as hypoacusis and persistent ear discharge (10).

Military shrapnel or drop weld injuries caused by hot sparks, molten slag or metal during welding have been known to perforate the TM. These can be retained in middle ear over a prolonged time and result in chronic inflammation and otorrhea.

### Dermatologic Disorders

Various cutaneous lesions involving the EAC and causing otorrhea may get overlooked in the ENT outpatient department. Conditions such as seborrheic dermatitis, contact dermatitis, atopic dermatitis and psoriasis can cause otorrhea. Common allergens or irritants include ear plugs, hearing aid moulds, metallic earrings, shampoo, hair dye and soaps. Topical application of Neomycin, Chloramphenicol, hydrocortisone or benzalkonium can incite a type IV hypersensitivity reaction and result in secondary contact OE (20).

These lesions can cause intense pruritus and prompt the use of cotton-tipped applicators, unsterile wooden sticks, hairpins or fingernails in order to relieve itching. Scratching can result in excoriation of EAC skin and transfer of pathogenic organisms, which causes superadded OE.

### EAC Lesions

Certain benign neoplastic and non-tumoral lesions can involve the EAC either primarily or as an extension of a lesion on the pinna. Seborrheic keratosis, actinic keratosis, squamous papilloma, ceruminous adenomas, osteoma or exostosis can present as mass lesions in the EAC and can give rise to non-specific symptoms such as otalgia, hearing loss or otorrhea if associated with retained infected debris (21, 22). A prompt biopsy is indicated in all cases of refractory otorrhea where slightest suspicion of mass lesion in EAC is evident.

### Malignant Tumours

Malignant neoplasms of the external ear are rare and include squamous cell carcinoma, basal cell carcinoma, malignant melanoma and adnexal carcinomas. They present as space occupying lesions in the EAC. Most of these lesions are diagnosed at a late stage as the initial presentation is non-specific, including otorrhea, otalgia and hearing loss. Biopsy from deeper tissues under microscopic visualization is necessary to differentiate it from chronic inflammatory lesions (23).

### Radiation-associated Otitis Externa

Radiation-induced injury can result in Temporal Bone (TB) necrosis. Purulent otorrhea, otalgia

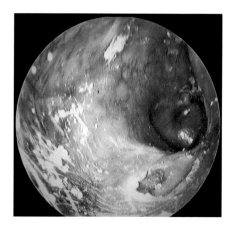

**Figure 5.5** Bony sequestrum involving the tympanic bone seen in a case of localized radiation-induced osteonecrosis of temporal bone. Associated granulations and osteitis in such a case can result in recurrent otorrhea (right ear).

and hearing loss are the common complaints (24). Obliterative endarteritis and consequent persistent hypoxia in an irradiated bone can result in soft tissue and bony necrosis. It is more common in diabetics, elderly and immunosuppressed individuals.

Ramsden et al. described a localized form which affects the EAC and a diffuse form in which there is extensive ischaemic necrosis of TB. The localized form occurs when Temporal Bone (TB) falls in the periphery of radiation field and presents with otorrhea and otalgia (25). A bony sequestrum involving the tympanic bone may be seen in the EAC (Figure 5.5). This variety can be managed conservatively with regular aural toileting and topical and oral antibiotics. The bony sequestrum may get spontaneously extruded over a period of time resulting in complete healing. The diffuse form is seen in cases when Temporal Bone (TB) or structures within it are directly irradiated. Deep boring pain, profuse ear discharge, distortion of Temporal Bone (TB) architecture with exposure of deep-seated structures and intracranial complications may occur. Extensive surgical debridement may be necessary to control the symptoms.

### Otoacariasis

Parasitic infestation by ticks and mites in the EAC can result in chronic ear discharge. Mites such as *Sarcoptes scabiei*, *Demodex* sp. can reside in the skin epithelium, hair follicles and sebaceous glands in the EAC. Such infestations are usually rare in immunocompetent individuals.

Intense pruritus can result in scratching and excoriation. Formation of granulation tissue, hyperaemia of skin and perforation of TM can result in otorrhea (10).

### Aural Myiasis

It is a condition caused by infestation of external or middle ear by dipteran larvae, which thrive on dead or alive host tissue. This condition is usually seen in debilitated or psychiatric patients staying in poor hygienic conditions. Certain flies (Sarcophagidae, Calliphoridae) can lay eggs after being attracted to the ear discharge or necrotic tissue in the EAC. Blood-tinged, foul-smelling discharge is the usual complaint. The maggots are visible on otoscopic examination. They may form burrowing channels and reach the underlying structures resulting in extensive damage (10).

### Management of Otorrhea Due to Causes in External Ear

Topical intervention along with adequate analgesia is the mainstay of treatment.

*Therapeutic Agents:* Ototopical agents can be used once aural toileting has been done. A number of antifungal and antibacterial ototopical agents are available either as single formulations or as combinations. No topical antifungal preparation is currently approved by USFDA for use in the ear (26). Certain formulations have steroids which are useful because of their anti-inflammatory action. Topical antibiotics achieve high concentration of the drug in the EAC and are able to eliminate most pathogens. Addition of steroids to the topical antibiotic formulations helps in reducing oedema, relieves pain and increases their efficacy (27).

The most commonly used topical antibiotics are fluoroquinolones. Clinical cure rates have been found to be comparable for all topical antibiotics (27). Topical preparations containing aminoglycosides such as gentamicin and neomycin are useful but have the potential for ototoxicity when used in presence of a TM perforation. Fluoroquinolones are active against most pathogens involved and are currently the only FDA-approved class of drug for use in presence of a perforation due to lack of ototoxic potential (2, 28).

Acidified solutions restore the acidic environment of the EAC and suppress the growth of bacterial and fungal pathogens (29). Two percent acetic acid is commercially available and useful as a primary therapy. Therapeutic outcomes have been found to be comparable to topical antibiotics. Acetic acid and isopropyl alcohol are also part of certain commercially available antibiotic preparations.

A number of antiseptic agents are also useful in managing resistant infections (Table 5.1). These preparations can be applied topically with a cotton-tipped applicator in the external canal. Their use must be refrained in the presence of perforated TM due to their ototoxic potential (1).

The granulations present in EAC can be mechanically or chemically debrided. Caustic agents such as phenol, trichloroacetic acid or silver nitrate crystals can be used to debulk the granulations.

Ichthammol glycerine containing ichthammol 10% (sulfonated shale oil) is a useful topical agent in chronic OE (30, 31). Glycerine is a hygroscopic agent and reduces oedema in the EAC. Ichthammol is known to have anti-inflammatory, antibacterial and weak fungicidal properties (32, 33). It is less active against *P. aeruginosa* and *Proteus mirabilis* (30). Soaked ear wicks can be placed in the EAC for prolonged action.

Boric acid solution has been found to be useful in chronic ear infections. Commercially available preparations are prepared in isopropyl alcohol or distilled water and available as 2–5% ear drops (34, 35). It is also available in powder form and can be used directly to achieve a higher concentration in EAC. As a keratolytic agent, it lowers the pH in the EAC and has bactericidal, fungicidal effect and anti-biofilm properties (36). Its role as a first-line therapy is unsubstantiated, but its concomitant use with antibiotics may help to curtail the overall duration of therapy and prevent development of microbial resistance. Clinical studies have found it to be safe even in ears with a perforated drum (34, 37). Some animal studies have reported ototoxic potential of boric acid drops prepared in alcohol when used in ears with a perforated drum (38, 39). As alcohol is known to be ototoxic, it may be safer to use dry powder or a solution prepared in distilled water in the presence of a TM perforation (36).

Burow's solution is an otological preparation available as a colourless liquid containing 13% aluminium acetate. Known for its astringent action and antimicrobial activity against *S. aureus*, *P. aeruginosa*, *P. mirabilis* and fungi, it is popular both as primary and second-line therapy. The clinical effect is due to both its acidic content and aluminium acetate. In vitro studies have shown that it disrupts the cell wall and causes bacteriolysis (40, 41). It has been found to be useful in resistant otorrhea due to OE and media, GM and discharging mastoid cavity (41, 42).

Benzocaine, lignocaine or dibucaine can be used as topical anaesthetics (otogesic 1.1% drops) or as a part of commercially available

**Table 5.1: Common Antiseptics and Acidifying Agents Available for Topical Application**

| S. No. | Brand Name | Constituent | Comment |
|---|---|---|---|
| 1 | Merchurochrome | Merbromin 2%* | Causes staining |
| 2 | Betadine | Povidone iodine* 5% | Antibacterial (G+, G–, anaerobes), sporicidal |
| 3 | Cresylate otic solution | Cresyl acetate*25% | Antibacterial, antifungal |
| 4 | Gentian violet | Gentian violet*1%, 2%, glycerine | Antibacterial and antifungal dye, causes staining, possible anti-biofilm effect |
| 5 | Silverex ionic gel, ionsil | Silver nitrate gel 0.2%, 0.5%, 1% | Antibacterial, antifungal effect, higher concentration (20%) used caustic action |
| 6 | BIPP paste or impregnated gauze | Bismuth iodine paraffin paste (BIPP)* | Astringent, antiseptic (103) |
| 7 | Castellani paint* | Carbol fuchsin, resorcinol, acetone, 95% ethyl alcohol, boric acid (104) | Acidifying agent, antifungal antibacterial, causes pink staining |
| 8 | Burow's solution | 13% aluminium acetate (aluminium sulfate, calcium carbonate, acetic acid, purified water) (41) | pH 3.06, astringent, antibacterial, antifungal, no ototoxic potential (42, 105) |
| 9 | Boro Spirit | Boric acid 2%, 4%, 5% | pH 4.7, acidifying agent, antifungal antibacterial, anti-biofilm effect |
| 10 | Vosol drops, acetic acid otic solution, Oticept, Acetasol HC | Acetic acid 2%* | pH 2.6, available with hydrocortisone, acidifying antibacterial and agent (29) |
| 11 | Vinegar | 1:1 dilution of commercially available vinegar | pH 3.5–4 |

\* Antiseptics with ototoxic potential.

antibiotic preparations. They help in reducing pain, though routine use should be discouraged as it may mask the symptoms in resistant cases.

Tacrolimus is derived from *Streptomyces tsukubaensis* and belongs to macrolide group. It is a calcineurin inhibitor and is known for its immunosuppressive effect. It is commonly used in dermatological practice for topical treatment of chronic inflammatory skin conditions. It reduces the levels of neuropeptide substance P and has an anti-pruritic effect. It is a well-tolerated topical agent. Ear wick soaked in 0.1% tacrolimus ointment has been found to be useful in non-infectious dry chronic otitis (43).

5-Fluorouracil (5-FU) is chemotherapeutic drug which is active against tumour cells by inhibiting DNA synthesis. It does not have any known ototoxicity and systemic absorption is negligible. Topical application of 5-FU has been tried in GM (44).

An ear wick soaked in Quadriderm® (betamethasone, gentamicin, tolnaftate, clioquinol) ointment is also effective in refractory cases (34).

Use of antiseptic ear drops was commonplace in the past. They have been found to be equally efficacious in resolution of symptoms (4). With emerging resistance to fluoroquinolones, they may once again find more acceptance in managing resistant cases of otorrhea.

*Mode of Use:* Topical antibiotics drops can be directly instilled in the EAC. Alternatively, an ear wick made of compressed cellulose can be soaked in the therapeutic agent of choice and left in situ for 5–7 days. It gradually expands in the EAC and helps to relieve the oedema. The drops can be instilled over it, thus increasing the contact time of the drug. Antiseptic agents can be smeared in the EAC with a cotton-tipped applicator or used as drops. Insufflation of boric acid in powdered form can be done using a powered device.

*Duration:* The usual requirement of topical drugs is for 7–14 days. If the symptoms do not subside by end of second week, it should be considered as treatment failure and modification of the therapy should be done. Common causes of treatment failure are poor patient compliance and improper instillation of drops. Therefore, all patients should be instructed about the proper usage of drops. They should be advised to lie down with the affected ear up and instil the drops in the canal to its brim and continue to be

## Table 5.2: Specific Management of External and Middle Ear Disorders Causing Otorrhea

| Disease | Management |
| --- | --- |
| Malignant otitis externa | Antibiotics (parenteral and oral) |
| Keratosis obturans | Microscopic assisted removal of desquamated epithelium topical steroid, surgical debridement |
| EAC Cholesteatoma | Stage I- topical application of salicylates, antibiotics and steroids (107) |
| | Stage II–IV surgical debridement (12) |
| Meatal stenosis | Congenital - canalplasty |
| | Post-inflammatory -wet stage- topical steroid antibiotic, dry stage- surgical excision of fibrous tissue |
| Radiation associated otorrhea | Localized - regular aural toilet, hydrogen peroxide lavage, steroid antibiotic drops, local tissue debridement) |
| | Diffuse – mastoidectomy, STP- MEO, lateral TB resection (108–110) |
| Dermatological disorders | Topical antifungals, corticosteroids, astringents for weeping lesions. |
| Tumours | Tumour specific treatment |
| Granulomatous conditions | OMAAV- steroids, immunosupressants |
| | TOM-ATT, sequestrectomy |
| Eosinophilic otitis media | Topical and systemic steroids, anti-IgE drugs |

TB = temporal bone, STP-MEO = subtotal petrosectomy-middle ear obliteration,
TCA = Trichloroacetic acid, SCC = squamous cell carcinoma,
RMS = rhabdomyosarcoma, ACC = adenoid cystic carcinoma,
CCRT = concurrent chemoradiotherapy, OMAAV = otitis media with
anti-neutrophilic cytoplasmic antibody, HPE = histopathologic examination,
TOM = tuberculous otitis media, ATT = anti tubercular treatment

in the position for 5–10 minutes. Patients should be reviewed in between for aural toileting.

*Systemic Treatment:* Oral antibiotics are not routinely indicated in uncomplicated OE (diabetes, immunocompromised state, prior radiotherapy, extension outside the EAC ruled out) (4). Specific treatment of systemic diseases such as tuberculosis, ANCA-associated vasculitis and Temporal Bone (TB) malignancy should be initiated once diagnosis is established (Table 5.2). Control of diabetes and immunosuppressed state are important for clinical effect of therapy. Pain relief can be achieved with acetaminophen, non-steroidal anti-inflammatory drugs. Opioids are rarely indicated.

### Diseases of Middle Ear
#### Acute Otitis Media

AOM is a common cause of otalgia and otorrhea. Rupture of the TM results in copious blood-stained mucopurulent otorrhea and is associated with relief of otalgia (Figure 5.6a and b). Discharge can be pulsatile when associated with a small perforation. Common organisms to be implicated are *S. pneumoniae*, *H. influenza* and *M. catarrhalis*. To a lesser extent, *Streptococcus pyogenes* and *S. aureus* are also known to cause infection (45). Chronic otorrhea can be due to recurrent episodes of AOM. However, the ear discharge may continue to persist even after a

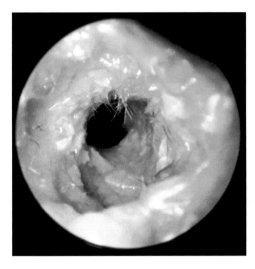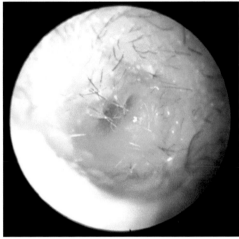

**Figure 5.6**  Post-perforation appearance of mucopurulent discharge in the external auditory canal in acute otitis media. (From Hawke Library. Dr Michael Hawke, Toronto, Canada.)

single episode of AOM. Recurrent episodes of AOM are usually seen in paediatric age group and are associated with certain risk factors such as age less than 3 years, genetic predisposition, parental smoking and attendance at day care centers. Persistence of infection and otorrhea or recurrence within a month can occur despite adequate antibiotics and is attributed to proliferation of certain resistant microbial strains once the antibiotic therapy is stopped (46).

### Chronic Otitis Media

Chronic inflammation of the middle ear cleft mucosa is associated with persistent ear discharge. Recurrent ear discharge can also be due to an existing defect in the TM which allows entry of water and microbes into the middle ear cleft. Adenoid tissue in the nasopharynx has been associated with presence of biofilms, microorganisms from these biofilms can ascend through the eustachian tube into the middle ear. Recent literature has implicated biofilms in the adenoid as a cause of initiation as well as persistence of infection in COM (47). Proliferation of goblet cells, epithelial hyperplasia, squamous metaplasia and biofilms in middle ear is also responsible for recalcitrance of infection (48).

Invasion of the middle ear space by epithelium from the EAC results in the formation of a cholesteatoma. It is associated with accumulation of keratin, osteitis, granulation tissue formation and bone destruction. Bothersome chronic otorrhea due to putrefaction of the keratinous debris can occur.

Otorrhea associated with mucosal disease is usually copious, non-foul smelling and occurs intermittently (Figure 5.7a). A cholesteatoma is associated with scanty, malodourous and persistent ear discharge, which may be occasionally bloodstained if associated with granulations in EAC or middle ear (Figure 5.7b and c). Frequently isolated organisms in COM are *P. aeruginosa*, *S. aureus*, *P. mirabilis*, *Escherichia coli* and *Klebsiella pneumoniae*. Certain anaerobes such as *Peptococcus*, *Peptostreptococcus*, *Bacteroides* and *Fusobacterium* are more frequently isolated in the presence of cholesteatoma and are responsible for the associated malodour and resistance to antibiotics (49).

### Post-ventilation Tube Otorrhea

Ventilation tube placement is a common surgical procedure carried out in children for recurrent AOM or persistent otitis media with effusion (OME). It is not uncommon for children with tympanostomy tubes to develop otorrhea (Figure 5.8a–c). The reported incidence is 3.4–74% and is the most common sequel of ventilation tube insertion (50, 51). Otorrhea occurring within 4 weeks of insertion has been classified as early post-postoperative and delayed if it occurs later than 4 weeks. When it persists for 3 months, it is chronic and recurrent if three or more episodes of otorrhea occur (51). When the otorrhea occurs within 4 weeks of insertion, infection may be due to causes associated with the surgical procedure itself (52).

Dried discharge can block the lumen of the grommet and may result in early extrusion. *S. aureus*,

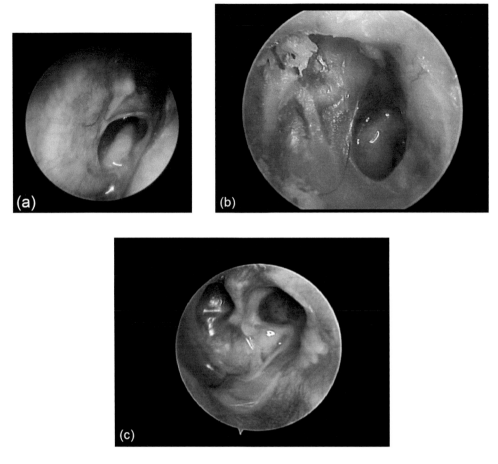

**Figure 5.7** (a) Copious mucopurulent discharge occurring due to acute infection in a case of long-standing perforation of tympanic membrane (right ear). (b) Otoendoscopic examination of left ear showing an attic cholesteatoma. Note that the posterior part of tympanic membrane is adherent to the promontory mucosa which appears to be inflamed and causing scanty otorrhea. The ossicles appear to be eroded. (c) Granulations in the pars tensa retraction pocket resulting in purulent otorrhea (left ear). ([a] From Hawke Library, Dr. Michael Hawke, Toronto, Canada.)

*P. aeruginosa* and *H. influenzae* are the usual pathogens isolated. *S. pneumoniae* and *M. catarrhalis* have been found to be less prevalent (51, 53).

Age less than 4 years, history of recurrent AOM, inadequate water entry precautions, parental smoking, design and material of the grommet and pathogenic colonization of the tube are some of the causes associated with the occurrence of ventilation tube otorrhea (54). Silicone tubes and grommets with narrow inner diameter are less prone to get infected (55). Human serum albumin or silver oxide coating on titanium tubes and phosphoryl-choline coating on fluoroplastic tubes help prevent formation of biofilm on the tube surface by preventing the binding of microorganisms (56, 57).

Currently, there is no compelling evidence to support routine water entry precautions (use of ear plugs, restriction of swimming activity) (52, 58). The pressure required at the TM to allow entry of water through the narrow tympanostomy tube is not generated during surface swimming (59). It may be advisable to avoid diving activities or contact with contaminated water, especially in at-risk children or children with persistent or recurrent otorrhea.

### Tuberculous Otitis Media

Tuberculosis is a common infectious disease in the developing world and can affect any organ in the body. The middle ear is an uncommon site

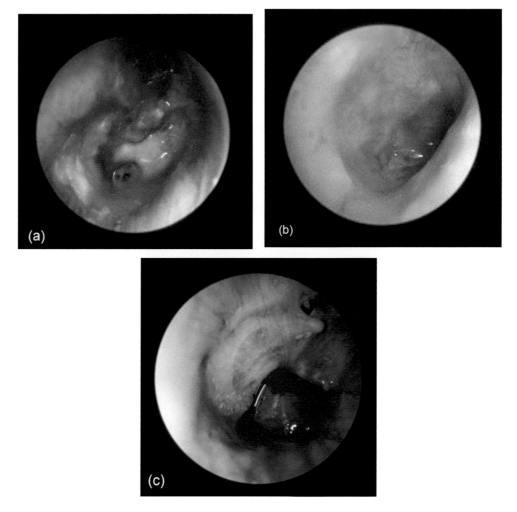

**Figure 5.8** (a and b) Otorrhea is a common sequalae of ventilation tube insertion. It can be due to recurrent episodes of acute otitis media, contact with contaminated water or causes related to surgical procedure itself. (c) Granuloma in the tympanic membrane completely engulfing the ventilation tube inserted into the tympanic membrane (right ear). (From Hawke Library, Dr. Michael Hawke, Toronto, Canada.)

of affliction by the acid-fast bacillus (AFB) and its incidence is as low as 0.9% of all COM cases (60). The middle ear can be infected primarily due to direct implantation through the EAC and a perforated TM. Secondary involvement via hematogenous spread or aspiration of infected upper airway secretions through the eustachian tube is more commonly reported. The classical clinical picture as described by Wallner in 1953 includes presence of painless odourless otorrhea, which is resistant to treatment, multiple TM perforations, pale granulation tissue in middle ear cleft, bone necrosis and disproportionate hearing loss (61). Friable hyperaemic granulations

have also been reported (62). Multiple TM perforations coalesce early in the course of disease and may be conspicuously absent. The incidence of complications such as mastoiditis, labyrinthitis, petrositis, facial paralysis, venous thrombosis and osteomyelitis is seemingly high for the innocuous-looking otorrhea.

Diagnosis is often delayed due to a low index of suspicion and non-specific symptoms and signs. AFB are difficult to demonstrate in the aural discharge and biopsied soft tissue due to pauci-bacillary content in middle ear cleft. Culture has a low yield due to fastidious nature of mycobacterium and interference in growth by other bacteria present in secretions (60). More often than not treatment initiation is done on the basis of characteristic histological findings such as caseating granulomas with Langerhans giant cells, epithelioid cells and histiocytes. GeneXpert test is a recently available useful test in the armamentarium of microbiologist to diagnose mycobacterial infections in suspicious cases (63). It is a fully automated PCR-based assay which can simultaneously detect *Mycobacterium tuberculosis* complex and rifampicin resistance within 2 hours.

Radiology is also helpful in diagnosing suspicious cases. A chest X-ray must be ordered to rule out coexisting pulmonary lesions. Findings of HRCT Temporal Bone (TB) are non-specific and may reveal soft tissue density completely filling the mastoid and middle ear along with diffuse bone erosion. Widespread bone erosion in the absence of aggressive clinical disease or presence of a cochlear promontory fistula in a patient with recurrent otorrhea and polypoid granulations must prompt diagnosis of tuberculous otomastoid infection (64). Though tuberculosis is an uncommon cause of otorrhea, it must always be considered as an important differential diagnosis in developing countries where it is endemic.

### ANCA-associated Otitis Media (OMAAV)

Anti-neutrophilic cytoplasmic antibodies against myeloperoxidase and proteinase-3 can give rise to systemic necrotizing vasculitis involving small- to medium-sized blood vessels. ANCA-associated vasculitis includes granulomatosis with polyangiitis, microscopic polyangiitis and eosinophilic granulomatosis polyangiitis (10). Otological symptoms such as otorrhea secondary to granulation tissue or OME refractory to treatment may be the initial presentation; however, diagnosis may remain elusive in the absence of systemic involvement. Insidious or sudden onset hearing loss, facial paralysis, tinnitus and vertigo are non specific associated symptoms. Diagnosis is mainly based on histological findings (necrotizing vasculitis involving small- and medium-sized vessels), positivity for serum MPO or PR3 ANCA, involvement of other organs such as kidney, lungs, eye and hypertrophic pachymeningitis seen on radiology. Other causes of intractable otorrhea such as tuberculosis, cholesteatoma, MOE, malignancy and Eosinophilic Otitis Media (EOM) should be ruled out by appropriate investigations prior to diagnosing a case of ANCA-associated otitis media (65, 66).

### Eosinophilic Otitis Media

Tomioka et al. have recently described this disease entity in patients with bronchial asthma. It is characterized by presence of viscous, eosinophil-rich otorrhea or middle ear effusion (67). This diagnosis must be considered in patients with intractable otorrhea or OME, which is viscous in consistency, rich in eosinophils who have a history of bronchial asthma or nasal polyposis. Depending upon the severity of disease, the condition of middle ear mucosa has been graded as normal looking, thickened or extensively granulating, which may give rise to viscid secretions (68, 69). Sudden or progressive hearing loss is common in patients who have granulations in the middle ear. Early diagnosis of this condition is essential for intervention and adequate treatment as these patients do not respond to conventional medical management with topical or oral antibiotics.

### Tumours of Middle Ear

Primary tumours of middle ear are rare, therefore otorrhea secondary to neoplastic lesions of the middle ear is rarely encountered. Malignant neoplasms of the middle ear and mastoid include primary adenocarcinoma, rhabdomyosarcoma, lymphoma, multiple myeloma and metastatic deposits. Metastatic deposits in the middle ear can occur through hematogenous spread, direct extension through eustachian tube, perineural spread or leukemic infiltration (70). The primary sources of these deposits are lungs, breast, kidney, thyroid and larynx (71). Leukemic infiltration of mastoid by immature granulocytes can present as post-aural swelling, bulging of TM and sagging of posterior canal wall, thus making it difficult to differentiate it from acute mastoiditis (72). These lesions can sometimes precede clinical leukaemia or may herald a relapse in a treated patient (73, 74).

Otalgia, hearing loss, peri-auricular swelling and facial paralysis are more common presenting complaints of TB metastasis (75, 76). Otorrhea is not common though otitic infections occurring in presence of metastasis are more severe and difficult to treat (72).

Clinically signs and symptoms of both primary and metastatic lesions can mimic COM. Diagnosis is challenging as otorrhea and associated granulations may mask the tumorous lesion. Intense and lancinating pain, blood-stained discharge, facial paralysis and periauricular swelling are highly suspect of malignancy and should warn the clinician to obtain biopsy prior to undertaking any definitive surgical or medical management (77).

### Radiation-associated Otitis Media

Temporal Bone (TB) radionecrosis can occur due to direct irradiation of the bone or when it falls in the periphery while irradiating nearby structures such as parotid gland, mandible, nasopharynx, oral cavity, oropharynx or maxilla. It is usually associated with doses greater than 60 Gy (78).

Otitis media secondary to irradiation, though a rare manifestation, can present several years later. The middle ear and mastoid usually get involved in diffuse form of osteo-radionecrosis of TB. Post-irradiation ischaemia, hypoxia and osteocyte loss result in bone resorption and sequestrum formation. Soft tissue involvement can cause mucosal thickening and ulceration, submucosal fibrosis, atrophic changes and bone exposure, which result in chronic foul-smelling otorrhea and otalgia. TM perforation, granulations and cholesteatoma may develop. Spontaneous resolution of symptoms does not occur. Antibiotics both oral and topical are not effective in altering the course of the disease. Bacterial biofilms associated with diseased and hypoxic tissue may be responsible for the recalcitrance of the otorrhea (79). The organisms associated with osteo-radionecrosis are *S. aureus*, *P. aeruginosa*, *Streptococcus viridians*, *Actinomyces* sp. and *Candida albicans* (80).

## Management of Otorrhea Due to Causes in Middle Ear and Mastoid

*AOM:* The condition of external ear and middle ear is noted after aural toileting. Oral amoxicillin should be started at a dose of 80–90 mg/kg/day in two divided doses. Additional β-lactamase coverage should be included in case the patient has received amoxicillin in the last 30 days or if history of recurrent AOM is present (45). High dose of amoxicillin yields drug levels in middle ear, which exceed the minimum inhibitory concentration required for resistant strains of *S. pneumoniae*. In case of penicillin allergy or treatment failure, second-generation (cefuroxime) or third-generation (cefdinir, ceftriaxone, cefpodoxime) cephalosporin or macrolide antibiotic (azithromycin) can be used for treatment. Duration of therapy should be 5–10 days, depending upon the severity (45).

*Chronic Otitis Media:* Non-surgical management of COM includes topical instillation of antibiotics with or without steroids and systemic antibiotics. Aural toileting is important and may sometimes be the only treatment offered to the patient (81). Topically administered antibiotics achieve a much higher concentration in the tissue without the undesirable side effects of systemic administration. Coverage for both Gram-positive (*S. aureus*) and Gram-negative (*P. aeruginosa*) organisms is required. Outcomes with topical quinolones have been found to be better than topical non-quinolones or systemic

antibiotics for short-term resolution of otorrhea (82). Inclusion of systemic antibiotic to topical fluoroquinolone regime does not seem to have any additional advantage (83).

Systemic route may be preferred when the topical drug may not be able to reach the middle ear tissue even with the tragal pump method such as presence of copious discharge or a small perforation in TM. Systemic antibiotics also have a distinct advantage in very young children or in the presence of oedema of EAC when topical administration is difficult. Overall duration of therapy in uncomplicated cases is 1–2 weeks (81).

*Tympanostomy Tube-related Otorrhea (TTO):* TTO can occur either due to recurrent middle ear infection, foreign body reaction or bacterial or fungal colonization of the tympanostomy tube. Topical administration of a broad-spectrum fluoroquinolone antibiotic with steroid for a period of 7–10 days is considered to be safe and effective in managing TTO due to recurrent middle ear infection (51, 84, 85). Dohar et al. have reported that topical ciprofloxacin with dexamethasone used for 7 days is superior to oral amoxicillin with clavulanic acid used for 10 days (86).

Meticulous ear toileting to ensure that the drops reach the middle ear through the ventilation tube is essential. The caregiver should be advised to use the tragal pump method for delivering the drug. Superior outcomes with topical administration are likely due to increased local drug concentration and better coverage of pathogens, especially *P. aeruginosa*. Systemic fluoroquinolones with activity against *Pseudomonas* are contraindicated in young children and can only be delivered topically. Placement of an ear wick in the EAC can improve the topical drug delivery (87). It may be a useful technique in patients with refractory TTO or in very young children in whom repeated delivery of topical drug is difficult.

Systemic antibiotics are indicated in TTO in the following conditions (13):

- Coexisting bacterial sinusitis, pharyngitis

- High-grade fever, severe otalgia

- Cellulitis of pinna or surrounding soft tissue

- Persistence or worsening of otorrhea despite topical therapy

- Immunocompromised state

- When effective topical administration is not possible – uncooperative child, EAC oedema

Presence of a biofilm on the tympanostomy tube may render the organisms resistant to topical and systemic therapy. Recalcitrant otorrhea despite medical management may resolve only after tympanostomy tube removal (87, 88).

### Discharging Postoperative Ear
#### *Discharging Mastoid Cavity*

Chronic or intermittent ear discharge from a mastoid cavity is troublesome and significantly affects the quality of life. The basic principle of cholesteatoma ear surgery is to achieve a disease-free and a dry ear. Poor surgical technique is one of the most important factors associated with postoperative ear discharge (89–91). Sino-dural angle, mastoid tip, retrosigmoid, peri-labyrinthine, peri-sinus, tegmen and retro-facial air cells may be incompletely exenterated. Partially exteriorized cells can harbour residual cholesteatoma resulting in persistent otorrhea (92). Retained epithelium or unhealthy mucosa in the air cells can be associated with granulation tissue resulting in formation of chronically discharging mucosal cysts and a wet cavity (93) (Figure 5.9a).

Predisposition to recurrent ear discharge in postoperative setting can be due to poor topography of mastoid bowl such as a high facial ridge, bony overhangs or a cavity with a sump in the mastoid tip. Mastoid tip cells below the level of the EAC result in gravity-dependent accumulation of epithelial debris, which has been described by Goldenberg as "the sink trap effect" (94). Inadequate meatoplasty can cause inadequate aeration and retention of debris, which acts as a nidus for infection (89).

Poorly vascularized epithelial lining of the mastoid bowl which breaks down often and causes formation of granulation tissue perpetuates infection and chronicity. Moisture and opportunistic organisms also predispose to recurrent infection (Figure 5.9b). Perforated TM and contamination of the cavity with water are other causes of intermittent ear discharge in mastoid cavity (93) (Figure 5.9c).

Patient factors such as poorly controlled glycaemic profile, immunodeficient state and

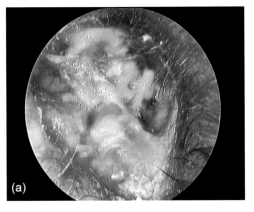
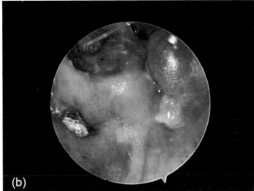
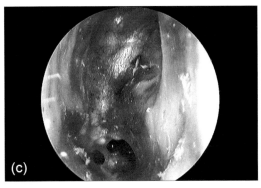

**Figure 5.9** (a) Appearance of cysts in the unhealthy lining epithelium of mastoid cavity in an operated case of chronic otitis media. In this patient, multiple cysts present in the sino-dural angle, facial ridge and tympanic membrane were causing recurrent ear discharge (right ear). (b) Fungal debris present in mastoid cavity (right ear). (c) Perforation of tympanic membrane in a patient who had undergone canal wall down mastoidectomy with partial obliteration of mastoid cavity for cholesteatomatous ear disease. Water entry through the perforation is a cause of recurrent otorrhea in such cases (left ear).

poor hygiene may also contribute to a chronically discharging mastoid cavity (95). *S. aureus* and *P. aeruginosa* are most commonly isolated microbes and may be associated with the formation of biofilms in the mastoid cavity (96, 97).

### Failed Tympanoplasty

Postoperative ear discharge after tympanoplasty is occasionally encountered. Otorrhea can be attributed to the following:

- Postoperative infection
- Graft failure
- Polypoid middle ear mucosa or middle ear granulation
- Re-perforation of TM
- Medialization of graft due to inadequate anchorage or poor eustachian tube function
- Granular myringitis
- Mucosalization of the TM
- Extrusion of prosthesis

### Management of Postoperative Otorrhea

*Discharging Mastoid Cavity:* Conservative management includes aural toileting, application of caustic agents such as silver nitrate or trichloroacetic acid to granulations, topical antibiotics or antiseptics (Table 5.1). Any transient cause of otorrhea in a well-done mastoid surgery must be identified and managed prior to opting for a revision surgery (98). Revision surgery may have to be resorted to only when the discharge persists despite adequate and appropriate medical management (99). If the initial management entailed a canal wall up procedure, recurrent discharge maybe due to residual cholesteatoma and may warrant a canal wall down procedure.

*Failed Tympanoplasty:* Revision surgery is indicated in most cases of failed tympanoplasty, conservative management may be tried in case of an unwilling patient/patient who is unfit to undergo surgery due to other medical conditions.

### Temporal Bone Defects

Aetiologically, Temporal Bone (TB) defects can be traumatic, iatrogenic, congenital or spontaneous in onset. They are most commonly located within or in close proximity to the otic capsule, tegmen plate or posterior fossa dural plate (100). The most common manifestation is in the form of recurrent meningitis, meningo-encephalic herniation, serous middle ear effusion, CSF otorrhea or rhinorrhoea. When associated with a perforation of TM, these defects can present as unrelenting watery ear discharge. Alternatively,

unremitting otorrhea may occur secondary to myringotomy, which has been inadvertently performed for persistent middle ear fluid (101).

Post-mastoidectomy Temporal Bone (TB) defects may be associated with meningoceles or meningo-encephaloceles, which may be associated with cholesteatoma, chronic ear discharge or intermittent CSF leakage. A high index of suspicion is required while evaluating post-mastoidectomy patients with chronic ear discharge. Any suspicious granulations or pulsating mass in the mastoid cavity should be evaluated with appropriate radiological investigations such as HRCT and MRI to rule out presence of Temporal Bone (TB) defects and meningo-encephaloceles (102).

### Management of CSF Otorrhea

Tegmen plate, post-fossa dural plate or otic capsule defects can cause CSF rhinorrhoea or CSF otorrhea when associated with a TM perforation. Both conditions are difficult to suspect clinically and the diagnosis may remain elusive. Radiology is important in diagnosing these defects. Once diagnosed, these defects need to be closed surgically. Trans-mastoid approach followed by two- or three-layered closure or a subtotal petrosectomy followed by middle ear obliteration, a middle cranial fossa approach or a combined approach for closure of these defects has been described (100).

## CONCLUSION

A large number of pathological processes can give rise to ear discharge and the clinician should be well-equipped to identify these pathologies in order to provide good medical care to the patients. The importance of good history taking, clinical examination to ascertain the cause of otorrhea prior to formulating a treatment plan for the patient cannot be over-emphasized in a patient presenting with otorrhoea. The goal of treatment is making the ear dry along with management of pain, infection and control of inciting factors. Specific management should be as per the pathology of disease causing otorrhea.

## REFERENCES

1. Roland PS, Marple BF. Disorders of external auditory canal. J Am Acad Audiol. 1997;8:367–78.

2. Roland PS, Belcher BP, Bettis R, et al. A single topical agent is clinically equivalent to the combination of topical and oral antibiotic treatment for otitis externa. Am J Otolaryngol. 2008;29:255–61.

3. Seedat RY. The discharging ear: a practical approach. Contin Med Educ. 2004;22:246–49.

4. Rosenfeld RM, Brown L, Cannon CR, Roland PS, et al. Clinical practice guideline: acute otitis externa. Otolaryngol Head Neck Surg. 2006;134(Suppl 4):S1–24.

5. Chander J, Maini S, Subrahmanyan S, Handa A. Otomycosis: a clinico-mycological study and efficacy of mercurochrome in its treatment. Mycopathologia. 1996;135:9–12.

6. Makino K, Amatsu M, Kinishi M, Mohri M. The clinical features and pathogenesis of myringitis granulosa. Arch Otorhinolaryngol. 1988;245:224–9.

7. Wolf M, Primov-Fever A, Barshack I, et al. Granular myringitis: incidence and clinical characteristics. Otol. Neurotol. 2006;27:1094–7.

8. Grandis JR, Branstetter BF, Yu VL. The changing face of malignant (necrotising) external otitis: clinical, radiological, and anatomic correlations. Lancet Infect Dis. 2004;4:34–9.

9. Chen JC, Yeh CF, Shiao AS, Tu TY. Temporal bone osteomyelitis: the relationship with malignant otitis externa, the diagnostic dilemma, and changing trends. Sci World J. 2014;2014:591714.

10. Magliocca KR, Vivas EX, Griffith CC. Idiopathic, infectious and reactive lesions of the ear and temporal bone. Head Neck Pathol. 2018;12:328–49.

11. Dubach P, Hausler R. External auditory canal cholesteatoma: reassessment of and amendments to its categorization, pathogenesis, and treatment in 34 patients. Otol Neurotol. 2008;29:941–8.

12. Naim R, Linthicum FJ, Shen T, Bran G, et al. Classification of the external auditory canal cholesteatoma. Laryngoscope. 2005;115:455–60.

13. Romdhoni AC. Keratosis obturans management. BHSJ. 2018;1:75–9.

14. Piepergerdes MC, Kramer BM, Behnke EE. Keratosis obturans and external auditory canal cholesteatoma. Laryngoscope. 1980;90:383–91.

15. Luong A, Roland PS. Acquired external auditory canal stenosis: assessment and management. Curr Opin Otolaryngol Head Neck Surg. 2005;13:273–6.

16. Yellon RF. Congenital external auditory canal stenosis and partial atretic plate. Int J Pediatr Otorhinolaryngol. 2009;73:1545–9.

17. Jahrsdoerter RA, Yeakley JW, Aguilar EA, et al. Grading system for the selection of patients with congenital aural atresia. Am J Otol. 1992;13:6–12.

18. Kim D, Bhimani M. Ramsay Hunt syndrome presenting as simple otitis externa. CJEM. 2008;10:247–50.

19. Sweeney CJ, Gilden DH. Ramsay Hunt syndrome. J Neurol Neurosurg Psychiatry. 2001;71:149–54.

20. Sood S, Strachan DR, Tsikoudas A, Stables GI. Allergic otitis externa. Clin Otolaryngol Allied Sci. 2002; 27:233–6.

21. Devaney KO, Boschman CR, Willard SC, Ferlito A, et al. Tumours of the external ear and temporal bone. Lancet Oncol. 2005;6:411–20.

22. Sand M, Sand D, Brors D, et al. Cutaneous lesions of the external ear. Head Face Med. 2008;4:2.

23. Zhen S, Fu T, Qi J. Diagnosis and treatment of carcinoma in external auditory canal. J Otol. 2014;9:146–50.

24. Yuhan B, Nguyen B, Svider P, et al. Osteoradionecrosis of the temporal bone: an evidence based approach. Otol Neurotol. 2018;39:1172–83.

25. Ramsden RT, Bulman CH, Lorigan BP. Osteoradionecrosis of the temporal bone. J Laryngol Otol. 1975;89:941–55.

26. Munguia R, Daniel SJ. Ototopical antifungals and otomycosis: a review. Int J Pediatr Otorhinolaryngol. 2008;72:453–9.

27. Kaushik V, Malik T, Saeed SR. Interventions for acute otitis externa. Cochrane Database Syst Rev. 2010; (1):Cd00474.

28. Noonan KY, Kim SY, Wong LY, Martin IW, et al. Treatment of ciprofloxacin-resistant ear infections. Otol Neurotol. 2018;39:e837–42.

29. Thorp MA, Kruger J, Oliver S, Nilssen EL, et al. The antibacterial activity of acetic acid and Burow's solution as topical otological preparations. J Laryngol Otol. 1998;112:925–8.

30. Nilssen E, Wormald PJ, Oliver S. Glycerol and ichthammol: medicinal solution or mythical potion? J Laryngol Otol. 1996;110:319–21.

31. Boyd AS. Ichthammol revisited. Int J Dermatol. 2010; 49:757–60.

32. Ahmed K, Roberts ML, Mannion PT. Antimicrobial activity of glycerine ichthammol in otitis externa. Clin Otolaryngol Allied Sci. 1995;20:201–3.

33. Kownatzki E, Uhrich S, Schopf E. The effect of a sulphonated shale oil extract (Ichthyol) on the migration of human neutrophilic granulocytes in vitro. Arch Dermatol Res. 1984;276:235–9.

34. Loock JW. A randomised controlled trial of active chronic otitis media comparing courses of eardrops versus one-off topical treatments suitable for primary, secondary and tertiary healthcare settings. Clin Otolaryngol. 2012;37:261–70.

35. Del Palacio A, Cuetara MS, Lopez-Suso MJ, Garau M. Randomized prospective comparative study: short-term treatment with ciclopiroxolamine (cream and solution) versus boric acid in the treatment of otomycosis. Mycoses. 2002;45:317–28.

36. Adriztina I, Adenin LI, Lubis YM. Efficacy of boric acid as a treatment of choice for chronic suppurative otitis media and its ototoxicity. Korean J Fam Med. 2018; 39:2–9.

37. Minja BM, Moshi NH, Ingvarsson L, Bastos I, et al. Chronic suppurative otitis media in Tanzanian school children and its effects on hearing. East Afr Med J. 2006;83:322–5.

38. Ozturkcan S, Dundar R, Katilmis H, Ilknur AE, et al. The ototoxic effect of boric acid solutions applied into the middle ear of guinea pigs. Eur Arch Otorhinolaryngol. 2009;266:663–7.

39. Aktas S, Basoglu MS, Aslan H, Ilknur AE, et al. Hearing loss effects of administering boric alcohol solution prepared with alcohol in various degrees on guinea pigs (an experimental study). Int J Pediatr Otorhinolaryngol. 2013;77:1465–8.

40. Hyo Y, Yamada S, Ishimatsu M, Fukutsuji K, et al. Antimicrobial effects of Burow's solution on *Staphylococcus aureus* and *Pseudomonas aeruginosa*. Med Mol Morphol. 2012;45:66–71.

41. Kashiwamura M, Chiba E, Matsumura M, Nakamura Y, et al. The efficacy of Burow's solution as an ear preparation for the treatment of chronic ear infections. Otol Neurotol. 2004;25:9–13.

42. Jinnouchi O, Kuwahara T, Ishida S, Okano Y, et al. Anti-microbial and therapeutic effects of modified Burow's solution on refractory otorrhea. Auris Nasus Larynx. 2012;39:374–7.

43. Caffier PP, Harth W, Mayelzadeh B, Haupt H, et al. Tacrolimus: a new option in therapy-resistant chronic external otitis. Laryngoscope. 2007; 117:1046–52.

44. Atef A.M, Hamouda MM, Mohamed AHA, Fattah AFA. Topical 5-fluorouracil for granular myringitis: a double-blinded study. J Laryngol Otol. 2010; 124:279–84.

45. Lieberthal AS, Carroll AE, Chonmaitree T, et al. The diagnosis and management of acute otitis media. Pediatrics. 2013;131:e964–99.

46. Granath A. Recurrent acute otitis media: what are the options for treatment and prevention? Curr Otorhinolaryngol Rep. 2017;5:93–100.

47. Jacquier H, Vironneau P, Dang H, et al. Bacterial biofilm in adenoids of children with chronic otitis media. Part II: a case–control study of nasopharyngeal microbiota, virulence, and resistance of biofilms in adenoids. Acta Otolaryngol. 2020;140:220–4.

48. Jensen RG, Johansen HK, Bjarnsholt T, et al. Recurrent otorrhea in chronic suppurative otitis media: is biofilm the missing link? Eur Arch Otorhinolaryngol. 2017;274:1–7.

49. Verhoeff M, van der Veen EL, Rovers MM, et al. Chronic suppurative otitis media: a review. Int J Pediatr Otorhinolaryngol. 2006;70:1–12.

50. Hochman J, Blakley B, Abdoh A, Aleid H. Post-tympanostomy tube otorrhea: a meta-analysis. Otolaryngol Head Neck Surg. 2006;135:8–11.

51. Rosenfeld RM, Schwartz SR, Pynnonen MA, et al. Clinical practice guideline: tympanostomy tubes in children. Otolaryngol Head Neck Surg. 2013; 149(Suppl 1):S1–35.

52. van Dongen TMA, Damoiseaux R, Schilder AGM. Tympanostomy tube otorrhea in children: prevention and treatment. Curr Opin Otolaryngol Head Neck Surg. 2018;26:437–40.

53. Van Dongen TM, Venekamp RP, Wensing AMJ, et al. Acute otorrhea in children with tympanostomy tubes: prevalence of bacteria and viruses in the post-pneumococcal conjugate vaccine era. Pediatr Infect Dis J. 2015;34:355–60.

54. Hannley MT, Denneny JC, Holzer SS. Use of ototopical antibiotics in treating 3 common ear diseases. Otolaryngol Head Neck Surg. 2000;122:934–40.

55. Knutsson J, Priwin C, Hessén-Söderman AC, et al. A randomized study of four different types of tympanostomy ventilation tubes: full-term follow-up. Int J Pediatr Otorhinolaryngol. 2018;107:140–4.

56. Kinnari TJ, Rihkanen H, Laine T, et al. Albumin-coated tympanostomy tubes: prospective, double-blind clinical study. Laryngoscope. 2004;114:2038–43.

57. Hong P, Johnson LB, Smith N, Corsten G. A randomized double-blind controlled trial of phosphorylcholine-coated tympanostomy tube versus standard tympanostomy tube in children with recurrent acute and chronic otitis media. Laryngoscope. 2011;121:214–9.

58. Steele DW, Adam GP, Di M, et al. Prevention and treatment of tympanostomy tube otorrhea: a meta-analysis. Pediatrics. 2017;139:e20170667.

59. Subtil J, Martins N, Nunes T, et al. Including auditory tube function on models is relevant to assess water exposure after tympanostomy tubes: multiphase computerized fluid dynamics model. Int J Pediatr Otorhinolaryngol. 2018;111:187–91.

60. Wallner LJ. Tuberculous otitis media. Laryngoscope. 1953;63:1058–77.

61. Singh B. Role of surgery in tuberculous mastoiditis. J Laryngol Otol. 1991;105:907–15.

62. Cho YS, Lee HS, Kim SW, et al. Tuberculous otitis media: a clinical and radiologic analysis of 52 patients. Laryngoscope. 2006;116:921–7.

63. Helb D, Jones M, Story E, et al. Rapid detection of *Mycobacterium tuberculosis* and rifampin resistance by use of on-demand, near-patient technology. J Clin Microbiol. 2010;48:229–37.

64. Hoshino T, Miyashita H, Asai Y. Computed tomography of the temporal bone in tuberculous otitis media. J Laryngol Otol. 1994;108:702–5.

65. Okada M, Suemori K, Takagi D, et al. Comparison of localized and systemic otitis media with ANCA-associated vasculitis. Otol Neurotol. 2017;38:e506–10.

66. Harabuchi Y, Kishibe K, Tateyama K, et al. Clinical features and treatment outcomes of otitis media with antineutrophil cytoplasmic antibody (ANCA)-associated vasculitis (OMAAV): a retrospective analysis of 235 patients from a nationwide survey in Japan. Mod Rheumatol. 2017;27:87–94.

67. Tomioka S, Kobayashi T, Takasaka T. Intractable otitis media in patients with bronchial asthma (eosinophilic otitis media). In: Sanna M., editor. Cholesteatoma and Mastoid Surgery. Rome: CIC Edizioni Internazionali, 1997, p. 851–853.

68. Nagamine H, Lino Y, Kojima C, Miyazawa T, Lida T. Clinical characteristics of so called eosinophilic otitis media. Auris Nasus Larynx. 2002;29:19–28.

69. Kanazawa H, Yoshida N, Yamamoto H, et al. Risk factors associated with severity of eosinophilic otitis media. Auris Nasus Larynx. 2014;41:513–7.

70. Cureoglu S, Tulunay O, Ferlito A, et al. Otologic manifestations of metastatic tumors to the temporal bone. Acta Otolaryngol. 2004;124:1117–23.

71. Gloria-Cruz TI, Schachern PA, Paparella MM, et al. Metastases to temporal bones from primary nonsystemic malignant neoplasms. Arch Otolaryngol Head Neck Surg. 2000;126:209–14.

72. Druss JG. Aural manifestations of leukemia. Arch Otolaryngol. 1945;42:267.

73. Andres E, Kurtz JE, Maloisel F, Dufour P. Otological manifestations of acute leukaemia: report of two cases and review of literature. Clin Lab Haematol. 2001;23:57–60.

74. Kurtz JE, AndreÁs E, Veillon F, et al. Hearing loss revealing acute leukemia. Am J Med. 2000;109:509–10.

75. Song K, Park KW, Heo J-H, et al. Clinical characteristics of temporal bone metastases. Clin Exp Otorhinolaryngol. 2019;12:27–32.

76. Maddox HE, 3rd. Metastatic tumors of the temporal bone. Ann Otol. 1967;76:149–65.

77. Stucker FJ, Holmes WF. Metastatic disease of the temporal bone. Laryngoscope. 1976;86:1136–40.

78. Huang XM, Zheng YQ, Zhang XM, et al. Diagnosis and management of skull base osteoradionecrosis after radiotherapy for nasopharyngeal carcinoma. Laryngoscope. 2006;116:1626–31.

79. Nason R, Chole RA. Bacterial biofilms may explain chronicity in osteoradionecrosis of the temporal bone. Otol Neurotol. 2007;28:1026–8.

80. Sharon JD, Khwaja SS, Drescher A, et al. Osteoradionecrosis of the temporal bone: a case series. Otol Neurotol. 2014;35:1207–17.

81. Chong LY, Head K, Richmond P, Snelling T, et al. Systemic antibiotics for chronic suppurative otitis media. Cochrane Database Syst Rev. 2018;3:CD005101.

82. Macfadyen C, Acuin J, Gamble C. Systemic antibiotics versus topical treatments for chronically discharging ears with underlying eardrum perforations. Cochrane Database Syst Rev. 2006;1:CD005608.

83. Onali MA, Bareeqa SB, Zia S, Ahmed SI, et al. Efficacy of empirical therapy with combined ciprofloxacin versus topical drops alone in patients with tubotympanic chronic suppurative otitis media: a randomized double-blind controlled trial. Clin Med Insights Ear Nose Throat. 2018;11:1179550617751907.

84. Roland PS, Anon JB, Moe RD, Conroy PJ, Wall GM, et al. Topical ciprofloxacin/dexamethasone is superior to ciprofloxacin alone in pediatric patients with acute otitis media and otorrhea through tympanostomy tubes. Laryngoscope. 2003;113:2116–22.

85. Venekamp RP, Javed F, van Dongen TM, Waddell A, et al. Interventions for children with ear discharge occurring at least two weeks following grommet (ventilation tube) insertion. Cochrane Database Syst Rev. 2016;11:CD011684.

86. Dohar J, Giles W, Roland P, Bikhaji N, et al. Topical ciprofloxacin/dexamethasone superior to oral amoxicillin/clavulanic acid in acute otitis media with otorrhea through tympanostomy tubes. Pediatrics. 2006;118:561–9.

87. Dedhia K, Choi S, Chi DH. Management of refractory tympanostomy tube otorrhea with ear wicks. Laryngoscope. 2015;125:751–3.

88. Bothwell MR, Smith AL, Phillips T. Recalcitrant otorrhea due to Pseudomonas biofilm. Otolaryngol Head Neck Surg. 2003;129:599–601.

89. Wormald PJ, Nilssen E. The facial ridge and the discharging mastoid cavity. Laryngoscope. 1998;108:92–6.

90. Jackson CG, Glasscock ME, Schwaber MK, et al. Open mastoid procedures: contemporary indications and surgical technique. Laryngoscope. 1985;95:1037–43.

91. Mastoidectomy FU. In: Fisch U, May J, editors. Tympanoplasty, Mastoidectomy and Stapes Surgery. New York: Thieme, 1994, p. 145–99.

92. Bhatia S, Karmarkar S, DeDonato G, Mutlu C, et al. Canal wall down mastoidectomy: causes of failure, pitfalls and their management. J Laryngol Otol. 1995;109:583–9.

93. Pillsbury H, Carrasco V. Revision mastoidectomy. Arch Otolaryngol Head Neck Surg. 1990;116:1019–22.

94. Goldenberg RA. Sink-trap effect as a cause of failure in mastoidectomy. Laryngoscope. 1988;98:1143–4.

95. Gluth MB, Metrailer AM, Dornhoffer JL, Moore PC. Patterns of failure in canal wall down mastoidectomy cavity instability. Otol Neurotol. 2012;33:998–1001.

96. Saunders J, Murray M, Alleman A. Biofilms in chronic suppurative otitis media and cholesteatoma: scanning electron microscopy findings. Am J Otolaryngol. 2011;32:32–7.

97. Lampikoski H, Aarnisalo AA, Jero J, Kinnari, TJ. Mastoid biofilm in chronic otitis media. Otol Neurotol. 2012;33:785–788.

98. Li S, Meng J, Zhang F, Li X, et al. Revision surgery for canal wall down mastoidectomy: intra-operative findings and results. Acta Otolaryngol. 2016;136:18–22.

99. Gulya AJ, Schweitzer L. Revision mastoid surgery. Oper Tech Otolaryngol Head Neck Surg. 1992;3:39–42.

100. Gupta A, Sikka K, Irugu DVK, Verma H, et al. Temporal bone meningoencephaloceles and cerebrospinal fluid leaks: experience in a tertiary care hospital. J Laryngol Otol. 2019;133:192–200.

101. Valtonen H, Geyer C, Tarlov E, Heilman CB, et al. Tegmental defects and cerebrospinal fluid otorrhea. ORL J Otorhinolaryngol Relat Spec. 2001;63:46–52.

102. García VE, Carratalá IL, Fernández JE, Marco J. et al. Management of cerebrospinal fluid otorrhea. Acta Otorrinolaringol Esp. 2013;64:191–6.

103. Nigam A, Allwood MC. BIPP: how does it work? Clin Otolaryngol Allied Sci. 1990;15:173–5.

104. Babakurban ST, Topal Ö, Aydin E, Hizal E, et al. Therapeutic effect of Castellani's paint in patients with an itchy ear canal. J Laryngol Otol. 2016;130:934–8.

105. Serin GM, Ciprut A, Baylancicek S, Sari M, et al. Ototoxic effect of Burow solution applied to the guinea pig middle ear. Otol Neurotol. 2007;28:605–8.

106. Anthony PF, Anthony WP. Surgical treatment of external auditory canal cholesteatoma. Laryngoscope. 1982;1:70–5.

107. Morrissey D, Grigg R. Incidence of osteoradionecrosis of the temporal bone. ANZ J Surg. 2011;81:876–9.

108. Kammeijer Q, Van Spronsen E, Mirck PG, Dreschler WA. Treatment outcomes of temporal bone osteoradionecrosis. Otolaryngol Head Neck Surg. 2015;152:718–23.

109. Prasad S, Janecka IP. Efficacy of surgical treatments for squamous cell carcinoma of the temporal bone: a literature review. Otolaryngol Head Neck Surg. 1994;110:270–80.

# APPROACH TO A PATIENT WITH OTALGIA

# 6 Approach to a Patient with Otalgia

*Rohit Singh, Amit Sood and N Ramakrishnan*

## CONTENTS

## INTRODUCTION

Otalgia is one of the cardinal symptoms of ear disease and the most distressing one which brings a patient to the Ear, Nose and Throat (ENT) Outpatient Department (OPD). The causes are numerous and can be broadly classified into Primary Otalgia and Secondary Otalgia. Primary otalgia results from diseases of the ear which may be infective in origin causing local inflammation. Secondary otalgia, also known as referred otalgia, occurs as a result of non-otological disease where the stimulation of nociceptors occurs at a distant site but pain is perceived in ear because of various head and neck structures sharing a common innervations with the ear (1). The ENT surgeon should be aware of various diseases causing otalgia and should be able to deduce the underlying cause using precise history, clinical examination and investigative modalities like imaging (2).

## SALIENT ANATOMIC FEATURES

The ear can be divided into the external, middle and inner parts. The external ear comprises the pinna, the external auditory canal and the lateral surface of the tympanic membrane. The middle ear structures consist of the medial surface of the tympanic membrane, the ossicles, the eustachian tube orifice, the hypotympanic air cells, the tympanic segment of the facial nerve and the promontory with the tympanic plexus on it. The inner ear consists of the membranous and bony labyrinths.

An understanding of complex pattern of innervation of ear is important to understand the likely source of referred otalgia. The sensory innervation of ear is provided by both cranial nerves and cervical nerves. Both somatic and branchial precursors innervate the skin overlying the pinna, which results in a significant overlap of sensory innervation. The Auriculo-Temporal nerve, a branch of the

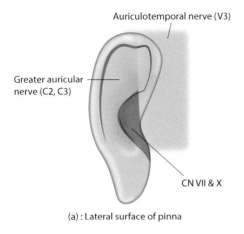

(a) : Lateral surface of pinna

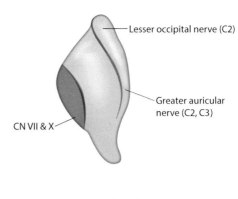

(b) : Medial surface of pinna

**Figure 6.1** Innervation of the pinna.

Mandibular division of Trigeminal nerve, gives sensory supply to the anterior aspect of helix and crus of the pinna, which includes the tragus along with the anterosuperior aspect of the external auditory canal along with the lateral aspect of the tympanic membrane (3). The Greater Auricular nerve derived from cervical roots C2 and C3 gives sensory innervation to the posterior and medial parts of the pinna. The lesser occipital nerve derived from C2 nerve rootlets supplies the posterosuperior aspect of pinna. However, the area near the conchal bowl is not supplied by any of these nerves and its sensory innervation is through the Facial and Vagus nerves. The corresponding region on the posterior aspect of the pinna is also supplied by the Facial and Vagus nerves. These cranial nerves also give sensory innervation to the posterior aspect of the external auditory canal and the posterolateral aspect of the tympanic membrane (Figure 6.1).

The middle ear receives its sensory input through Jacobson's branch of the Glossopharyngeal nerve as a part of the tympanic plexus. The inner ear does not have a dedicated sensory supply, and this is the reason many inner ear pathologies develop without presenting with otalgia (4).

## DIFFERENTIAL DIAGNOSIS

Otalgia can be divided into two broad types based on its aetiology:

**Primary Otalgia**: It is defined as pain in and around the ear, which is due to any inflammatory, neoplastic or traumatic condition of the ear.

**Secondary Otalgia:** It is defined as pain in ear, which is not attributed to ear pathology but is due to any pathology or lesion of head and neck that shares common innervations with the ear. This also forms the basis of convergence – projection theory (5).

Various causes of otalgia are listed in Table 6.1 (6).

### PRIMARY OTALGIA
### Diseases of External Ear
#### *Otitis Externa*

It is also known as "Swimmer's ear". It is characterized by inflammation and oedema of external auditory canal. The otalgia of otitis externa is mediated through sensory innervations of external auditory canal and pinna. There is usually a prior history of water entry into ears. Other predisposing factors include a narrow external auditory meatus, atopy, dermatological conditions like seborrheic dermatitis, immunocompromised states and trauma to the ear. Otitis externa has a varied clinical course and can be divided into the following three stages.

- Stage 1: Pre-inflammatory stage
- Stage 2: Acute inflammatory stage
- Stage 3: Chronic inflammatory stage

The underlying pathology is the disruption of normal protective lipid/acid balance of the ear (normal pH: 4–5). This leads to oedema of the stratum corneum layer resulting in the blockage of apocrine and sebaceous glands leading to itching and aural fullness. As oedema increases, there is disruption of the epithelial layers and invasion by microorganisms. The most common microorganism seen in otitis externa is *Pseudomonas* sp. Other less commonly observed

## Table 6.1: Causes of Otalgia

**A. Primary Otalgia**
**Pinna**: Perichondritis, chondritis, trauma, skin lesion
**External auditory canal**: Otitis externa, furunculosis, otomycosis, Herpes zoster oticus (Ramsay Hunt syndrome), malignant otitis externa, malignant neoplasm, foreign bodies, bullous myringitis, impacted wax, trauma
**Middle ear**: Acute otitis media, complication of otitis media (mastoiditis, subperiosteal abscess, mastoid abscess, petrous apicitis), middle ear barotrauma, eustachian tube catarrh, malignancy of middle ear

**B. Secondary Otalgia**
1. Area supplied by Trigeminal nerve (cranial nerve V):
    a. Dental and periodontal diseases like carried tooth, impacted tooth, erupting dentition, malocclusion and apical abscess
    b. Lesions of oral cavity like any infection, trauma, aphthous ulcers or malignancy of oral cavity
    c. Inflammatory and malignant disorders of parotid and submandibular salivary gland
    d. Inflammatory disorders of temporomandibular joint, Costen's syndrome
    e. Trauma, infection and inflammatory disorders of nose and paranasal sinuses
    f. Trigeminal neuralgia and Sluder's neuralgia
    g. Atypical facial pain, including tension-type headache
2. Area supplied by Glossopharyngeal nerve (cranial nerve IX):
    a. Infections and inflammatory lesions of oropharynx like acute tonsillitis and peritonsillar abscess
    b. Eagle's syndrome
    c. Glossopharyngeal neuralgia
3. Area supplied by Vagus nerve (cranial nerve X):
    a. Malignancy or ulcerative lesions of oropharynx, hypopharynx and larynx
    b. Subacute thyroiditis
    c. Gastro-oesophageal reflux disease
    d. Aneurysmal dilatation of great vessels
4. Area supplied by spinal nerves C2 and C3:
    a. Cervical spondylosis
    b. Cervical spine trauma
5. Ramsay Hunt syndrome (herpes zoster oticus)
6. Bell's palsy
7. Psychogenic causes

microorganisms are *Staphylococcus aureus* and *Streptococcus* sp.

Otitis externa is diagnosed on the basis of characteristic history of otalgia and pruritis. Clinical examination of ear shows oedema, hyperaemia and tenderness while manipulating the pinna. There could be a purulent discharge in EAC, which should be sent for culture and antibiotic sensitivity (7).

Management options in otitis externa include regular aural toileting, topical medications to the external auditory canal with the help of a wick and analgesia. The single most effective treatment remains aural toileting; however, some resistant cases may require culture-directed systemic antibiotics. Glycerol and ichthammol (90%:10%) soaked aural wick is commonly used to reduce oedema (8).

Otitis externa generally shows a good response to aural toileting and topical medications. However, some complications are known to occur (more commonly in immunocompromised host), which range from erysipelas, cellulitis or perichondritis of pinna and EAC. A severe complication noticed in immunocompromised individuals is malignant otitis externa (skull base osteomyelitis), which has significant associated morbidity and mortality.

### Otomycosis

This is also known as fungal otitis externa and this condition is seen in hot and humid climates. Diabetes mellitus and other immunocompromised conditions predispose individuals for this condition. The commonest fungal organisms implicated are *Aspergillus niger* and *Candida albicans*. The patient generally presents with complaints of otalgia and itching in the ear. Clinical findings may include black and white discharge with debris from the EAC, which resembles a "wet newspaper".

Repeated aural toileting forms the mainstay of treatment. Analgesics can be given for otalgia and topical antifungal drops may be added to accelerate recovery (9).

### Perichondritis of External Ear

This term strictly refers to inflammation of perichondrium of the external ear, including pinna and EAC. However, it is commonly described as a spectrum of conditions of external ear, which are as follows:

- Erysipelas of external ear (infection of the overlying skin)

- Cellulitis of the external ear (infection of the soft tissue)

- Perichondritis (infection and inflammation of the perichondrium)

- Chondritis (infection and inflammation of cartilage itself)

The most common aetiology is trauma, which may include laceration of the pinna, surgery of the external ear, hematoma of pinna, piercing of cartilage of pinna, frostbite, burns, and chemical injuries. The most common microorganisms isolated are *Pseudomonas aeruginosa*, *Streptococcus* sp., *S. aureus*, and Gram-negative organisms like *Proteus* and *Enterococcus*.

The pathogenesis of perichondritis involves thickening and inflammation of perichondrium because of intense infiltration of polymorphonuclear cells. This leads to destruction of the cartilage as a result of phagocytosis by macrophages.

The diagnosis is generally clinical with the patient presenting with a dull aching pain and the classical signs of erythema and inflammation involving the cartilaginous pinna. Generally, there is an underlying history of trauma that needs to be brought out.

The management options include analgesics and broad-spectrum antibiotics to cover common organisms, and *P. aeruginosa* in particular. In the presence of fluctuant sub-perichondrial abscess, intervention in the form of incision and drainage may be required (10). If pus is drained/aspirated, it should be sent for culture and antibiotic sensitivity and the area should be thoroughly washed with a solution of antibiotics and steroids. However, if only a hematoma is drained, transfixation sutures should be placed to obliterate the dead space to prevent the recurrence of hematoma. Resistant cases may require excision of the necrotic cartilage followed by secondary reconstruction.

### Ramsay Hunt Syndrome or Herpes Zoster Oticus

Varicella zoster virus is the causative agent of this condition, which remains latent in the geniculate ganglion for decades. The virus reaches the geniculate ganglion as a result of a previous attack of chicken pox (11). The virus first replicates in geniculate ganglion following which it travels to involve the facial nerve. It may also involve the vestibulo-cochlear nerve and its ganglia.

Various physical and psychological stressors and underlying immunosuppressive states act as stimuli for reactivation of the virus. The patient presents with complaints of severe otalgia associated with painful vesicles with an erythematous base, which appears in the external auditory canal, concha, and behind the pinna

(12). These vesicles then rupture to form crusts. There is also lower motor neuron-type facial paralysis, which usually recovers in up to 90% of cases over course of few weeks (13). Few patients also present with vestibular symptoms, and sensorineural hearing loss is known to occur in 5–6% of the cases.

Diagnosis is generally clinical; however, Varicella zoster virus DNA can be assessed by PCR of the vesicle fluid or cerebrospinal fluid. Histopathological examination of vesicle scrapings show multinucleate giant cells. Gadolinium-enhanced MRI of temporal bone shows enhancement at geniculate ganglion. Oral antivirals (Acyclovir/Famciclovir/Valacyclovir) and oral prednisolone along with eye care and analgesics form the mainstay of treatment.

### Malignant Otitis Externa

Malignant otitis externa is a rare complication of otitis externa. The term malignant is a misnomer here and the term necrotizing is used for aggressive soft tissue infection without any bony involvement. If underlying bone is involved, it represents a more severe clinical entity known as "skull base osteomyelitis". Skull base osteomyelitis most frequently affects the elderly and diabetics. It is proposed that diabetic microangiopathy and endarteritis of small vessels along with decreased immunity in elderly predispose them to this condition. Other immunosuppressed states such as HIV, steroid therapy, chemotherapy, leukaemia and organ transplant recipients are also predisposed for this condition.

*P. aeruginosa* is the most common etiological agent. It causes infection of the soft tissue of the external auditory canal, which further spreads to the skull base through the fissures of Santorini. The infection further spreads medially along the tympano-mastoid suture along various fascial planes and venous channels invading connective tissue, bone, cartilage, and nerves. There occurs an intense inflammatory reaction and the compact bone is converted to granulation tissue. The infection further progresses to involve multiple skull base foramina and the cranial nerves exiting through it. The facial nerve is the most commonly affected due to its close proximity to the external auditory canal. Further medial spread of the disease along Jugular foramen can involve the lower cranial nerves. Spread along the petrous apex, it can involve the abducens, the trigeminal nerve and the optic nerve. Septic thrombosis of the sigmoid sinus and the internal Jugular vein can also occur.

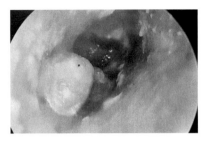

**Figure 6.2** Otoendoscopy showing granulation tissue present over floor of EAC in a case of malignant otitis externa.

Patients are usually elderly diabetics who present with severe continuous otalgia, purulent otorrhoea and hearing loss. Often, there is an associated history of ear canal trauma, which could be self-inflicted. The most common presenting symptom is otalgia, which is nocturnal, lancinating, boring and is resistant to analgesics. The next most common presenting symptom is otorrhoea, which is purulent and is seen on examination of an extremely tender and oedematous external auditory canal. The floor of the bony external auditory canal may reveal granulation tissue, polyp or bare bone. There could be associated hearing loss, which is generally conductive in nature due to obstruction of external auditory canal by granulation tissue or oedema. If the disease has progressed medially involving foramina of skull base, then there can be associated cranial neuropathies. The first nerve to get involved is the facial nerve followed by cranial nerves IX, X, XI, XII and then V and VI. Sigmoid sinus thrombosis and Jugular venous thrombosis are late signs and are associated with a poor prognosis (Figures 6.2 and 6.3).

Diagnosis is based on clinical features, microbiology, radiological findings of the skull base and histopathological examination showing inflammation in absence of neoplasia (14).

*P. aeruginosa* is most commonly isolated, other organisms implicated in the pathogenesis of this disease are *S. aureus, Staphylococcus epidermidis, Proteus* and *Klebsiella*. Certain fungi such as *Aspergillus, Malassezia* and *Scedosporium* have also been isolated in certain cases.

A high-resolution computed tomography of the temporal bone can detect bony erosion of the skull base. However, it has limitations in detecting bone demineralization of more than 30%. Magnetic resonance imaging (MRI) has a good soft tissue differentiation and can detect bone marrow oedema in skull base osteomyelitis. However, it cannot assess response to treatment and disease resolution. Nuclear imaging is a useful tool in diagnosis of this disease, determining extent of the disease, assessing response of the treatment and resolution of infection. Technetium-99 is a radiotracer which accumulates in area of high osteoblastic activity and Tc-99 scintigraphy has almost 100% sensitivity in diagnosis of skull base osteomyelitis. Another radiotracer Gallium-67 accumulates in leukocytes in areas of active inflammation and acts as a reliable tool for assessment of response to treatment. Indium-111 is a radiotracer that detects neutrophil-mediated inflammation. 18-Fluorodeoxyglucose Positron Emission Tomography (FDG-PET) is also accurate in detection of presence or absence of skull base osteomyelitis (15).

Aggressive control of underlying hyperglycaemic state is one of the most crucial management strategies. Aural toileting is helpful in control of pain and it reduces granulation and debris. Systemic antibiotics with targeted antipseudomonal therapy are the mainstay of treatment. Fluoroquinolones (oral Ciprofloxacin 750 mg twice daily) are standard first-line agents. Cephalosporins and aminoglycosides either as monotherapy or in combination are useful in resistant cases. In case of fungal osteomyelitis, Amphotericin B and oral Itraconazole may be considered. Hyperbaric oxygen and surgical debridement of necrotic tissue are adjuncts to systemic antimicrobial therapy.

### Bullous Myringitis

It is an acute, painful, inflammatory condition of the tympanic membrane which is characterized by presence of vesicles or bullae on the surface of tympanic membrane. The proposed pathology is that bullae develop because of extravasation of serum or blood between outer epithelial

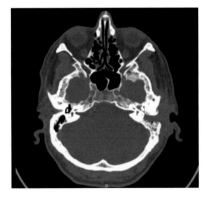

**Figure 6.3** HRCT temporal bone shows significant erosion of bony EAC.

layer and middle fibrous layer of tympanic membrane. Underlying pathogens are *Streptococcus pneumoniae, Haemophilus influenzae*, β-haemolytic streptococci and certain respiratory viruses like respiratory syncytial virus, enteroviruses and rhinoviruses. More often than not, this disease is seen to occur in conjunction with acute otitis media. Although this disease can occur at any age, it is more prevalent in paediatric age group (16).

Diagnosis is mainly clinical, and a typical patient presents with sudden onset severe otalgia in presence of upper respiratory tract infection. Otoscopic examination reveals presence of bullae on tympanic membrane and rupture of these bullae can lead to self-limiting, serosanguinous otorrhea. In most of cases, this disease is self-limiting with spontaneous resolution of all symptoms. Treatment is generally symptomatic with oral analgesics; however, if involvement of inner ear is suspected (presence of sudden SNHL or vertigo), broad-spectrum antibiotics are advocated along with a short course of oral steroids.

### Diseases of Middle Ear
#### Acute Otitis Media

This disease refers to acute painful inflammation of the middle ear, which is mediated by certain respiratory viruses and bacteria such as *S. pneumoniae, H. influenzae* and β-haemolytic streptococci. The disease is known to occur in all age groups; however, it is more prevalent in the paediatric population. A typical patient presents with otalgia, mucopurulent otorrhea if perforation occurs and conductive hearing loss on audiological evaluation. Diagnosis is based on history and characteristic otoscopic findings showing a bulging, inflamed tympanic membrane or mucopurulent otorrhea in the external auditory canal if the tympanic membrane has perforated (Figure 6.4).

Most cases recover spontaneously and only symptomatic treatment in form of analgesics

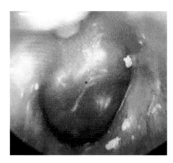

**Figure 6.4** Otoendoscopy showing bulging and inflamed tympanic membrane in a case of acute otitis media.

is required. A Cochrane review conducted showed administration of antibiotics reduces chances of tympanic membrane perforation in children; however, it showed no proven efficacy in adults (17).

#### Complicated Otitis Media

Most of the extracranial complications of otitis media manifest with otalgia as one of the presenting features. These complications include acute mastoiditis, subperiosteal abscess and mastoid abscess to name but a few. Intracranial extension of infection can lead to otalgia because of involvement of dura as it is a pain-sensitive structure (18). Perimeningeal foci of infection as seen in epidural abscess can result in unremitting otalgia because of involvement of nociceptive afferents from the trigeminal and vagus nerves.

#### Temporal Bone Malignancy

These are rare head and neck tumours with no definite causative association identified. However, exposure to sunlight, radiation and presence of cholesteatoma are postulated risk factors. The disease presents with non-specific signs and symptoms which mimic chronic otitis media (squamous). The main symptoms are otalgia, otorrhea and hearing loss. The clinician needs to have high index of suspicion if these symptoms are of long duration, and not responding to standard therapy.

### SECONDARY OTALGIA (REFERRED OTALGIA)

Various theories have been proposed for referred pain.

**Convergent-projection theory:** Ruch in 1961 proposed that sensory fibres from different tissues, such as skin, viscera, muscles and joints, converge onto common spinal neurons, which could lead to a misinterpretation of the source of nociceptive activity. The source of pain in one tissue can be misinterpreted as originating from some other structure. The convergent-projection theory would explain the segmental nature of referred pain and the increased referred pain intensity when local pain is intensified. This theory, however, does not explain the delay in the development of referred pain following the onset of local pain, like otalgia in glossopharyngeal neuralgia, trigeminal neuralgia and carcinoma of oral cavity and oropharynx.

**Convergence-facilitation theory:** This theory was proposed by Graven-Nielsen. The somatosensory sensitivity changes which are reported in referred pain areas could be explained by sensitization mechanisms in the dorsal horn and brainstem neurons, while the delay in appearance of referred pain could be explained by the time required for creation of central sensitization (19).

### Dental Causes

Dental disorders are one of the most common causes of referred otalgia. The commonest cause of inflammation of the dental pulp (pulpitis) is dental caries. The pain in dental caries is often poorly localized as the sensory innervation is mainly via non-myelinated type C pain fibres. Pain associated with acute apical periodontitis and acute apical abscess tends to be severe, throbbing and localized to the affected tooth. Partially erupted or impacted wisdom teeth can lead to inflammation of the surrounding soft tissue (pericoronitis). Chronic pericoronitis can present as poorly localized facial/jaw pain with referred otalgia (20).

### Temporomandibular Joint Dysfunction Syndrome (Costen's Syndrome)

The typical features of TMJ dysfunction are diffuse pain felt in or around the joint, crepitus and trismus. Pain is the most common and prevalent symptom. The true prevalence of TMJ dysfunction is not certain. Sufferers of referred otalgia from TMJ dysfunction are more likely to be female, with statistically significant elevated levels of physical comorbidity and psychological stress. Bruxism is found to be a major aetiological factor and has been reported to be present in more than 50% of cases. Pain from the TMJ, or from related tissues, is common, but there is often no definable organic disease.

The most reliable diagnostic clinical finding in TMJ dysfunction is tenderness of the masticatory muscles, with tenderness of the lateral pterygoid reported in 85%. Tenderness of the joint itself was reported in 67% of patients and 38% had crepitus on auscultation. Intraoral palpation of the lateral and medial pterygoids frequently reveals tenderness, and this finding is more commonly seen in patients with referred otalgia.

MRI can demonstrate joint effusion or internal derangement of the joint. The mainstay of treatment for TMJ dysfunction is conservative. Application of local heat and massage can be of benefit. Benzodiazepines or low-dose tricyclic antidepressants can help symptoms for more refractory symptoms, but there is risk of dependence (21). A small proportion of patients may require further investigation and treatment by maxillofacial surgeons; TMJ surgery is generally considered only as a last resort.

### Neuralgias

Otalgia can present as one of the features of various cranial neuralgias. The mechanism of pain begins in demyelinated fibres which become hyper-excitable and generate high-frequency discharges. Trigeminal neuralgia and postherpetic neuralgia are the commonest forms of craniofacial-neuralgia. Trigeminal neuralgia is defined as a sudden, usually unilateral, brief stabbing recurrent pain in the distribution of one or more of the branches of the V cranial nerve. Because of this classic mode of presentation, otalgia is rarely reported as a symptom of trigeminal neuralgia.

Glossopharyngeal neuralgia as defined by the International Headache Society is a severe transient stabbing pain experienced in the ear, base of tongue, tonsillar fossa or beneath the angle of the jaw (22). Glossopharyngeal neuralgia has been described as of two clinical types based on the distribution of the pain: a tympanic type which mainly affects the ear, and an oropharyngeal type which affects the throat (23).The onset of pain is commonly provoked by swallowing and on occasion by coughing, yawning or talking. Symptoms are paroxysmal and last for seconds to minutes and remission periods occur. Glossopharyngeal neuralgia usually occurs without any evident lesion affecting the Glossopharyngeal nerve. However, most authors implicate vascular compression of the nerve at the root entry zone as the main cause of "idiopathic" Glossopharyngeal neuralgia (24). The posterior inferior cerebellar artery is the most frequent vessel responsible for compressing the Glossopharyngeal nerve (25).

Patients with neuralgia do not respond to conventional analgesic drugs because of its mechanism of pain production as described above. The ideal drugs are those which are able to limit the discharge frequency. The first-line medical treatment of neuralgia is with Carbamazepine. Surgery for Glossopharyngeal neuralgia most commonly involves microvascular decompression. Nerve section can also be performed, either through a posterior fossa approach or through a trans-cervical approach (26).

### Malignancy

Malignancy is not the commonest cause of referred otalgia, but its importance as a potential cause warrants this differential being high on the assessing clinician's list. Malignant tumours of the upper aerodigestive tract can present with referred otalgia as part of a symptom complex. The presence of otalgia, dysphagia, nodal metastasis and weight loss have all been shown to be independent predictors of duration of survival of patients with head and neck cancer (27). Carcinoma of oral cavity (tongue), oropharynx and hypopharynx and even some supraglottic cancers can cause otalgia. The nasopharynx is not usually a subsite referring pain to the ear, but otalgia has been reported as being the presenting symptom in up to 14% of patients with nasopharyngeal carcinoma (28).

### Stylohyoid (Eagle's) Syndrome

The condition was first reported by Eagle in 1937 and subsequently came to bear his name. The normal styloid process is approximately 2.5 cm long and is generally accepted to be elongated if its length exceeds 4 cm (Figure 6.5). The stylohyoid syndrome results in neuralgia secondary to an elongated Styloid process or mineralization of the stylohyoid ligament. Symptoms are postulated to occur due to compression of the Hypoglossal nerve, impingement of the Carotid vessels or inflammatory changes at the insertion of the stylohyoid ligament. The symptoms are classically a dull pharyngeal pain, often located within the tonsillar fossa, with radiation to the ipsilateral ear, odynophagia and a foreign body sensation (29).

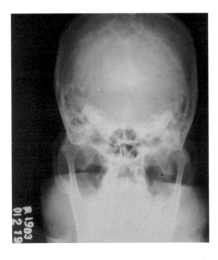

**Figure 6.5** Imaging showing elongated styloid process in a case of Eagle's syndrome.

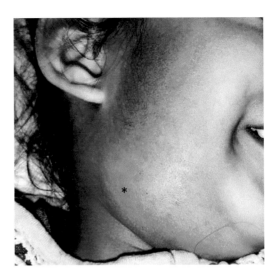

**Figure 6.6** Parapharyngeal abscess.

### Laryngopharyngeal Reflux (LPR)

LPR describes retrograde flow of gastric contents beyond the upper oesophageal sphincter and into the larynx and pharynx. Irritation of the respiratory epithelium by gastric acid stimulates the glossopharyngeal and vagus nerves producing ear pain (30).

### Cervical Spine

Skeletal conditions such as osteoarthritis, trauma and tumours of the cervical spine can cause pain over the pinna and mastoid region by nerve root irritation (31). Sensory fibres from C2 and C3 are also distributed to skin and muscles of the scalp and neck, and, as a result, cervical lymphadenitis and infections of the scalp can occasionally produce mild earache.

### Infections

Upper airway infections, particularly tonsillitis, peritonsillar abscess (quinsy) and pharyngitis, refer pain to the ear by means of the Glossopharyngeal nerve (Figure 6.6). Infections of the deep neck spaces, such as a parapharyngeal or retropharyngeal abscess, may also present in similar way.

### Parotid Gland

Otalgia can precede facial swelling in cases of mumps par otitis; this is most commonly observed in children (Figure 6.7). Bacterial infections of the parotid gland may also be responsible for ear pain (32).

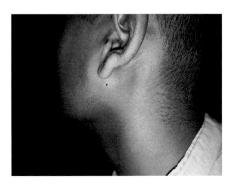

**Figure 6.7** Inflammation of parotid gland (parotitis).

## CLINICAL EVALUATION AND MANAGEMENT OF A PATIENT WITH OTALGIA

### History

A detailed history will help the clinician to narrow down towards possible few causes from a long list of diseases with otalgia as its presenting feature. Key points in the history include character of otalgia and other associated cardinal features like otorrhea, hearing loss, tinnitus and vertigo (33).

- **Age**: Patient's age at presentation is also important in deciding likely aetiology. Diseases like acute otitis media are common in the paediatric age group and malignancy is more commonly seen in the geriatric age group.

- **Location**: Asking the patient to locate the exact site of pain will help the clinician to differentiate between localized pain and diffuse pain. For example, eliciting three-point tenderness is helpful in suspected cases of acute mastoiditis, whereas referred pain is usually dull and non-localizing.

- **Onset:** Usually acute onset severe/moderate pain is result of an acute infection/inflammatory conditions like AOM, otitis externa, myringitis and acute inflammation of TM joint.

- **Radiation**: Pain in migraine is unilateral and involves temporal area which radiates towards occipital area, whereas in trigeminal neuralgia patient experiences pain in half face/oral cavity/tongue, which may radiate to ipsilateral ear or vice versa. In cases like hypopharyngeal tumours, patient may/may not experience radiating pain but patient say he has pain in throat and ear. Similarly, in case of acute follicular tonsillitis, patient can experience otalgia.

- **Associated symptoms**: Otalgia associated with other otological symptoms like otorrhea, hearing loss, tinnitus and aural fullness/local trauma indicates a local cause. Whereas symptoms like trismus, dysphagia, odynophagia, pain during mastication, throat pain/irritation in throat/swelling in throat/neck will indicate a distant (secondary) cause and warrant further investigation. Dental caries is also common cause of secondary otalgia.

- **Aggravating/relieving factors**: In TM joint dysfunction syndrome, chewing aggravates the pain. Pain on movement of pinna, tragal tenderness are seen in otitis externa.

- **Risk factors**: Elderly age group with history of tobacco/alcohol consumption and people who work in wood-cutting industries should raise the suspicion of malignancies. Patients with history of air travel/professional divers should also raise the suspicion of barotrauma.

### Clinical Examination

It includes not only otological examination but also comprehensive ENT examination. Key components of the physical examination include inspection of the auricle and periauricular regions and a thorough otoscopic examination with visualization of complete Pars tensa and Pars flaccida. Tenderness that occurs with traction on the auricle or pressure on the tragus indicates inflammation of external ear; usually otitis externa. Examination of nose and throat is carried out to look for any source of secondary otalgia. Temporomandibular joint and surrounding musculature is palpated to rule out any TMJ dysfunction. Thorough examination of cervical spine and complete examination of cranial nerves are done to look for any likely aetiology. Further, investigations like otomicroscopy, nasopharyngo-laryngoscopy, X-ray of temporomandibular joint and cervical spine and orthopantomogram can be used by clinician to come to a conclusion.

In view of vast array of diseases manifesting as otalgia, it is difficult to make a diagnostic algorithm for it. Figure 6.8 depicts an attempt to make diagnosis part easier by means of a flowchart.

### CONCLUSION

Otalgia is common symptom encountered by an ENT surgeon in OPD and emergency setting. The patient presenting with otalgia presents a diagnostic challenge for which a diligent and systematic evaluation plan and management protocol has to be followed. A detailed history

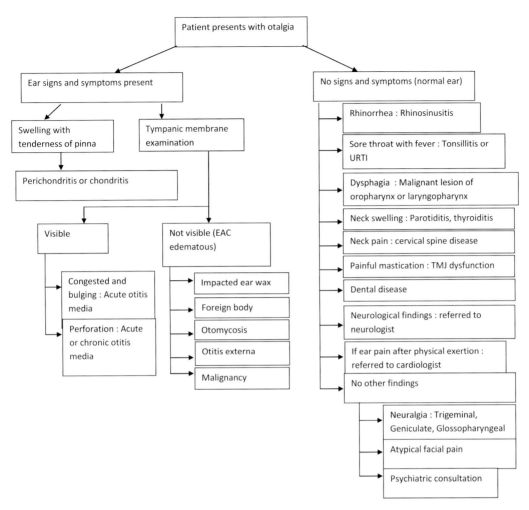

**Figure 6.8** Algorithm for Evaluation of Otalgia.

and an elaborate ENT examination along with appropriately directed studies are a must to uncover the underlying pathology.

## REFERENCES

1. Olsen KD. The many causes of otalgia: infection, trauma, cancer. Postgrad Med. 1986;80(6):50–63.

2. Leonetti JP, Li J, Smith PG. Otalgia: an isolated symptom of malignant infratemporal tumors. Am J Otol. 1998;19(4):496–8

3. Hollinshead WH. The nose and paranasal sinuses. Anatomy for Surgeons: The Head and Neck. Philadelphia, PA: Lippincott Williams & Wilkins, 1982, p. 259–63.

4. Majumdar S, Wu K, Bateman ND, Ray J. Diagnosis and management of otalgia in children. Arch Dis Child Educ Pract Ed. 2009;94(2):33–6.

5. Fernández-de-las-Peñas C, Dommerholt J. Basic concepts of myofascial trigger points (TrPs). Trigger Point Dry Needling: An Evidence and Clinical-Based Approach, Elsevier, 2013, vol. 1, p. 3–19.

6. Reiss M, Reiß G. Differential diagnosis of otalgia. Schmerz (Berlin, Germany). 1999;13(6):392–7.

7. Kaushik V, Malik T, Saeed SR. Interventions for acute otitis externa. Cochrane Database Syst Rev. 2010(1): CD004740.

8. Agius AM, Pickles JM, Burch KL. A prospective study of otitis externa. Clin Otolaryngol Allied Sci. 1992;17(2):150–4.

9. Kaur R, Mittal N, Kakkar M, Aggarwal AK, Mathur MD. Otomycosis: a clinicomycologic study. Ear Nose Throat J. 2000;79(8):606–9.

10. Martin R, Yonkers AJ, Yarington Jr CT. Perichondritis of the ear. Laryngoscope. 1976;86(5):664–73.

11. Robillard RB, Hilsinger RL, Adour KK. Ramsay Hunt facial paralysis: clinical analyses of 185 patients. Otolaryngol Head Neck Surg. 1986;95(3 Pt 1):292–7.

12. Adour KK. Otological complications of herpes zoster. Ann Neurol. 1994;(35 Suppl):S62–4.

13. Kinishi M, Amatsu M, Mohri M, Saito M, Hasegawa T, Hasegawa S. Acyclovir improves recovery rate of facial nerve palsy in Ramsay Hunt syndrome. Auris Nasus Larynx. 2001;28(3):223–6.

14. Ismail H, Hellier WP, Batty V. Use of magnetic resonance imaging as the primary imaging modality in the diagnosis and follow-up of malignant external otitis. J Laryngol Otol. 2004;118(7):576–9.

15. Berenholz L, Katzenell U, Harell M. Evolving resistant pseudomonas to ciprofloxacin in malignant otitis externa. Laryngoscope. 2002;112(9):1619–22.

16. McCormick DP, Saeed KA, Pittman C, et al. Bullous myringitis: a case-control study. Pediatrics. 2003; 112(4):982–6.

17. Venekamp RP, Sanders SL, Glasziou PP, Del Mar CB, Rovers MM. Antibiotics for acute otitis media in children. Cochrane Database Syst Rev. 2015(6):CD000219.

18. Vikram BK, Khaja N, Udayashankar SG, Venkatesha BK, Manjunath D. Clinico-epidemiological study of complicated and uncomplicated chronic suppurative otitis media. J Laryngol Otol. 2008;122(5):442–6.

19. Graff-Radford SB. Myofascial pain: diagnosis and management. Curr Pain Headache Rep. 2004;8(6):463–7.

20. Kreisberg MK, Turner J. Dental causes of referred otalgia. Ear Nose Throat J. 1987;66(10):398–408.

21. Kuttila SJ, Kuttila MH, Niemi PM, et al. Secondary otalgia in an adult population Arch Otolaryngol Head Neck Surg. 2001;127(4):401–5.

22. Classification and diagnostic criteria for headache disorders, cranial neuralgia, and facial pain. Headache Classification Committee of the International Headache Society. Cephalgia. 1988;8:1–96.

23. Soh KB. The glossopharyngeal nerve, glossopharyngeal neuralgia and the Eagle's syndrome: current concepts and management. Singapore Med J. 1999;40(10):659–65.

24. Teixeira MJ, de Siqueira SR, Bor-Seng-Shu E. Glossopharyngeal neuralgia: neurosurgical treatment and differential diagnosis. Acta Neurochir (Wien). 2008;150(5):471–5; discussion 475.

25. Fischbach F, Lehmann TN, Ricke J, Bruhn H. Vascular compression in glossopharyngeal neuralgia: demonstration by high-resolution MRI at 3 tesla. Neuroradiology. 2003;45(11):810–11.

26. Patel A, Kassam A, Horowitz M, Chang YF. Microvascular decompression in the management of glossopharyngeal neuralgia: analysis of 217 cases. Neurosurgery. 2002;50(4):705–10; discussion 710–11.

27. Pugliano FA, Piccirillo JF, Zequeira MR, et al. Symptoms as an index of biologic behaviour in head and neck cancer. Otolaryngol Head Neck Surg. 1999; 120(3):380–6.

28. Scarbrough TJ, Day TA, Williams TE, et al. Referred otalgia in head and neck cancer: a unifying schema. Am J Clin Oncol. 2003;26(5): e157–62.

29. Fini G, Gasparini G, Filippini F, Becelli R, Marcotullio D. The long styloid process syndrome or Eagle's syndrome. J Cranio-Maxillofacial Surgery. 2000; 28(2): 123–7.

30. Tutuian R, Castell DO. Diagnosis of laryngopharyngeal reflux. Curr Opin Otolaryngol Head Neck Surg. 2004;12:519–24.

31. Hatton P, Abbott RJ, Mitchell SCM, Holland IM. A cervical cord tumour presenting with earache. Br J Hosp Med. 1988;39:72.

32. 10 Leung AKC, Fong JHS, Leong AG. Otalgia in children. J Natl Med Assoc. 2000;5:254–60.

33. Siddiq NM, Samra MJ. Otalgia. BMJ. 2008; 336(7638):276–7.

# CLINICAL DECISION-MAKING IN THE VERTIGINOUS PATIENT: DIFFERENTIAL DIAGNOSIS AND MANAGEMENT

# 7 Vertigo in Children and Adults

*Anupam Kanodia and Hitesh Verma*

## CONTENTS

## INTRODUCTION

Dizziness is one of the common complaints in the outpatient department, especially for a family physician, neurologist or an otorhinolaryngologist (1). Vertigo is defined as a perception of movement when there is none. It is important to ascertain its nature, i.e. episodic or not, rotatory or non-rotatory nature and the duration of each episode. While history often leads to the diagnosis in adults, vertigo in paediatric age group is difficult to diagnose and manage. A meticulous physical examination and laboratory evaluation is important to reach the diagnosis.

### Vestibular Anatomy and Physiology

Labyrinths on the either side are mirror images of each other. Each labyrinth consists of three semicircular canals (SCCs) and two otolith organs each: the saccule and the utricle. While the semicircular canals give us an angular orientation of movement, the utricle and the saccule orient us to the horizontal linear and vertical linear motion, respectively (2).

Each SCC has a dilated end known as the ampulla. The ampulla has an elastic membrane across its cross section known as cupula. As the head moves, creating an angular movement in the plane of a canal, the endolymph in the canal moves in the opposite direction due to its inherent inertia. This stretches the cupula, leading to a change in the basal firing rate of the vestibular end organ.

The baseline firing gives property of bidirectionality to the vestibule; the firing increases for the vestibular afferents in the excitatory direction, while the contralateral vestibular afferents' firing decreases. This modulation of sensory input from the bilateral vestibular system reaches the cerebellum and other central pathways where it is processed and appropriate actions are initiated. These actions include reflexes like vestibulo-ocular reflex (to maintain stable vision), vestibulo-spinal reflex (to stabilize the body and prevent it from falling) and vestibulocollic reflex (to maintain head posture). The semicircular canals follow the three laws stated by Ewald (3). The macula of the utricle and saccule are in the horizontal and vertical plane, respectively. This gives the otolithic organs specificity in detecting the direction of movement.

## REVIEW OF LITERATURE
### Paediatric Age Group

a. *Prevalence*
The prevalence of vertigo in the paediatric age group ranges from less than 1% to 5% (4).

b. *Evaluation*
The following points must be asked to the parent while evaluating a child (5):

- Loss of consciousness or change in appearance suggest seizures or syncopal episode.

- Gait disturbance is suggestive of a vestibular or cerebellar lesion.

- Regression in motor milestones is indicative of a cerebral or cerebellar lesion.

- Delayed motor milestones may occur in vestibular pathology.

- Nystagmus rules out a psychogenic cause of vertigo, and the intensity, direction and type of nystagmus help to diagnose the cause.

### Adult Age Group

a. *Prevalence*

The prevalence in adults aged 40 or above varies from 0.71% to 35% and they face some form of balance dysfunction (6, 7).

b. *Evaluation*

#### HISTORY

A good history forms the mainstay of diagnosis. The points to be covered are as follows:

- *Timing of the initial spell.*

- *Frequency and duration of symptoms:* Ask for the frequency of episodes in a week or month and the average duration that an episode lasts (Table 7.1).

- *Precipitating factors:* BPPV is often related to a change in head posture while lying down or getting up. Migraine may be precipitated by lack of sleep, loud sounds, bright light, anxiety, change in weather and menstruation. Seizure activity in children may be precipitated by stress or flickering light.

- *Family history:* Benign Paroxysmal Vertigo of Childhood (BPVC) and migraine-related vertigo are often associated with a positive family history of migraine.

- *Associated medical conditions:* Patients with comorbidities like anaemia, cardiovascular disorders, hypothyroidism and diabetes experience a higher number of episodes of dizziness. Hypothyroidism has been found to be associated with Ménière's disease (MD) and otitis media with effusion (OME) (8). Anxiety and panic disorders are associated with non-specific dizziness (psychogenic vertigo).

### CLINICAL EXAMINATION

Clinical examination begins with a general physical examination, neuro-otological, audiological and head and neck examination.

### VESTIBULAR EVALUATION

Nystagmus is classified into two broad subtypes: pendular and jerk. In pendular nystagmus, ocular swing velocity is almost equal in both directions, whereas in jerky it is faster in one direction. Jerk nystagmus is the most common nystagmus seen in peripheral vestibular disorders.

- *Spontaneous or elicited nystagmus:* Labyrinthine nystagmus is unidirectional, more prominent while looking towards fast component, enhanced by removing eye fixation and associated with a feeling of rotation. The fast component of the nystagmus beats towards hyperactive labyrinth or normal labyrinth if the diseased labyrinth is hypoactive. Vertical nystagmus may be seen in central lesions.

- *Fistula test:* Application of pressure to the middle ear causes fluid displacement inside the lateral canal in the presence of a fistula, hence generating nystagmus. Pneumatic otoscopy can be used to apply this pressure. Apart from perilymphatic fistulas, this test is also positive in cases of otosyphilis, MD and superior semicircular canal dehiscence.

- *Head Impulse Test (HIT)/Head Thrust Test (HTT):* This test is performed by rapidly turning the patient's head to one side by 10–15°, while the patient fixates on the examiner's eyes. The manoeuvre is to be done on both the sides, in a random manner. The other way is to ask the patient to look to one side and then rapidly bringing the head to midline.

This tests the Angular Vestibulo-Ocular Reflex (aVOR), which causes an equal and opposite movement of the eyeball when compared to the movement of the head. This reflex is expected to

### Table 7.1: Differential Diagnosis of Vertigo on the Basis of Duration of Symptoms

| Seconds to Minutes | Few Minutes to Hours | More Than 24 Hours to 3–4 Weeks |
| --- | --- | --- |
| • Benign paroxysmal positional vertigo<br>• Hypoglycaemia<br>• Labyrinthine fistula<br>• Semicircular canal dehiscence<br>• Caloric effect<br>• Cervical vertigo<br>• Post-concussion syndrome<br>• Alternobaric and vertebrobasilar insufficiency | • Ménière's disease, delayed endolymphatic hydrops<br>• Migraine-related vertigo<br>• Following middle ear surgery<br>• Seizures related vertigo | • Vestibular neuritis<br>• Iatrogenic or accidental trauma<br>• Labyrinthitis<br>• Cerebellopontine angle tumours |

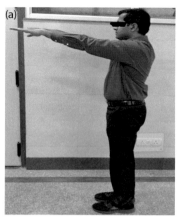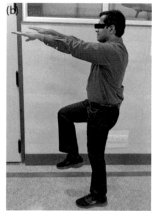

**Figure 7.1** Fukuda stepping test.

be impaired in the presence of a unilateral vestibular lesion. This will result in the generation of a low-amplitude saccadic movement (corrective or catch-up saccades) of the eye towards the normal side when the head is thrust towards the lesioned labyrinth. Although this test is to be done in all the three planes of the three semicircular canals, horizontal canal is most commonly and conveniently tested with this test.

- *Head Shake Test (HST):* HST tests inadequacy in dynamic vestibular function. Rapidly shaking the head in the plane of the horizontal canal for 20–30 cycles is suggested. In the presence of a lesioned labyrinth, unequal input from both the sides accumulates in the central velocity storage areas. Hence, once the head-shaking is stopped suddenly, a vigorous nystagmus follows. Use of Frenzel's glasses is suggested to improve the sensitivity of this test.

- *Positional (sustained) or positioning (transient) manoeuvres:* These manoeuvres are best observed with patient wearing Frenzel's glasses. Although there are multiple manoeuvres described, the two most commonly used ones are the Dix-Hallpike and supine roll test. These tests are described in the segment on vertigo in elderly.

- *Fukuda stepping test:* The patient steps in place with eyes closed and arms outstretched outwards for 30 seconds to 1 min. An angular deviation of more than 30° points towards an ipsilateral vestibular lesion. This test along with Romberg and sharpened Romberg test assesses the vestibulo-spinal reflex (Figure 7.1a and b).

- *Romberg test:* The patient is asked to stand with feet together. Sway is checked with eyes open and closed. A lesion in labyrinth or

cerebellum causes sway to the ipsilateral side (Figure 7.2a).

- *Sharpened Romberg test:* Patient stands with feet one behind the other and arms folded in an "X" to let the hands touch the opposite shoulder. Presence of sway is checked, which indicates an ipsilateral vestibular or cerebellar lesion (**Figure 7.2**b).

- *Gait test:* The patient is instructed to walk along a straight line and then rapidly turn and return along the same path. Deviation towards the ipsilateral side is seen in

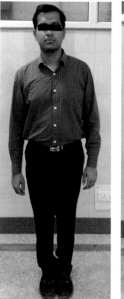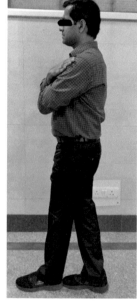

**Figure 7.2** (a) Romberg's test. (b) Sharpened Romberg's test.

labyrinthine lesions, whereas gross imbalance is seen in cerebellar lesions.

■ *Skew deviation and ocular tilt reaction:* Skew deviation refers to a vertical misalignment of eyes resulting from abnormal ocular-otolithic reflexes. An ocular palsy needs to be ruled out before one considers the finding of ocular skew deviation. Alternate card cover test is used to reveal the vertical corrective movement which confirms the finding. The site of the lesion is either towards the lower eye if it affects the peripheral nerve or vestibular nucleus or, more commonly, on the side of the higher eye due to the lesions in medial longitudinal fasciculus. The head is tilted towards the lower eye, causing an ocular tilt reaction. Skew deviations can also be seen in cerebellar lesions.

### Cerebellar Examination

■ Nystagmus

■ Finger-nose test

■ Heel-shin test

■ Tandem walking test

■ Romberg test

■ Sharpened Romberg test

■ Fukuda stepping test

■ Check for dysdiadochokinesia – asymmetric pronation and supination of hand on the side of lesion

■ Check for muscle tone

### Cranial Nerve Examination

It is recommended that a patient with unexplained vertigo, syncopal episodes or oscillopsia undergoes a thorough ophthalmological and cardiovascular examination (9). Syncopal disorders require a thorough history along with haematological and cardiovascular examination to reach a diagnosis.

### INVESTIGATIONS

■ *Air caloric testing:* The patient's head is positioned 30° elevated from the supine position to bring the horizontal SCC perpendicular to gravity with its ampulla at the top (Figure 7.3). The ear is then irrigated for about 60 seconds sequentially with warm air (44°C) and then with cold air (30°C). Warm irrigation of air reduces the density of the endolymph in the now superior part of the HC, i.e. the ampulla. This causes a convective flow of endolymph from the canal to the ampulla causing deflection of the cupula and generation of vestibular input. The opposite occurs for cold irrigation. Jongkee's formula is then applied to the values of the slow-phase velocities hence generated to calculate directional preponderance (DP) and unilateral weakness (UW):

$$UW = \frac{(RW + RC) - (LW + LC)}{(RW + RC + LW + LC)} \times 100\%$$

$$DP = \frac{(RW + LC) - (LW + RC)}{(RW + RC + LW + LC)} \times 100\%$$

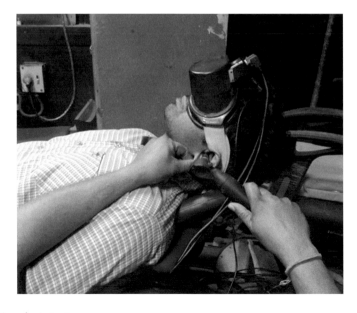

**Figure 7.3**  Air caloric test.

Here, R and L refer to the right and left labyrinth, respectively. W and C refer to the warm and cold irrigation, respectively. One needs to clearly document the tympanic membrane status before doing the test, and check for wax in the ear canal which may preclude recording of the correct values.

- *Electronystagmography:* It supports the clinical diagnosis and also helps in assessing the progression of disease by providing the quantitative information of the affected vestibulo-ocular reflex. The corneo-retinal potentials generated by eye movement are recorded electrically by electrodes fixed around the eyes and are expressed graphically. Smooth pursuit, saccadic and optokinetic are the most commonly studied stimuli. Videographic recording of the responses is known as videonystagmography (VNG) (Figure 7.3).

- *Posturography:* It evaluates the effect of each element of balance component by computer direct moveable platform with movable visual input.

## DIFFERENTIAL DIAGNOSIS
### Chronic Vertigo

Benign Paroxysmal Positional Vertigo (BPPV) This is the most common cause of peripheral vertigo in adults. The postulated causes of BPPV include head trauma, vitamin D deficiency, viral labyrinthitis or just increasing age (10). Females are more commonly affected. Although BPPV can affect all the three canals, the posterior canal is the most commonly affected accounting for 80% of the cases. The pathophysiology behind posterior SCC-BPPV is the migration of otoliths into the ampullary end of posterior canal. During positioning of head to the right, the ampullofugal movement of these otoliths causes excitatory input to the vestibular afferents. This causes an intense sensation of vertigo. Dix-Hallpike manoeuvre is used to diagnose ipsilateral posterior canal or contralateral anterior canal canalolithiasis (11). Supine roll manoeuvre is used to diagnose lateral SCC-BPPV. These diagnostic manoeuvres may become inconclusive if the patient is on vestibular suppressants. Details of these positional tests are discussed in section on Vertigo in Elderly.

**Treatment:** Particle repositioning manoeuvres (PRM) like Epley's manoeuvre and Semont's manoeuvre can be used to treat PC-BPPV. Epley's manoeuvre remains the most popular (12). Persons with debris stuck in posterior canal

cupula (cupulolithiasis) are better treated with Semont's manoeuvre (13). Brandt-Daroff exercises are advised to habituate the brain to the offending position. It also serves to dislodge the otolithic debris from cupula. It is a type of vestibular rehabilitation. A log roll repositioning manoeuvre (Barbecue manoeuvre) or Gufoni manoeuvre can be used to treat lateral SCC-BPPV (14). The patient can also be advised to sleep in the contralateral position for a long duration for posterior limb canalolithiasis. Appiani or Vanucchi-Asprella manoeuvre has been described to treat cupulolithiasis or anterior arm canalolithiasis (15). The patient is advised to avoid driving, travel and jerky head movement after the manoeuvres have been performed.

Benign paroxysmal vertigo of childhood (BPVC) is considered to be a relatively rare peripheral vestibular disorder in children that is often misdiagnosed. It is usually seen in the age group of 2–5 years. The clinical picture is similar to adult BPPV but with several adjuncts (16). The child may even express fear and parents may report clumsiness or poor balance. The diagnostic criteria include at least five documented vertigo attacks with a normal clinical examination with one of the following symptoms – pallor, fearfulness, nystagmus, ataxia or vomiting (17).

*Vestibular Migraine (Migraine-associated Vertigo – MAV)* MAV, better known as vestibular migraine (VM), is a common cause of vertigo in paediatric age group and adults (18). The attacks of vertigo may or may not be provoked by certain factors like change of place, change of weather, menstruation, stress, lack of sleep and hunger. Head banging, diaphoresis, pallor, abdominal pain and vomiting maybe seen in such cases (19). To streamline the management of VM, diagnostic criteria have been laid down by the HIS Classification Committee and Committee for Classification of Vestibular Disorders of the Bárány Society (Table 7.2).

*Notes:* Vestibular symptoms are rated as moderate when they do not interfere with the routine activity; severe if the daily activities have to be discontinued.

**Treatment:** It consists of three aspects:

i. *General measures:* Avoidance of triggers.

ii. *Acute episodic treatment:* Sumatriptan nasal spray has been found effective in adolescents. Zolmitriptan 2.5 mg and rizatriptan 10 mg have been found effective in adult age group (20). Antiemetics, ibuprofen and paracetamol have been found effective in all age groups.

## Table 7.2: Diagnostic Criteria for Classification of Vestibular Disorders

### Vestibular Migraine

At least five episodes with moderate to severe intensity vestibular symptoms, each lasting 5 minutes to 72 hours

Current or previous history of migraine with or without aura

Presence of one or more features of migraine with at least half of the vestibular episodes:

- Photophobia and phonophobia
- Visual aura
- Headache with at least two of the following characters: unilateral, throbbing in nature, moderate to severe pain, aggravation by routine physical activity

Not better accounted for by another vestibular or ICHD diagnosis

### Probable Vestibular Migraine

At least five episodes with moderate to severe intensity vestibular symptoms, each lasting 5 minutes to 72 hours

Only one of these criteria for vestibular migraine is fulfilled (migraine history or features of migraine during the episode)

Not better accounted for by another vestibular or ICHD diagnosis

---

iii. *Prophylactic treatment:* Adult patients with disabling symptoms or with a symptom frequency of three or more episodes in a month should receive prophylactic treatment on the same lines as migraine with or without aura. Options for adults include propranolol 80–240 mg, metoprolol 50–200 mg, bisoprolol 5–10 mg, sodium valproate 500–600 mg, topiramate 25–100 mg or flunarizine 5–10 mg daily (20). An RCT has also suggested venlafaxine as a treatment option (21). For paediatric age group, propranolol, topiramate, flunarizine and valproate are safe options (22).

*MD and Secondary Endolymphatic Hydrops* It is primarily seen in adults, and is extremely rare in children. Two diagnostic categories of MD have been made – probable and definite MD (23).

i. Definitive MD requires at least two or more documented attacks of vertigo lasting >= 20 minutes but <=12 hours, low- to medium-frequency sensorineural hearing loss documented audiometrically on at least one occasion, fluctuating hearing, tinnitus and/or fullness in the diseased ear as well which cannot be better accounted by any other vestibular diagnosis.

ii. Probable MD requires at least two or more documented attacks of vertigo lasting >= 20 minutes but <=24 hours, fluctuating hearing, tinnitus and/or fullness in the diseased ear as well which cannot be better accounted by any other vestibular diagnosis.

There are two other variants of MD: otolithic crisis of Tumarkin, which manifests as falls or drop attacks; and Lermoyèz attacks, where the hearing attacks and tinnitus, if present, improve during attacks of vertigo (24).

**Investigations:** Pure tone audiometry reveals unilateral sensorineural hearing loss, which in the early stages is more pronounced in the lower frequencies. Glycerol test has been traditionally described to improve hearing in three consecutive octaves by 5–10 dB on testing 30 minutes after administration of oral glycerol at 1–1.5 mg/kg wt (25). MRI of the inner ear is recommended to rule out any central lesions that mimic MD. Electrocochleography can be done, which shows a SP/AP ratio of >0.4. Vestibular evoked myogenic potentials (VEMP) detect the sacculocolic reflex and measures the ipsilateral sternocleidomastoid muscle relaxation when a sound stimulus is presented to the saccule. The amplitude of the response may be decreased in MD and can be increased in the recovery phase of MD (26).

Please note that except audiometry, none of the investigations is necessary to make a diagnosis of MD.

**Treatment:**

1. Acute attack – vestibular suppressants (thiazides, anti-histamines, benzodiazepines) are well-established pharmacotherapy to control vertigo and related symptoms.

2. Prophylaxis in between episodes –

   i. *Lifestyle management:* Patients are advised to reduce their salt intake, follow a regular lifestyle, avoid stimulants like tea, coffee, nicotine or alcohol and ensure adequate sleep. However, these measures have no proven role yet (27). Vestibular rehabilitation exercises help to restore balance and to train the visual and proprioception inputs.

ii. *Drugs for prophylaxis:* Diuretics have been suggested as the first-line treatment. Chlorthalidone and thiazides have been shown to reduce the intensity of episodes and the need for surgical intervention. A Cochrane review suggests that there is no concrete evidence that proves the benefit of diuretics (28). Betahistine is another commonly used drug in doses of 48–144 mg/day. It is a weak H1 agonist and a stronger H3 antagonist. It mainly acts by improving cochlear microcirculation (29). A Cochrane review suggests its benefit in reducing the frequency of attacks and improving the quality of life (30). One should however keep in mind the possibility of exacerbation of asthma and peptic ulcer disease due to its H1 agonist action. Steroids and cytotoxic drugs have a therapeutic effect on autoimmunity-induced cases.

iii. *Intratympanic treatment:* Intratympanic dexamethasone administration has been advised when there is unsatisfactory improvement with oral medications. However, there is limited evidence to support its use. Intratympanic gentamicin to chemically ablate the labyrinth can be used when no oral treatment and intratympanic dexamethasone has been found effective and hearing is either poor or needs to be sacrificed for vertigo control (31).

iv. *Surgical treatment:* Endolymphatic sac surgery renders no significant benefit as per a Cochrane review. Labyrinthectomy and vestibular neurectomy are the other options that have been described (32).

*Seizure Disorder* It is predominantly a childhood cause of dizziness. It is usually associated with syndromic patients or patients who have suffered head trauma. This disorder presents as short spells of reported giddiness with or without loss of consciousness. There may be accompanying autonomic symptoms like nausea, vomiting or pallor. EEG and MRI are also indicated for patients with focal neurological deficits and absence of any psychiatric complaints (33).

*Otitis Media (With or Without Effusion)* It is an uncommon cause of vertigo in children, even rarer in adults. Serous labyrinthitis or change of pressure within the middle ear causing displacement of oval or round window is thought to be the underlying cause (34).

Otoscopy helps to establish this diagnosis. Antihistamines and decongestants are the mainstay of treatment for acute otitis media. Persistent cases may require myringotomy with or without placement of a ventilation tube. OME is usually caused by eustachian tube dysfunction or adenoiditis (35).

*Complications due to Otitis Media* Both acute and chronic otitis media can cause complications leading to vertigo or disequilibrium. These complications chiefly include cerebellar abscess, labyrinthitis and meningitis (36).

i. *Cerebellar abscess* (Figure 7.4): This presents with acute onset vomiting, vertigo and signs of raised intracranial tension. Cerebellar signs are positive and MRI clinches the diagnosis. They require intravenous antibiotics, intracranial pressure lowering agents, drainage of the abscess and canal wall down mastoidectomy.

ii. *Labyrinthitis:* This presents with acute onset sensorineural hearing loss along with vertigo. It causes an irritated hyperactive labyrinth in the acute stage, whereas long-lasting labyrinthitis causes a hypoactive or a dead labyrinth. Otogenic labyrinthitis can be either serous or suppurative, and it is a retrospective clinical diagnosis. Meningitic labyrinthitis occurs in children less than 2 years of age, and usually occurs bilaterally. It is notorious to leave residual labyrinthitis ossificans, which makes the process of cochlear implantation difficult (37).

Vertigo in labyrinthitis is to be treated with sedatives like benzodiazepines, vestibular suppressants, antiemetics, intravenous fluid administration and absolute rest. Steroids are considered for prevention of hearing impairment. If acute otitis media is the underlying cause, then an urgent myringotomy is to be done. For chronic otitis media squamous, canal wall down mastoidectomy is to be done following stabilization of the patient, while in mucosal disease a cortical mastoidectomy may suffice.

*Tumours* Benign or malignant tumours of middle ear, internal acoustic canal, endolymphatic sac, cerebellopontine (CP) angle, cerebellum, brainstem or even spinal cord can present with vertigo. CP angle tumours are the most common in this list (Figure 7.5) (38).

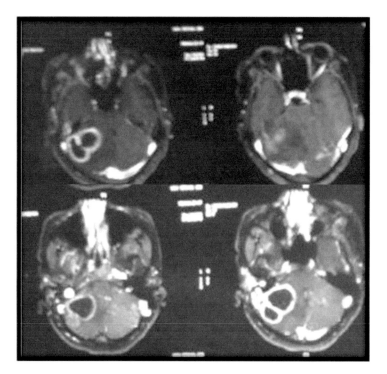

**Figure 7.4** MRI brain T2 image showing hyperintense mass in left middle ear cleft with hypointense mass in cerebellar region with peripheral enhancement.

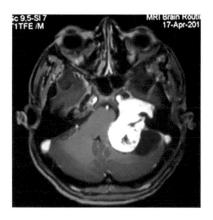

**Figure 7.5** MRI showing hypointense to hyperintense SOL in right CP angle.

A good otological examination with cerebellar and cranial nerve assessment might point towards such pathology. Baseline audiometry for hearing assessment and radiology in the form of MRI is needed. Surgical excision if possible is the treatment of choice.

*Psychogenic Dizziness (Panic and Anxiety Disorders)* They are the most common cause of dizziness in teenagers. A fraction of dizzy adults also fall in this category. Classic vertigo symptoms are not seen. The patient complains of light-headedness or syncope. Such patients need a referral to a psychiatrist. The clinical examination is usually non-contributory (39).

*Chemical Vestibulopathy* Chemical vestibulopathy usually occurs in patients on chronic aminoglycoside treatment (gentamicin and streptomycin) or other vestibulotoxic medications. It is usually bilaterally symmetrical. Recently, amiodarone has also been implicated. The patients complain of oscillopsia or disequilibrium rather than vertigo (40).

*Motion Sickness* It is a physiological form of giddiness experienced by some people in the wake of real or perceived motion, and causes gastrointestinal, autonomic and neurological symptoms.

The brain relies on visual, vestibular and somatosensory cues to form an estimate of the motion and orientation of the body in space. During travelling, there occurs a mismatch between these inputs, which confuses the brain. There are behavioural modifications suggested to minimize or prevent motion sickness. One should not fixate his/her gaze on a stationary object which is close, like reading a book, texting on mobile or watching a movie in a moving vehicle. Instead, it is advisable to sit on the front

**117**

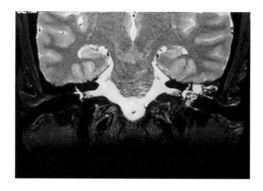

**Figure 7.6** MRI T2 image depicting hyperintense mass similar to fluid of inner ear on left side.

seat in the car and fixate the gaze on the horizon so as to keep the visual input in sync with the vestibular input (41).

For patients with severe symptoms, medications like transdermal scopolamine and orally administered antihistamines like meclizine and dimenhydrinate are advised, but the sedation they cause limits their routine use (42).

*Perilymphatic Fistula* This refers to an abnormal communication between the membranous labyrinth and middle ear (Figure 7.6). This is an infrequent complication of barotrauma, heavy weightlifting or a head injury. Sensorineural hearing loss, tinnitus and ear fullness are the other symptoms. Fistula test and flood audiological test are positive. Radiology may reveal a pneumo-labyrinth, presence of fluid in the dependent part of middle ear and the possible site of the leak (43). Treatment consists of conservative measures to avoid loud sounds and sudden pressure changes, failing which surgical patch repair needs to be considered.

*Superior Semicircular Canal Dehiscence (SSCD)* This refers to an abnormal communication between the membranous part of superior semicircular canal with the dura above, due to the erosion and absence of the bone overlying the superior SCC. This allows transfer of the intracranial pressure to the middle ear. Vertigo is induced by coughing, sneezing or Valsalva manoeuvre. Diagnosis is made by high-resolution CT (HRCT) scan of the temporal bone and by VEMP test. Surgical repair of the bony defect and round window reinforcement may be of benefit to the patient (44).

*Cervical Vertigo* It is a controversial diagnosis. The coordination of head, eye and body posture is supported by proprioception feedback of neck. The diagnosis is based on tally of the vertigo symptoms with neck pain and eliminating other vestibular diagnosis. Four hypotheses that could possibly explain the cervical origin of vertigo are sympathetic dysfunction, vertebral artery rotation, proprioceptive and migraine-associated cervical vertigo (45).

*Nutritional Causes* Vitamin B12, iron, folate and vitamin D deficiency can contribute to vague symptoms of dizziness (15, 46, 47).

*Trauma* Head trauma can independently cause vertigo and the duration may vary from seconds to days. It has also been implicated as a contributing factor in labyrinthine concussion, BPPV, perilymphatic fistula and delayed endolymphatic hydrops.

*Other Causes*

i. *Drugs:* Alcohol, barbiturates, anticonvulsants and tranquillizers overdose can cause vertigo.

ii. *Ocular:* Macular lesion can induce spontaneous pendular nystagmus. Amblyopia and central lesions affecting ocular pathway may present with ocular nystagmus.

iii. *Congenital:* Nystagmus is usually spontaneous horizontal, pendular or jerky. Patients are present with positive family history and vertigo from childhood.

iv. The extremely rare causes of vertigo include genetic ataxia, demyelinating disorders, mal de debarquement syndrome, Cogan syndrome, Susac syndrome, vestibular paroxysmia, otosphilis and granulomatous diseases (48, 49). Even presence of ear wax has been known to rarely cause imbalance (50).

**Acute Vertigo**

*Vestibular Neuritis* It has been postulated that vestibular neuritis is viral in origin, especially herpes simplex virus. The patient presents with severe giddiness, vomiting and nystagmus. Hearing is usually normal; aural fullness may be reported by some patients. Vestibular neuritis needs to be differentiated from a posterior circulation stroke. HINTS (Head Impulse test, Nystagmus, Testing for Skew deviation) and postural instability are an important clinical exam to achieve this differentiation (51).

The nystagmus usually beats towards the contralateral (healthy) ear. The acute phase of illness lasts 48–72 hours following which the symptoms gradually resolve; however, the symptom of disequilibrium may persist for 4–6 weeks. This is the time duration required for the contralateral normal vestibule to compensate for the lost function of the affected vestibule (52).

Treatment is often symptomatic in adults (vestibular suppressants and benzodiazepines), but it is to be used for short term only as it delays the onset of compensation. Antibiotics can be used in the presence of an active bacterial infection. Non-infective neuritis can be treated with steroids. Vestibular rehabilitation therapy is the mainstay of therapy.

*Posterior Circulation Stroke*  An insult to the posterior inferior cerebellar artery (PICA) can cause cerebellar infarction leading to imbalance, nystagmus and the cerebellar signs. Skew deviation of the eyes may be present (53). These stroke disorders need to be swiftly identified to enable a timely referral to a neurologist.

## CONCLUSION

Vertigo is a common but vaguely understood domain. It is important to pinpoint the exact complaint and elicit a good history to achieve a guided examination and laboratory diagnosis. It often requires a multi-specialty approach involving neurology, otorhinolaryngology and sometimes, psychiatry.

## TAKE HOME MESSAGE

The detailed history and relevant clinical examination is the key for diagnosing the aetiology of vertigo.

## REFERENCES

1. Kovacs E, Wang X, Grill E. Economic burden of vertigo: a systematic review. Health Econ Rev. 2019;9(1):37.

2. Batu ED, Anlar B, Topçu M, Turanlı G, Aysun S. Vertigo in childhood: a retrospective series of 100 children. Eur J Paediatr Neurol. 2015;19(2):226–32.

3. Murofushi T, Curthoys IS. Physiological and anatomical study of click-sensitive primary vestibular afferents in the guinea pig. Acta Otolaryngol. 1997;117(1):66–72.

4. Li C-M, Hoffman HJ, Ward BK, Cohen HS, Rine RM. Epidemiology of dizziness and balance problems in children in the United States: a population-based study. J Pediatr. 2016;171:240–3. doi:10.1016/j.jpeds.2015.12.002

5. Gans R. Equilibrium-Vestibular assessment for infants. Audiol Today. 2012;(Jan-Feb):25–31.

6. Agrawal Y, Ward BK, Minor LB. Vestibular dysfunction: prevalence, impact and need for targeted treatment. J Vestib Res. 2013;23(3):113–17.

7. Abrol R, Nehru VI, Venkatramana Y. Prevalence and etiology of vertigo in adult rural population. Indian J Otolaryngol Head Neck Surg. 2001;53(1):32–6.

8. Santosh UP, Rao MSS. Incidence of hypothyroidism in Meniere's disease. J Clin Diagn Res. 2016;10(5):MC01–3.

9. Damodaran O, Rizk E, Rodriguez J, Lee G. Cranial nerve assessment: a concise guide to clinical examination. Clin Anat. 2014;27(1):25–30.

10. AlGarni MA, Mirza AA, Althobaiti AA, Al-Nemari HH, Bakhsh LS. Association of benign paroxysmal positional vertigo with vitamin D deficiency: a systematic review and meta-analysis. Eur Arch Otorhinolaryngol. 2018;275(11):2705–11.

11. Nuti D, Zee DS, Mandala M. Benign paroxysmal positional vertigo: what we do and do not know. Semin Neurol. 2020;40(1):49–58.

12. Pérez-Vázquez P, Franco-Gutiérrez V. Treatment of benign paroxysmal positional vertigo: a clinical review. J Otol. 2017;12(4):165–73.

13. Levrat E, van Melle G, Monnier P, Maire R. Efficacy of the Semont manoeuvre in benign paroxysmal positional vertigo. Arch Otolaryngol Neck Surg. 2003;129(6):629–33.

14. Casani A Pietro, Nacci A, Dallan I, Panicucci E, Gufoni M, Sellari-Franceschini S. Horizontal semicircular canal benign paroxysmal positional vertigo: effectiveness of two different methods of treatment. Audiol Neurootol. 2011;16(3):175–84.

15. Yacovino DA, Hain TC, Gualtieri F. New therapeutic manoeuvre for anterior canal benign paroxysmal positional vertigo. J Neurol. 2009;256(11):1851–5.

16. Lindskog U, Ödkvist L, Noaksson L, Wallquist J. Benign paroxysmal vertigo in childhood: a long-term follow-up. Headache J Head Face Pain. 1999;39(1):33–7.

17. Lempert T, Olesen J, Furman J, et al. Vestibular migraine: diagnostic criteria. J Vestib Res. 2012; 22: 167–72.

18. Neuhauser HK, Radtke A, von Brevern M, et al. Migrainous vertigo: prevalence and impact on quality of life. Neurology. 2006;67(6):1028–33.

19. Spiri D, Rinaldi VE, Titomanlio L. Pediatric migraine and episodic syndromes that may be associated with migraine. Ital J Pediatr. 2014;40:92.

20. Obermann M, Strupp M. Current treatment options in vestibular migraine. Front Neurol. 2014;5:257.

21. Salviz M, Yuce T, Acar H, Karatas A, Acikalin RM. Propranolol and venlafaxine for vestibular migraine prophylaxis: a randomized controlled trial. Laryngoscope. 2016;126(1):169–74.

22. Teleanu RI, Vladacenco O, Teleanu DM, Epure DA. Treatment of pediatric migraine: a review. Maedica (Buchar). 2016;11(2):136–43.

23. Lopez-Escamez JA, Carey J, Chung W-H, et al. Diagnostic criteria for Meniere's disease. J Vestib Res. 2015;25(1):1–7.

24. Shen K-C, Young Y-H. Lermoyez syndrome revisited: 100-year mystery. Acta Otolaryngol. 2018;138(11): 981–6.

25. Yen PT, Lin CC, Huang TS. A preliminary report on the correlation of vestibular Meniére's disease with electrocochleography and glycerol test. Acta Otolaryngol Suppl. 1995;520(Pt 2):241–6.

26. Rauch SD, Zhou G, Kujawa SG, Guinan JJ, Herrmann BS. Vestibular evoked myogenic potentials show altered tuning in patients with Ménière's disease. Otol Neurotol. 2004;25(3):333–8.

27. Hussain K, Murdin L, Schilder AGM. Restriction of salt, caffeine and alcohol intake for the treatment of Ménière's disease or syndrome. Cochrane Database Syst Rev. 2018;12(12):CD012173.

28. Thirlwall AS, Kundu S. Diuretics for Ménière's disease or syndrome. Cochrane Database Syst Rev. 2006;(3):CD003599.

29. Motamed H, Moezzi M, Rooyfard AD, Angali KA, Izadi Z. A comparison of the effects and side effects of oral betahistine with injectable promethazine in the treatment of acute peripheral vertigo in emergency. J Clin Med Res. 2017;9(12):994–7.

30. Murdin L, Hussain K, Schilder AGM. Betahistine for symptoms of vertigo. Cochrane Database Syst Rev. 2016;(6):CD010696.

31. Phillips JS, Westerberg B. Intratympanic steroids for Ménière's disease or syndrome. Cochrane Database Syst Rev. 2011;(7):CD008514.

32. Pullens B, Verschuur HP, van Benthem PP. Surgery for Ménière's disease. Cochrane Database Syst Rev. 2013;(2):CD005395.

33. Davis KS, Byrd JK, Mehta V, et al. Occult primary head and neck squamous cell carcinoma: utility of discovering primary lesions. Otolaryngol Head Neck Surg. 2014;151(2):272–8.

34. Suzuki M, Kitano H, Yazawa Y, Kitajima K. Involvement of round and oval windows in the vestibular response to pressure changes in the middle ear of guinea pigs. Acta Otolaryngol. 1998;118(5):712–16.

35. Arman S, Amlani A, Doshi J. Glue ear management & deprivation: a retrospective study of 89 patients. Clin Otolaryngol. 2020;45(4):616–18.

36. Duarte MJ, Kozin ED, Barshak MB, et al. Otogenic brain abscesses: a systematic review. Laryngoscope Investig Otolaryngol. 2018;3(3):198–208.

37. Xu HX, Joglekar SS, Paparella MM. Labyrinthitis ossificans. Otol Neurotol. 2009;30(4):579–80.

38. de Albuquerque Maranhão AS, Godofredo VR, de Oliveira Penido N. Suppurative labyrinthitis associated with otitis media: 26 years' experience. Braz J Otorhinolaryngol. 2016;82(1):82–7.

39. Szirmai A. Vestibular disorders in childhood and adolescents. Eur Arch Otorhinolaryngol. 2010;267(11):1801–4.

40. Gurkov R, Manzari L, Blodow A, Wenzel A, Pavlovic D, Luis L. Amiodarone-associated bilateral vestibulopathy. Eur Arch Otorhinolaryngol. 2018;275(3):823–5.

41. Furman JM, Marcus DA, Balaban CD. Rizatriptan reduces vestibular-induced motion sickness in migraineurs. J Headache Pain. 2011;12(1):81–8.

42. Brainard A, Gresham C. Prevention and treatment of motion sickness. Am Fam Physician. 2014;90(1):41–6.

43. Casselman JW. Diagnostic imaging in clinical neuro-otology. Curr Opin Neurol. 2002;15(1):23–30.

44. Belden CJ, Weg N, Minor LB, Zinreich SJ. CT evaluation of bone dehiscence of the superior semicircular canal as a cause of sound- and/or pressure-induced vertigo. Radiology. 2003;226(2):337–43.

45. Ahmed W, Rajagopal R, Lloyd G. Systematic review of round window operations for the treatment of superior semicircular canal dehiscence. J Int Adv Otol. 2019;15(2):209–14.

46. Li Y, Peng B. Pathogenesis, diagnosis, and treatment of cervical vertigo. Pain Physician. 2015;18(4):E583–95.

47. Beitzke M, Pfister P, Fortin J, Skrabal F. Autonomic dysfunction and hemodynamics in vitamin B12 deficiency. Auton Neurosci. 2002;97(1):45–54.

48. Kingston M, French P, Goh B, et al. UK National Guidelines on the Management of Syphilis 2008. Int J STD AIDS. 2008;19(11):729–40.

49. Girasoli L, Cazzador D, Padoan R, et al. Update on vertigo in autoimmune disorders, from diagnosis to treatment. J Immunol Res. 2018;2018:5072582.

50. McCarter DF, Courtney AU, Pollart SM. Cerumen impaction. Am Fam Physician. 2007;75(10):1523–8.

51. Batuecas-Caletrío Á, Yáñez-González R, Sánchez-Blanco C, et al. [Peripheral vertigo versus central vertigo: application of the HINTS protocol]. Rev Neurol. 2014;59(8):349–53.

52. Jeong S-H, Kim H-J, Kim J-S. Vestibular neuritis. Semin Neurol. 2013;33(3):185–94.

53. Krishnan K, Bassilious K, Eriksen E, et al. Posterior circulation stroke diagnosis using HINTS in patients presenting with acute vestibular syndrome: a systematic review. Eur Stroke J. 2019;4(3):233–9.

# 8 Vertigo in Elderly

*Gunjan Dwivedi and Uma Patnaik*

## CONTENTS

## INTRODUCTION

Vertigo in elderly is an important clinical condition and a burdensome public health issue. The symptoms can range from disorders of orientation in space to motion perception, such as the illusion of spinning or the feeling of imbalance, which can affect the ability to achieve a stable gaze, posture and gait. Thus, dizziness in elderly is a multifactorial geriatric syndrome manifesting in multiple ways and involving several organ systems, such as sensory, neural and cardiovascular (1).

The prevalence of dizziness and imbalance ranges from approximately 20% to 30%, depending on the definition of dizziness and the population being studied. Generally the prevalence of dizziness increases with an increase in age (1–3). A U.S. population-based study found that 24% of people older than 72 years reported an episode of dizziness within the previous 2 months (1). Another population-based study in the United Kingdom reported that 30% of people older than 65 years had dizziness (2). A cross-sectional study in Sweden reported that the number of adults with dizziness increased up to approximately 50% in people older than 85 years (4).

### Disability Burden Secondary to Vertigo in Elderly

Dizziness in the elderly is a strong predictor of falls, and injuries secondary to falls cause restriction of movement leading to loss of independence (5, 6). The presence of impaired balance function increases the risk of hip and upper limb fractures (7). Fall is the leading cause of accidental death in individuals older than 65 years, and dizziness is one of the strongest contributors to the disability burden after the age of 65 (8, 9).

### Why Is Vertigo More Common in Elderly?

A peculiarity of balance disorders in elderly is that these patients rarely complain of rotatory vertigo, but with more of non-specific unsteadiness and dizziness compared to younger people with similar disease (10). The underlying process for this is the gradually progressive multimodal impairment of balance, including the loss of vestibular and proprioceptive functions associated with the impairment of central integration of these and other sensory inputs associated with ageing. This is called as presbystasis, presbyequilibrium or at times multisensory dizziness (7, 11, 12).The skeletal muscle strength and mass are also reduced with ageing, which increases the risk of fall-related injuries in elderly patients (13).The aetiology of dizziness in the elderly is most frequently benign; however, a few of these patients may harbour a serious, potentially life-threatening disease, such as stroke (14, 15).

Barin and Dodson (5) have broadly divided the causes of disequilibrium and dizziness in the elderly into the following three types:

a. Age-related decline of acuity in the sensory and motor pathways plus deterioration of central integration mechanisms.

b. Pathologies that cause dizziness in any age group but become more prevalent in older individuals, either because the age-related changes noted above make the elderly more susceptible to these pathologies or because the cumulative probability of exposure to these pathologies increases with time.

c. An assortment of environmental and lifestyle factors that increase the chance of dizziness and balance problems in the elderly.

### Pathophysiology of Imbalance in Elderly

Postural stability in elderly is maintained by integration of several factors: somatosensory, vestibular, visual and proprioceptive inputs to central nervous system. These sensory inputs are processed accurately at motor centres and cerebellum, which is followed by requisite output from the brain to the musculoskeletal system to maintain the balance of the body. With ageing, there is structural and functional deterioration of all these systems.

1. *Age-associated changes in vestibular system:* Loss of neurons and hair cells of otolith organs and the Semicircular Canals (SCCs) are a part of ageing. Hair cell degeneration has been reported within the maculae of the saccule and utricle and the cristae/ampullae of the SCCs (16, 17). Studies have confirmed age-related loss of hair cells in the labyrinth, but the sites affected (SCCs, utricle, saccule) and types (type I/II) of hair cells have been variable (18, 19). The structural integrity of vestibular nerve is also affected due to ageing. In Scarpa's ganglion, the number of primary vestibular neurons is reduced by nearly 25% in a person's life span (20, 21). Study on brainstem specimens in different age groups has documented a decrease in the number of secondary vestibular neurons within the vestibular nuclei (22). It is well-understood that age-related degeneration of peripheral and central vestibular structures is similar to that of the auditory system and is most likely caused by subtle changes of blood flow to the inner ear (23). Microvascular changes related to ageing have been reported in human and animal studies. Any reduction in blood flow can

have profound effect as inner ear arteries are end arteries and lack collaterals and anastomoses (24, 25).

2. *Age-associated changes in visual system:* The main concept involved with visual vertigo is that one's idea of one's posture in space is based on inputs from the eyes, the inner ear, the feet and the idea of where one should be in space. These inputs are integrated to make an assessment of where one is and where one will be in the near future, and this information is used to base actions designed to avoid falling over. Bronstein (1995) used the term "visual vertigo" for "visually induced vertiginous symptoms". He described a heterogeneous group of 15 patients, including several with brain disorders and several with weakness or misalignment of their eyes, and reported that typical triggers were "walking in supermarket aisles", visual moving surroundings during travelling in cars or trains, disco lights, people walking, cars passing by or even simple movement of eyes. He also discussed the idea of visual dependence, where visually dependent people orient their posture according to information from their eyes to a greater extent than others (26).

Visual acuity, accommodation, depth perception, contrast sensitivity and the ability to suppress nystagmus by visual fixation are diminished due to ageing of the oculomotor system with increased saccade latency and reduced eye tracking velocity (5, 27, 28). Contrast sensitivity and depth perception have been found to be the most important visual impairments that contribute to falls (28). Reduced dynamic visual acuity (where the subject or the target are moving) has a correlation with stability of gait and posture in elderly; however, static visual acuity has not been definitely proven to be so (28, 29). Ocular muscles also undergo degenerative changes which increase the saccade latency, reduce the gain of smooth pursuit and the ability to suppress vestibular nystagmus by fixation (30, 31). The gain of optokinetic responses also declines in elderly, especially for higher target velocities (30).

3. *Age-associated changes in proprioceptive system:* The proprioceptive system comprises afferents from sensors in muscles, joints and tendons. The information regarding orientation of each part of the body with respect to others and information regarding the contact areas of body with ground is provided by them. Proprioception from neck helps to detect the position of head. All this

information plays a key role in maintaining posture and balance. Vibration and touch thresholds deteriorate in elderly, adversely affecting tactile information which arises from the feet at their point of contact with the ground (32). The ability to detect the position and direction of joint movements also reduces with age (33).

4. *Age-associated changes in motor system:* Balance and postural stability are maintained by action of muscles once they receive commands from motor centres after the brain processes the inputs received from visual, vestibular and proprioceptive systems. The characteristics of muscles changes with ageing (34). There are changes in central motor command centres and also there is reduction in the number and size of muscle fibres, which leads to reduction in muscle strength (35). There is also decline in the speed by which the muscle can be contracted (36).

5. *Age-associated changes in central integration mechanisms:* With senile degeneration of central nervous system, there is decline in the number of neurons, supporting cells and myelination (37). There are degenerative changes in the areas responsible for postural stability and balance such as brainstem, cerebellum and other higher cortical centres. Consequently, there is disturbance in the mechanisms which receive and process the sensory inputs from various parts of body and give out signals for motor system for maintenance of balance. This leads to difficulty in compensating once the vestibular/visual or proprioceptive systems are affected and the vertigo lasts much longer and is more disabling (38).

### DIFFERENTIAL DIAGNOSIS

Vertigo in elderly can be caused by peripheral vestibular disorders as well as by central nervous system pathology. These are causes of vertigo which can present in any age group but become more prevalent in elderly due to age-related changes in the body. A summary of these is presented in Table 8.1. A few of these diseases which an otolaryngologist is faced with routinely will be discussed in this chapter.

### Peripheral Vertigo

*Benign Paroxysmal Positional Vertigo (BPPV)*

BPPV is by far the commonest diagnosis in patients of dizziness who are referred to otolaryngology clinics, especially the elderly, and

### Table 8.1: Aetiology of Vertigo and Dizziness in Elderly

| | |
|---|---|
| Vestibular causes | Benign paroxysmal positional vertigo |
| | Late-onset Ménière's disease |
| | Vestibular neuritis |
| | Labyrinthitis |
| Central nervous system causes | Vestibular migraine |
| | Brainstem vertigo |
| | Transient ischaemic attacks |
| | Stroke |
| | Neurodegenerative disorders |
| Cardiovascular causes | Postural hypotension |
| | Arrhythmia |
| | Heart failure |
| Medication | Benzodiazepines, antihypertensive, anxiolytics hypnotics, antiepileptic |
| Miscellaneous | Presbystasis |
| | Neoplastic diseases with metastases to brain |
| | Psychiatric dizziness |
| | Proprioception disorders |
| | Somatosensory impairments |

has been reported in 33–40% cases of elderly presenting with giddiness (39–41). Idiopathic BPPV is more common in elderly. It may be associated with otosclerosis, osteopenia or Ménière's Disease (MD) and at times may follow head trauma, Vertebro-basilar ischaemia or Vestibular Neuritis (VN).

BPPV is characterized by rotational vertigo caused by changes in head position. There are two accepted theories for pathophysiology of BPPV – cupulolithiasis and canalolithiasis. In 1969, Schuknecht postulated that BPPV was the result of "cupulolithiasis" of the posterior SCC (42). According to cupulolithiasis theory, the otoconia from the utricle and saccule get detached and move to ampullae of SCCs to adhere to the cupula, most commonly the posterior SCC. The otoconia are three times denser than the endolymph. So the cupula becomes sensitive to gravity and moves inappropriately with change in head position, causing movement of the endolymph and firing of inappropriate vestibular stimuli. This leads to a pathological Vestibulo-Ocular Reflex (VOR) leading to development of nystagmus and vertigo.

In 1979, Hall et al. proposed the canalolithiaisis theory as cupulolithiasis theory could not explain the fatiguability of nystagmus on repetitive position testing (43). According to this theory, there is accumulation of dislodged otoconia in the SCC and once they reach a particular critical mass, they are able to move the hair cells of cupula on movement of endolymph due to changes in head position. An inappropriate stimulus is generated from the cupula leading to inappropriate VOR, nystagmus and vertigo.

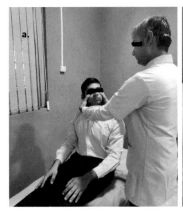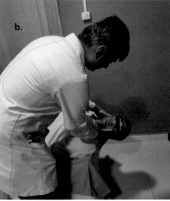

**Figure 8.1** Dix-Hallpike manoeuvre. (a) Patient seated on couch with head turned 45°. (b) Patient put in supine position with head hanging 30° below horizontal keep it turned 45° from central position.

In both the theories, the common pathogenic factor is dislodgement of otoconia. This is a degenerative process which is more common in the elderly. With ageing, the number and volume of otoliths decline progressively and the interconnecting fibres between the otoliths weaken leading to their separation and dislodgement from the otolithic membrane on the maculae of utricle and saccule. Thereafter they move freely in endolymph and reach SCCs through their non-ampullated ends. The otoconia most commonly enter the posterior SCC due to its orientation.

The patient typically presents with episodic vertigo associated with changes in head position which lasts for a few seconds to a few minutes. The episodes may be associated with nausea and vomiting, but there is no change in hearing status or tinnitus. Various positional tests can be done to diagnose BPPV. For posterior SCC BPPV, the Dix-Hallpike manoeuvre (Figure 8.1) has been described in which the patient is seated on an examination couch and the head is rotated 45° to one side. The patient is then brought into supine position with the head hyper-extended to reach the head-hanging position about 20–30° below horizontal. The head of patient is supported by the examiner and position maintained for 20–30 seconds. Appearance of geotropic torsional nystagmus with a severely giddy patient is a positive test. For horizontal SCC BPPV, supine roll test (Figure 8.2) can be done. The patient is made supine with head 30° elevated in central position first. Then the head is turned to 90° on one side and the position is maintained for 30 seconds and then to opposite side again keeping the position for 30 seconds. A positive test is the appearance of nystagmus and

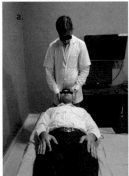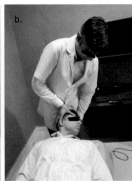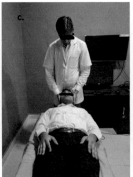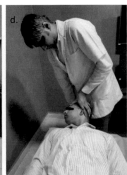

**Figure 8.2** Supine Roll test with head elevated by 30° while in neutral position. (a) Head in neutral position. (b) Head turned 90° to one side. (c) Head brought back to central position. (d) Head turned 90° to opposite side.

giddiness on any one or both sides. For superior or anterior SCC, BPPV patient is put in supine position with head to one side. The test is considered positive if there is downbeat nystagmus with contra-torsion to downside and appearance of upbeat nystagmus on upright position.

For the treatment for BPPV, there are various Particle Repositioning Manoeuvres (PRM) (44). Most commonly performed manoeuvre for posterior canal BPPV is the modified Epley's PRM (Figure 8.3), for lateral canal it is 360° barbeque roll (Figure 8.4) and for anterior canal it is the Kim's manoeuvre or the deep head hanging manoeuvre (Figure 8.5). The basic concept of these manoeuvres is to move the particles in the SCCs in such a way that they move towards the non-ampullated end of the affected SCC and get repositioned into the vestibule. The condition may also be managed by Brandt-Daroff exercises (Figure 8.6), which help to keep otoliths in motion in the endolymph and do not allow a critical mass to form, thus preventing cupular stimulation. BPPV is a self-limiting disorder and may resolve with conservative management.

### Ménière's Disease

Prosper Ménière, a French physician, first described this condition as an inner ear disorder in 1961. MD is an idiopathic inner ear disorder which is characterized by recurrent spontaneous vertigo accompanied with fluctuating or progressive Sensorineural Hearing Loss (SNHL), tinnitus and aural fullness in the affected ear (45). The pathological correlate of this disease is the endolymphatic hydrops which have been seen in temporal bones of patients with this syndrome (46–48).

The age of onset of MD is most commonly reported between second and sixth decades of life. However, in a large case series, Ballester et al. reported that 15% of patients with MD are more than 65 years of age (49). A multi-centre survey in Japan reported the proportion of cases of MD inpatients older than 60 years had increased during the last 30 years (50).

Episodes of vertigo in MD last for at least 20 minutes in duration, but it may last for several hours. The vertigo is generally associated with nausea and vomiting. Horizontal or rotatory nystagmus is present during the definitive episodes. Patients can at times have sudden falls without warning and without loss of consciousness. Such a sudden fall is called "otolithic crisis of Tumarkin" (51–53).

SNHL is one of the components of the classic triad of symptoms of MD. It must be confirmed audiometrically on at least one occasion in the affected ear. Hearing loss primarily affects the

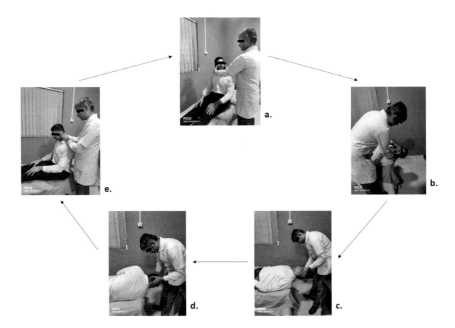

**Figure 8.3**  Epley's manoeuvre for right posterior SCC BPPV. (a) Head turned 45° towards the examiner while seating the patient on the couch. (b) Pt made supine and head hung 30° below horizontal continuing the 45° head turned position. (c) Head turned by 90° to opposite side continuing to keep head 30° below horizontal. (d) Patient turned to opposite side with head turned further 45° so that it faces the floor. (e) Patient slowly brought to sitting position with head slightly down by 20–30°.

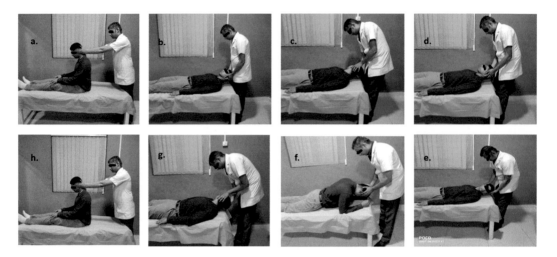

**Figure 8.4** 360° barbeque roll for right horizontal canal BPPV. (a) The patient is put in long-sitting position. (b) Patient placed in a supine position with the head elevated 30°. (c) Patient's head is rotated 90° to the right side and maintained for 30 seconds or until the nystagmus and vertigo cease. (d) Next the head is rotated back to neutral. (e) Next head is turned 90° to left. (f) Patient is put in prone position with head 30° down (achieved by patient supporting upper part of body on elbows). (g) Then patient's head turned 90° to the right side with patient in supine position. (h) Finally, patient put in long-sitting position. Each of these positions is maintained for 30 seconds or until the nystagmus and vertigo cease.

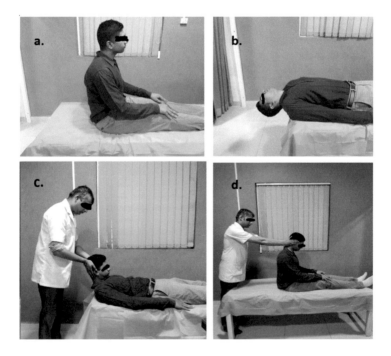

**Figure 8.5** Deep head hanging. (a) The patient is in the sitting position. (b) The head is brought to at least 30°below the horizontal with the head hung as deep as possible and kept so till the nystagmus induced by this step is over. (c) Next the head is brought up quickly to touch the chest while the patient is still supine. (d) After 30 seconds of previous step, the patient is brought back to a seated position with head flexion maintained.

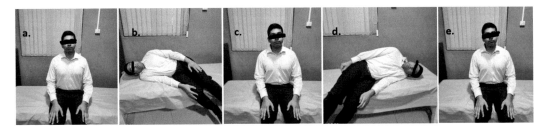

**Figure 8.6** Brandt-Daroff exercises. (a) The patient begins in a seated position with legs hanging by the side of bed. (b) Moves to a side-lying position with the head angled upward by 45°. This position is held for 30 seconds or until dizziness subsides. (c) Back to the seated position. (d) The side-lying position is then initiated to opposite side with 45° head up and maintained in the same way. (e) Patient moves back to the seated position.

low frequencies during initial phase of disease. It may recover after the episode, although with repeated episodes, this may become irreversible. The third classical symptom of this disease is a feeling of pressure within the ear which precedes the spell of vertigo and may be associated with tinnitus.

The most recent guidelines for the diagnosis in patients with MD were issued in 2015 by the Classification Committee of the Barany Society, the Japan Society for Equilibrium Research, the European Academy of Otology and Neurotology, the Equilibrium Committee of the American Academy of Otolaryngology–Head and Neck Surgery (AAO–HNS) and the Korean Balance Society (54). According to these guidelines, the diagnosis of MD in a patient of vertigo is based on clinical symptoms and exclusion of identifiable other aetiologies, making MD idiopathic. They have defined two types: definite and probable MD (Table 8.2). In the 2015 guidelines, diagnostic criteria have been suggested without providing minimal outcome criteria for use in clinical practice due to the absence of a gold standard test. Therefore, minimal outcome reporting is still based on the 1995 criteria issued by the AAO–HNS (Table 8.3).

## Table 8.2: Diagnostic Criteria for Ménière's Disease (Other Causes Excluded)

| Diagnosis | Criteria |
| --- | --- |
| Definite Ménière's disease | ≥Two definitive spontaneous episodes of vertigo lasting 20 minutes to 12 hours |
| | + |
| | Audiometrically documented low- to medium-frequency sensorineural hearing loss in the affected ear on at least one occasion before, during or after one of the episodes of vertigo |
| | + |
| | Fluctuating aural symptoms (hearing, tinnitus or fullness) in the affected ear |
| Probable Ménière's disease | ≥Two episodes of vertigo or dizziness, each lasting 20 minutes to 24 hours |
| | + |
| | Fluctuating aural symptoms (hearing, tinnitus or fullness) in the reported ear |

## Table 8.3: AAO-HNS 1995 Criteria for Diagnosis of Ménière's Disease

| Diagnosis | Criteria |
| --- | --- |
| Certain Ménière's disease | Certain Ménière's disease is "definite" disease with histopathological confirmation |
| Definite Ménière's disease | Definite Ménière's disease requires two or more definitive episodes of vertigo with hearing loss plus tinnitus and/or aural fullness |
| Probable Ménière's disease | Probable Ménière's disease needs only one definitive episode of vertigo and the other symptoms and signs |
| Possible Ménière's disease | Possible Ménière's disease is defined as definitive vertigo with no associated hearing loss or hearing loss with non-definitive disequilibrium |

An average of five attacks of MD occur per year in a patient at diagnosis; however, the frequency generally reduces over time and at 15 years less than two episodes occur per year. The patient is usually asymptomatic between the attacks (55). At presentation, the disease usually is unilateral, but it becomes bilateral in 50% of cases at 30 years, with hearing loss being the other main disability (56).

*Pathophysiology:* The exact pathophysiology of this disease is unknown. In 1938 Hallpike and Cairns had suggested the endolymphatic hydrops theory however, this is not universally accepted as in temporal bone studies, endolymphatic hydrops has been found in a number of patients of hearing loss who did not have symptoms of MD (57). Delayed Magnetic Resonance Imaging (MRI) after intratympanic injection of gadolinium contrast has revealed bilateral hydrops in cases with unilateral MD and diuretics administration in these patients do not always resolve the symptoms of MD (58). Membrane rupture theory was also proposed for acute episodes however could not be demonstrated histologically in temporal bone studies in all cases. Based on a large human temporal bone study, Merchant et al. suggested that the endolymphatic hydrops observed in MD might be a marker for disordered inner ear homeostasis in which some unknown factors produces both the clinical symptoms of Ménière's syndrome as well as endolymphatic hydrops. The implicated precipitating causes include autoimmune, vascular, allergic, genetic, dietary, infective and endocrine factors.

*Evaluation:* MD is by far a clinical diagnosis and a diagnosis of exclusion. Clinical examination during the attack reveals nystagmus towards the affected ear in the initial part (acute phase) of the vestibular attack, however it changes and beats towards the non-affected ear towards the end of the episode (recovery phase) (59).

For assessing cochlear function, a Pure Tone Audiometry (PTA) is done. In cases of MD, generally, during its early stages, the hearing loss mainly involves the lower frequencies also called the "rising audiogram". As the disease progresses, the higher frequencies are affected and then the patient may have an inverted V to downward sloping to nearly flat audiogram (60). To get an objective assessment for MD an Electrocochleography (ECochG) may be done which shows an increase in the ratio of Summating Potential (SP) to action potential (AP). An Auditory Brainstem Response (ABR) can be carried out to rule out retro-cochlear pathology. Central causes of vertigo need to be ruled out in these patients and MRI of brain may be done if there is suspicion of central pathology.

*Differential Diagnosis:* There is considerable overlap between MD and some other clinical conditions: Vestibular migraine, Vestibular Paroxysmia (VP), and Chronic Subjective Dizziness (CSD):

a. *Vestibular migraine:* Consensus document of the Barany Society and the International Headache Society gives the diagnostic criteria for vestibular migraine (Table 8.4) (61).

The pathophysiology of vestibular migraine is poorly understood; however, the large overlap between migraine pathways and vestibular pathways may be the reason for the view that vestibular migraine is a migraine variant with vestibular manifestations. Randomized controlled treatment trials are missing in vestibular migraine. Therefore, the treatment recommendations

## Table 8.4: Criteria for Diagnosis of Vestibular Migraine

| | |
|---|---|
| Vestibular migraine | A. At least five episodes with vestibular symptoms of moderate or severe intensity, lasting 5 minutes to 72 hours |
| | B. Current or previous history of migraine with or without aura according to the International Classification of Headache Disorders (ICHD) |
| | C. One or more migraine features with at least 50% of the vestibular episodes:<br>• Headache with at least two of the following characteristics: one-sided location, pulsating quality, moderate or severe pain intensity, aggravation by routine physical activity<br>• Photophobia and phonophobia<br>• Visual aura |
| | D. Not better accounted for by another vestibular or ICHD diagnosis |
| Probable vestibular migraine | A. At least five episodes with vestibular symptoms of moderate or severe intensity, lasting 5 minutes to 72 hours |
| | B. Only one of the criteria B and C for vestibular migraine is fulfilled (migraine history or migraine features during the episode) |
| | C. Not better accounted for by another vestibular or ICHD diagnosis |

## Table 8.5: Criteria for Diagnosis of Vestibular Paroxysmia

| | |
|---|---|
| Definite vestibular paroxysmia (each point needs to be fulfilled) | A. At least ten attacks of spontaneous spinning or non-spinning vertigo<br>B. Duration less than 1 minute<br>C. Stereotyped phenomenology in a particular patient<br>D. Response to a treatment with carbamazepine/ oxcarbazepine<br>E. Not better accounted for by another diagnosis |
| Probable vestibular paroxysmia (each point needs to be fulfilled) | A. At least five attacks of spinning or non-spinning vertigo<br>B. Duration less than 5 minutes<br>C. Spontaneous occurrence or provoked by certain head movements<br>D. Stereotyped phenomenology in a particular patient<br>E. Not better accounted for by another diagnosis |

for VM are at present based on the guidelines of migraine.

b. *Vestibular paroxysmia:* VP is characterized by recurrent, spontaneous, short attacks of spinning or non-spinning vertigo which generally last less than 1 minute and occur in a series of up to 30 or more per day. Criteria for vertigo episodes of VP were defined by International Classification of Vestibular Disorders (ICVD) in 2016 and they are presented in Table 8.5 (62).

The proposed pathophysiology of VP is the segmental cross-compression of the vestibulo-cochlear nerve by a vascular loop at the cerebellopontine angle which leads to its demyelination. The pulsatile compression subsequently leads to ephaptic spreading of action potentials which trigger vertigo attacks. Surgical decompression has been reported with success and these patients respond well to medication with carbamazepine/oxcarbazepine (63, 64).

c. *Chronic subjective dizziness:* CSD is a diagnosis that has gained wide acceptance today. It is believed that the pathophysiology of this disorder is that the balance function and emotion share common neurological pathways; therefore, the balance disorder can provoke fear and vice versa, giving rise to the impairment in perception of space and motion. Anxiety

contributes to space and motion phobias in these patients. Staab and Ruckenstein have given insight into psychophysiological dizziness and have helped to define its characteristics, which are presented in Table 8.6 (65).

*Treatment:* The management of MD has to be holistic and needs to achieve control of acute attacks, prevent more attacks, preserve hearing and prevent development of bilateral MD.

In acute attacks, vestibular sedatives such as prochlorperazine or cinnarizine are used to relieve the patient of severe incapacitating vertigo. Betahistine has been used in doses up to 48 mg daily with good patient tolerance. It has been suggested that betahistine improves the microcirculation of vestibule and thus helps in preventing development of endolymphatic hydrops by regulating the formation of inner ear fluids and also increasing the reabsorption of inner ear fluids. There is also increasing evidence to support the effect of betahistine on central vestibular pathways which helps in vestibular compensation (66, 67).

Diuretics like acetazolamide, hydrochlorothiazides and triamterene have been used with the aim to reduce the endolymphatic hydrops. However, there is insufficient evidence according to a *Cochrane Systematic Review* regarding their efficacy in control of symptoms of MD (68). Dietary restrictions like low sodium (salt) and

## Table 8.6: Criteria for Diagnosis of Chronic Subjective Dizziness

| | |
|---|---|
| Chronic subjective dizziness | 1. *Subjective unsteadiness or dizziness:* Persistent (≥3 months) sensations of unsteadiness or non-vertiginous dizziness that are present on most days. These symptoms may be described as follows:<br>  a. Rocking, swaying or wobbling that is usually not apparent to others<br>  b. A feeling that the floor is moving or wavy<br>  c. Light-headed, foggy or cloudy in the head<br>  d. Heavy-headed or full in the head<br>  e. Spinning 'inside the head' without a perception of movement of the visual surround<br>  f. A feeling of dissociation from the environment<br>2. *Hypersensitivity to motion:* Chronic (≥3 months) hypersensitivity to one's own motion, which is not direction-specific, and to the movement of objects in the environment<br>3. *Visual dizziness (also known as visual vertigo):* Exacerbation of symptoms in settings with complex visual stimuli, such as displays in grocery stores or shopping malls, or when performing precision visual tasks (e.g. reading or working on a computer) |

caffeine intake are advised to prevent development of endolymphatic hydrops (69).

If intractable vertigo persists despite adequate medical management for adequate period, salvage therapy in the form of intratympanic injections of dexamethasone can be used (70). Intratympanic gentamicin has also been shown to give good vertigo control in 87.5% of patients; however, it is associated with the development of SNHL in 0–38.7% patients (71). A study comparing intratympanic gentamicin with intratympanic dexamethasone showed good vertigo control (93.5%) of patients in gentamicin arm at 2 years follow-up. In the dexamethasone arm, it showed good vertigo control in 61% of patients (72). Intratympanic gentamicin gives good control of vertigo in Tumarkin's crisis.

Surgical intervention in the form of selective Vestibular nerve section (VNS) has been proposed for cases where the above treatment fails. VNS has been shown to have higher efficacy and higher rates of hearing preservation as compared in intratympanic gentamicin (73). Transtympanic low-pressure therapy with Menniett device has little evidence to support its use for MD (74). Endolymphatic sac surgery for MD in medical therapy refractory cases has been supported in a 2014 meta-analysis. However, in a 2010 Cochrane review, this was not found to be effective (75, 76). Therefore, there is insufficient evidence to support the use of endolymphatic sac surgery for MD. The proposed treatment algorithm for MD is as depicted in Figure 8.7.

### Vestibular Neuritis

VN is a common cause of vertigo. It is caused by selective inflammation of vestibular end organs and the nerve. Its onset can be between 30 and 60 years; however, it is more common between 40 and 50 years (77).

The aetiology is considered to be viral in origin. This theory gets support from the fact that VN patients generally have a preceding history of upper respiratory tract infections with flu-like symptoms. Reactivation of Herpes Simplex Type 1 Virus (HSV) infection in vestibular ganglia and vestibular nuclei is also considered a possibility. There is evidence of other viral infections too in VN such as Epstein-Barr virus, Rubella virus, Cytomegalovirus, Adenovirus and Influenza viruses. Various other mechanisms such as vascular and immunological have also been proposed, which are supposed to be the more likely in elderly though not proven. Head trauma leading to vestibular nerve damage can also lead to VN. Again, falls are more common in elderly and can contribute to development of VN in elderly.

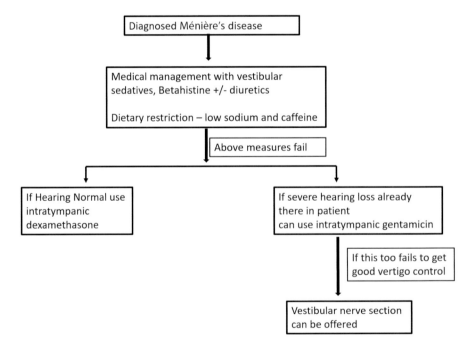

**Figure 8.7** Treatment algorithm for Ménière's disease.

VN patients present with sudden unilateral loss of vestibular function. Generally, in majority of cases, the Superior Vestibular nerve (SVN) and the end organs that it innervates (the superior and lateral SCCs and the utricle) are affected, while the function of the Inferior Vestibular nerve (IVN) and the end organs that it innervates (the posterior SCC and the saccule) are spared (78). However, in some cases, even the IVN may be affected (79). The reason for this more common SVN involvement is unclear, but it may be explained by the anatomical differences between the two divisions of the vestibular nerve. The commonest characteristic histopathology of VN found in the human temporal bone is degeneration of the SVN and vestibular ganglion with variable involvement of the neuroepithelium of the end organs and a deficiency in the population of the nerve fibres and microscopic findings of myelin degeneration. Temporal bone studies have revealed that the lateral bony channel of the SVN is seven times longer than the IVN and is three times longer than the singular nerve channel. In addition, the SVN courses through a longer area of severe narrowing compared with the inferior or singular nerves and a larger number of bony spicules occupy the superior vestibular channel. This renders the superior division of the vestibular nerve more susceptible to entrapment and possible ischaemic labyrinthine changes (80, 81).

The patient presents with acute onset of vertigo, nausea and vomiting in the absence of hearing loss or tinnitus. Typically, the vertigo of VN develops over a period of hours, remains severe for a few days and then resolves over next few weeks. Some patients can have residual imbalance that lasts for months. Mild transitory episodes of dizziness may recur over a period of 12–18 months.

On examination, the hallmark horizontal nystagmus beating to unaffected side is seen which reduces in intensity with optic fixation. Head Impulse Test (HIT) is positive for these patients. To perform HIT, the patient is asked to fix his or her eyes on a target such as examiner's nose. The examiner then generates a rapid head impulse of the patient while monitoring the patient's eyes for a Corrective Saccade (CS) response. A CS is a rapid eye movement generated by the brain to re-fixate the patient's eyes on the target. Subjects with normal vestibular function do not generate a CS after a head impulse (the eyes remain fixed on the target). Subjects with vestibular hypofunction may generate a CS after the head is quickly rotated towards the hypofunctional side and this is considered a positive HIT.

Hearing assessment does not reveal any deterioration in hearing. If hearing is reduced, then the diagnosis of labyrinthitis or the first episode of MD or a sudden bleed/cystic degeneration in a pre-existing vestibular schwannoma should be entertained. Such a patient should definitely undergo an MRI of brain to rule out retrocochlear pathology like a CP angle tumour.

The acute stage of VN should be treated with vestibular sedatives, antiemetics and vertigo precautions. Vestibular sedatives should be withdrawn as early as possible, preferably in 3 days so as to allow the vestibular system and its connections to compensate for the mismatched vestibular stimuli from each side. To help faster compensation, vestibular rehabilitation exercises should be advised to the patient. Vestibular rehabilitation exercises are effective, though may be less so in elderly (82).

As VN is an inflammatory condition, corticosteroids have been used in treating it. However, no significant advantage has been seen when compared to placebo in the recovery and there is insufficient evidence in literature at present to support use of corticosteroids for this (83). VN has also been considered to be of viral aetiology. However, no benefit with antivirals has been shown in acute phase (84).

## Posterior Circulation Stroke (PCS) and Vertigo

Posterior circulation is the blood supply to posterior brain which comprises the brainstem, thalamus, cerebellum, medial temporal lobes and occipital lobes (Figure 8.8). It comprises two vertebral arteries which join to form the basilar artery, two posterior cerebral arteries and their branches. PCS differ from strokes in anterior circulation with respect to clinical features. They can present with acute vestibular syndrome (AVS), which comprises acute onset vertigo, ataxia, vomiting and headache.

In the elderly, vertebrobasilar ischaemia or PCS is common and comprises 20% of all strokes (85). It needs to be differentiated from AVS due to VN/labyrinthitis. Evaluation for stroke is particularly important in patients who are older and have comorbidities like hypertension, ischaemic heart disease and diabetes or are on anticoagulants.

Dizziness is the presenting complaint in almost 47–75% of patients having PCS (85, 86). When vertigo occurs as a symptom of vertebrobasilar ischemic strokes, it is usually accompanied by other neurological symptoms or signs. Differentiating this vertigo from peripheral vestibular vertigo can be challenging at times, when the presentation

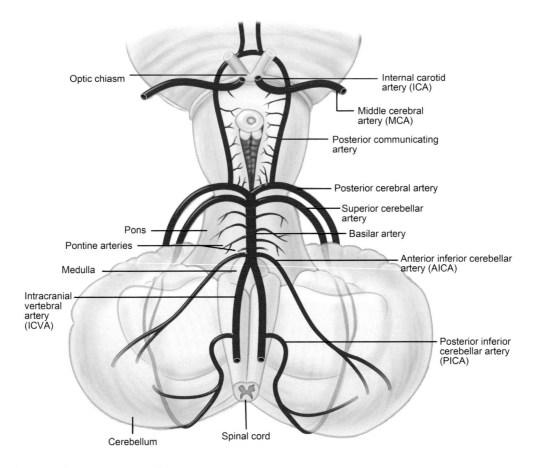

**Figure 8.8** Posterior circulation.

includes only an episode of isolated vertigo without any other symptoms or differentiating specific signs. Theoretically, a small infarct localized to structures such as the nodulus, root entry zone of the eighth nerve at the pontomedullary junction and vestibular nucleus can cause vertigo without other accompanying neurological symptoms or signs as all of these structures receive afferent vestibular inputs from the inner ear. Cerebellar infarction in the territory of posterior inferior cerebellar artery (PICA) is also known to cause isolated vestibular syndrome (Figure 8.9) (87–92).

The clinician thus needs to entertain the diagnosis of PCS while evaluating patients of AVS, especially in elderly with comorbidities. A useful clinical tool for assessing such a patient is a three-step bedside oculomotor examination (Head-Impulse-Nystagmus-Test-of-Skew [HINTS]) which can help differentiate benign peripheral AVS from a more sinister central AVS.

HINTS has the following three components:

1. *Horizontal head impulse test (h-HIT):* It can detect a deficient VOR function which has been shown to be the best clinical predictor of stroke in a setting of vertigo (93). This test was first described in 1988 by Halmagyi and Curthoys as a bedside clinical test for peripheral vestibular disease (94). If this test is positive, i.e. catch up saccades are seen on h-HIT, then AVS is due to peripheral aetiology. If it is negative, then it is a pointer towards stroke.

2. *Nystagmus:* Characteristic nystagmus of a peripheral vestibular pathology is a predominantly horizontal beating unidirectional nystagmus which increases in intensity when the patient looks in the direction of fast phase of the nystagmus. Vertical/direction changing/torsional nystagmus points towards a central pathology.

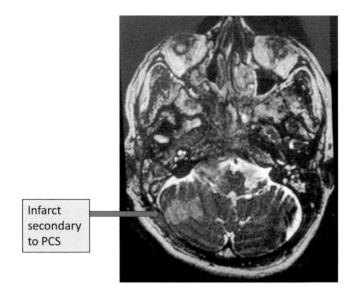

Infarct secondary to PCS

**Figure 8.9** Right side cerebellar infarct secondary to PCS. Patient presented with giddiness with initial nystagmus to left, which later evolved to direction-changing nystagmus.

3. *Skew deviation:* It is the vertical ocular misalignment seen on alternate cover test. It occurs because of mismatched right-left vestibular tone. Though it has been seen in patients with peripheral vestibulopathy, it has been primarily identified as a sign of pathology in the posterior cranial fossa. It is most commonly seen in cases of brainstem stroke.

Therefore, when HINTS is positive, it points to peripheral vestibular pathology; if it is negative, central pathology needs to be ruled out. HINTS has been shown to be more sensitive than the combined presence of all other traditional neurological signs for identifying stroke as a cause of AVS. Also a benign HINTS examination result at the bedside "rules out" stroke better than a negative diffusion-weighted MRI of brain in the first 24–48 hours after onset of symptom with acceptable specificity (96%) as the stoke may be evolving and may not be picked up in early MRI (95).

## CONCLUSION

The aetiology of dizziness in older patients differs significantly from that of younger patients due to their comorbidities, age-related degenerative changes in the body and usage of various medications. In elderly, presbyvertigo should be entertained in diagnosis and an adequate approach for dizziness at this age range should include the evaluation of cardiologic, neurological, visual and proprioceptive systems apart from the vestibular system. Revision of drugs that suppress vestibular function may be required. Hence, a holistic approach is a must for management of vertigo in elderly.

## KEY LEARNING POINTS

1. Falls are common in elderly patients leading to severe injuries and in many of them falls are related to vertigo.

2. Vertigo in elderly most of the time are benign peripheral in aetiology; however, a few of these patients may harbour a serious, potentially life-threatening cause, such as stroke.

3. Elderly patients need to be evaluated comprehensively with adequate evaluation of their vestibular, cardiovascular and central nervous system functions. It should be kept in mind that visual problems and proprioceptive function decline can be contributory. Presbyvertigo should also be entertained in the diagnosis.

4. HINTS is a useful bedside tool to differentiate peripheral from central vertigo.

5. Early imaging should be considered whenever there is a doubt of central pathology.

## ACKNOWLEDGEMENT

We acknowledge Maj Pavitra (Junior Resident ENT, AFMC) for making anatomical diagrams.

# REFERENCES

1. Tinetti ME, Williams CS, Gill TM. Dizziness among older adults: a possible geriatric syndrome. Ann Intern Med. 2000;132(5):337–44.

2. Colledge NR, Wilson JA, Macintyre CC, MacLennan WJ. The prevalence and characteristics of dizziness in an elderly community. Age Ageing. 1994;23(2):117–20.

3. Sloane PD, Coeytaux RR, Beck RS, Dallara J. Dizziness: state of the science. Ann Intern Med. 2001;134(9 Pt 2): 823–32.

4. Jonsson R, Sixt E, Landahl S, Rosenhall U. Prevalence of dizziness and vertigo in an urban elderly population. J Vestib Res. 2004;14(1):47–52.

5. Barin K, Dodson EE. Dizziness in the elderly. Otolaryngol Clin North Am. 2011;44:437–54.

6. Agrawal Y, Carey JP, DellaSantina CC, Schubert MC, Minor LB. Disorders of balance and vestibular function in US adults: data from the national health and nutrition examination survey, 2001–2004. Arch Intern Med. 2009;169:938–44.

7. EkvallHansson E, Magnusson M. Vestibular asymmetry predicts falls among elderly patients with multi-sensory dizziness. BMC Geriatr. 2013:13:77.

8. Kannus P, Parkkari J, Koskinen S, et al. Fall-induced injuries and deaths among older adults. JAMA. 1999;281:1895–9.

9. Mueller M, Strobl R, Jahn K, Linkohr B, Peters A, Grill E. Burden of disability attributable to vertigo and dizziness in the aged: results from the KORA-Age study. Eur J Public Health. 2014;24:802–7.

10. Piker EG, Jacobson GP. Self-report symptoms differ between younger and older dizzy patients. Otol Neurotol. 2014;35(5):873–9.

11. Tuunainen E, Jantti P, Poe D, Rasku J, Toppila E, Pyykko I. Characterization of presbyequilibrium among institutionalized elderly persons. Auris Nasus Larynx. 2012;39:577–82.

12. Tuunainen E, Poe D, Jantti P, et al. Presbyequilibrium in the oldest old, a combination of vestibular, oculomotor and postural deficits. Aging Clin Exp Res. 2011;23:364–71.

13. Woo N, Kim SH. Sarcopenia influences fall-related injuries in community-dwelling older adults. Geriatr Nurs. 2014;35:279–82.

14. Saber Tehrani AS, Kattah JC, Mantokoudis G, et al. Small strokes causing severe vertigo: frequency of false-negative MRIs and nonlacunar mechanisms. Neurology. 2014;83(2):169–73.

15. Dagan E, Wolf M, Migirov LM. Why do geriatric patients attend otolaryngology emergency rooms? Isr Med Assoc J. 2012;14:633–6.

16. Rosenhall U, Rubin W. Degenerative changes in the human vestibular sensory epithelia. Acta Otolaryngol. 1975;79(1/2):67–80.

17. Richter E. Quantitative study of human Scarpa's ganglion and vestibular sensory epithelia. Acta Otolaryngol. 1980;90(3/4):199–208.

18. Merchant S, Velázquez-Villaseñor L, Tsuji K, et al. Temporal bone studies of the human peripheral vestibular system: normative vestibular hair cell data. Ann Otol Rhinol Laryngol Suppl. 2000;181:3–13.

19. Ishiyama G. Imbalance and vertigo: the aging human vestibular periphery. Semin Neurol. 2009;29(5): 491–9.

20. Ishiyama A, Lopez I, Ishiyama G, et al. Unbiased quantification of the microdissected human Scarpa's ganglion neurons. Laryngoscope. 2004;114(8): 1496–9.

21. Lopez I, Ishiyama G, Tang Y, et al. Estimation of the number of nerve fibers in the human vestibular end organs using unbiased stereology and immuno-histochemistry. J Neurosci Methods. 2005;145(1/2): 37–46.

22. Tang Y, Lopez I, Baloh R. Age-related change of the neuronal number in the human medial vestibular nucleus: a stereological investigation. J Vestib Res. 2001;11(6):357–63.

23. Lyon M, Davis J. Age-related blood flow and capillary changes in the rat utricular macula: a quantitative stereological and microsphere study. J Assoc Res Otolaryngol. 2002;3(2):167–73.

24. Lyon M, Wanamaker H. Blood flow and assessment of capillaries in the aging rat posterior canal crista. Hear Res. 1993;67(1/2):157–65.

25. Johnsson L, Hawkins J. Vascular changes in the human inner ear associated with aging. Ann Otol Rhinol Laryngol. 1972;81(3):364–76.

26. Adolfo MB. Visual vertigo syndrome: clinical and posturography findings. J Neurol Neurosurg Psychiatry. 1995;59:472–6.

27. Lord S, Clark R, Webster I. Visual acuity and contrast sensitivity in relation to falls in an elderly population. Age Ageing. 1991;20(3):175–81.

28. Lord S. Visual risk factors for falls in older people. Age Ageing. 2006;35(Suppl 2):ii 42–5.

29. Ishigaki H, Miyao M. Implications for dynamic visual acuity with changes in aged and sex. Percept Mot Skills. 1994;78(2):363–9.

30. Kerber K, Ishiyama G, Baloh R. A longitudinal study of oculomotor function in normal older people. Neurobiol Aging. 2006;27(9):1346–53.

31. Moschner C, Baloh R. Age-related changes in visual tracking. J Gerontol. 1994;49(5):M235–8.

32. Wiles P, Pearce S, Rice P, et al. Vibration perception threshold: influence of age, height, sex, and smoking, and calculation of accurate centile values. Diabet Med. 1991;8(2):157–61.

33. Sturnieks D, St George R, Lord S. Balance disorders in the elderly. Neurophysiol Clin. 2008;38(6):467–78.

34. Larsson L, Ramamurthy B. Aging-related changes in skeletal muscle: mechanisms and interventions. Drugs Aging. 2000;17(4):303–16.

35. Faulkner J, Larkin L, Claflin D, et al. Age-related changes in the structure and function of skeletal muscles. Clin Exp Pharmacol Physiol. 2007;34(11):1091–6.

36. Roos M, Rice C, Vandervoort A. Age-related changes in motor unit function. Muscle Nerve. 1997;20(6): 679–90.

37. McPherson D, Whitaker S, Wrobel B. DDX: Disequilibrium of aging. In: Goebel JA, editor. Practical Management of the Dizzy Patient. Philadelphia: Lippincott Williams & Wilkins, 2008, p. 297–344.

38. O'Connor K, Loughlin P, Redfern M, et al. Postural adaptations to repeated optic flow stimulation in older adults. Gait Posture. 2008;28(3):385–91.

39. Neuhauser HK, von Brevern M, Radtke A, et al. Epidemiology of vestibular vertigo: a neurotologic survey of the general population. Neurology. 2005;65(6):898–904.

40. Sogebi OA, Ariba AJ, Otulana TO, Osalusi BS. Vestibular disorders in elderly patients: characteristics, causes and consequences. Pan Afr Med J. 2014;19:146.

41. Katsarkas A. Dizziness in aging: the clinical experience. Geriatrics. 2008;63:18–20.

42. Cupulolithiasis SHF. Arch Otolaryngol. 1969;90:765–8.

43. Hall SF, Ruby RF, Mcclure JA. The mechanics of benign paroxysmal vertigo. J Otolaryngol. 1979;8:151–8.

44. Gold DR, Morris L, Kheradmand A, Schubert MC. Repositioning maneuvers for benign paroxysmal positional vertigo. Curr Treat Options Neurol. 2014;16(8):307.

45. Committee on Hearing and Equilibrium guidelines for the diagnosis and evaluation of therapy in Meniere's disease. Otolaryngol Head Neck Surg. 1995;113(3):181–5.

46. Lindsay JR. Labyrinthine dropsy and Ménière's disease. Arch Otolaryngol. 1942;35:853–67.

47. Altmann F, Fowler EP Jr. Histological findings in Ménière's symptom complex. Ann Otol Rhinol Laryngol. 1943;52:52–80.

48. Cawthorne T. Meniere's disease. Ann Otol Rhinol Laryngol. 1947;56:18–38.

49. Ballester M, Liard P, Vibert D, Hausler R. Meniere's disease in the elderly. Otol Neurotol. 2002;23(1):73–8.

50. Shojaku H, Watanabe Y, Yagi T, et al. Changes in the characteristics of definite Meniere's disease over time in Japan: a long-term survey by the Peripheral Vestibular Disorder Research Committee of Japan, formerly the Meniere's Disease Research Committee of Japan. Acta Otolaryngol. 2009;129(2):155–60.

51. Paparella MM, Costa SS, Fox R, Yoo TH. Meniere's disease and other labyrinthine diseases. In: Paparella MM, Shumrick DA, Gluckmann J, Meyerhoff WL, editors. Otolaryngology, Vol. II: Otology, 3rd ed. Philadelphia: WB Saunders, 1991, p. 1689–714.

52. Paparella MM. The natural course of Meniere's disease. In: Filipo R, Barbara M, editors. Proceedings of the Third International Symposium on Meniere's Disease. Amsterdam: Kugler, 1994, p. 9–20.

53. Paparella MM. Pathogenesis of Meniere's disease and Meniere's syndrome. Acta Otolaryngol (Stockh). 1984;(Suppl 406):10–25.

54. Lopez-Escamez JA, Carey J, Chung WH, et al. Diagnostic criteria for Meniere's disease. J Vestib Res. 2015;25(1):1–7.

55. Perez-Garrigues H, Lopez-Escamez JA, Perez P, et al. Time course of episodes of definitive vertigo in Ménière's disease. Arch Otolaryngol Head Neck Surg. 2008;134:1149–54.

56. Stahle J, Friberg U, Svedberg A. Long term progression of Meniere's disease. Acta Otolaryngol Suppl. 1991;485:78–83.

57. Merchant SN, Adams JC, Nadol JB Jr. Pathophysiology of Meniere's syndrome: are symptoms caused by endolymphatic hydrops? Otol Neurotol. 2005;26(1):74–81.

58. Pyykko I, Nakashima T, Yoshida T, et al. Menieres disease: a reappraisal supported by a variable latency of symptoms and the MRI visualisation of endolymphatic hydrops. BMJ Open. 2013;3(2):pii:e001555

59. McClure JA, Copp JC, Lycett P. Recovery nystagmus in Ménière's disease. Laryngoscope. 1981;91(10):1727–37.

60. Zhang Y, Liu B, Wang R, Jia R, Gu X. Characteristics of the cochlear symptoms and functions in Meniere's disease. Chin Med J (Engl). 2016;129(20):2445–50.

61. Lempert T, Olesen J, Furman J, et al. Vestibular migraine: diagnostic criteria. J Vestib Res. 2012; 22(4):167–72.

62. Strupp M, Lopez-Escamez JA, Kim J-S, et al. Vestibular paroxysmia: diagnostic criteria. J Vestib Res. 2016;26(5–6):409–15.

63. Moller MB, Moller AR, Jannetta PJ, Jho HD, Sekhar LN. Microvascular decompression of the eighth nerve in patients with disabling positional vertigo: selection criteria and operative results in 207 patients. Acta Neurochir (Wien). 1993;125:75–82.

64. Hufner K, Barresi D, Glaser M, et al. Vestibular paroxysmia: diagnostic features and medical treatment. Neurology 2008;71(13):1006–14.

65. Staab JP, Ruckenstein MJ, Amsterdam JD. A prospective trial of sertraline for chronic subjective dizziness. Laryngoscope. 2004;114(9):1637–41.

66. Bergquist F, Ruthven A, Ludwig M, Dutia MB. Histaminergic and glycinergic modulation of GABA release in the vestibular nuclei of normal and labyrinth ectomised rats. J Physiol. 2006;577(Pt 3):857–68.

67. Tighilet B, Léonard J, Watabe I, Bernard-Demanze L, Lacour M. Betahistine treatment in a cat model of vestibular pathology: pharmacokinetic and pharmacodynamic approaches. Front Neurol. 2018;9:431.

68. Thirlwall AS, Kundu S. Diuretics for Meniere's disease or syndrome. Cochrane Database Syst Rev. 2006;(3):CD003599.

69. Luxford E, Berliner KI, Lee J, Luxford WM. Dietary modification as adjunct treatment in Meniere's disease: patient willingness and ability to comply. Otol Neurotol. 2013;34(8):438–43.

70. Phillips JS, Westerberg B. Intratympanic steroids for Meniere's disease or syndrome. Cochrane Database Syst Rev. 2011;(7):CD008514.

71. Huon LK, Fang TY, Wang PC. Outcomes of intratympanic gentamicin injection to treat Meniere's disease. Otol Neurotol. 2012;33(5):706–14.

72. Casani AP, Piaggi P, Cerchiai N, et al. Intra tympanic treatment of intractable unilateral Meniere disease: gentamicin ordexamethasone? A randomized controlled trial. Otolaryngol Head Neck Surg. 2012;146(3):430–7.

73. Hillman TA, Chen DA, Arriaga MA. Vestibular nerve section versus intratympanic gentamicin for Meniere's disease. Laryngoscope. 2004;114(2):216–22.

74. Van Sonsbeek S, Pullens B, van Benthem PP. Positive pressure therapy for Meniere's disease or syndrome. Cochrane Database Syst Rev. 2015;(3):CD008419.

75. Sood AJ, Lambert PR, Nguyen SA, Meyer TA. Endolymphatic sac surgery for Meniere's disease: a systematic review and meta-analysis. Otol Neurotol. 2014;35(6):1033–45.

76. Pullens B, Giard JL, Verschuur HP, vanBenthem PP. Surgery for Meniere's disease. Cochrane Database Syst Rev. 2010;(1):CD005395.

77. Sekitani T, Imate Y,Noguchi T, Inokuma T. Vestibular neuronitis: pidemiological survey by questionnaire in Japan. Acta Oto-Laryngol Suppl. 1993;(503):9–12.

78. Aw ST, Fetter M, Cremer PD,Karlberg M,Halmagyi GM. Individual semicircular canal function in superior and inferior vestibular neuritis. Neurology. 2001;57(5):768–74.

79. Monstad P, Økstad S, Mygland Å. Inferior vestibular neuritis: 3 cases with clinical features of acute vestibular neuritis, normal calorics but indications of saccular failure. BMC Neurol. 2006;6:45.

80. Goebel JA, O'Mara W, Gianoli G. Anatomic considerations in vestibular neuritis. Otol Neurotol. 2001;22(4):512–8.

81. Gianoli G, Goebel J, Mowry S, Poomipannit P. Anatomic differences in the lateral vestibular nerve channels and their implications in vestibular neuritis. Otol Neurotol. 2005;26(3):489–94.

82. Michelle NM, Hillier SL. Vestibular rehabilitation for unilateral peripheral vestibular dysfunction. Cochrane Syst Rev. 2015;1:CD005397.

83. Fishman JM, Burgess C, Waddell A. Corticosteroids for the treatment of idiopathic acute vestibular dysfunction (vestibular neuritis). Cochrane Database Syst Rev. 2011;(5):D008607.

84. Strupp M, Zingler VC, Arbusow V, et al. Methylprednisolone, valacyclovir, or the combination for vestibular neuritis N Engl J Med. 2004;351:354–61.

85. Savitz SI, Caplan LR. Vertebrobasilar disease. N Engl J Med. 2005;352:2618–26.

86. Searls DE, Pazdera L, Korbel E, Vysata O, Caplan LR. Symptoms and signs of posterior circulation ischemia in the New England Medical Center posterior circulation registry. Arch Neurol. 2012;69:346–51.

87. Choi KD, Lee H, Kim JS. Vertigo in brainstem and cerebellar strokes. Curr Opin Neurol. 2013;26:90–5.

88. Grad A, Baloh RW. Vertigo of vascular origin: clinical and electronystagmographic features in 84 cases. Arch Neurol. 1989;46:281–4.

89. Kim HA, Lee H. Recent advances in central acute vestibular syndrome of a vascular cause. J Neurol Sci. 2012;321:17–22.

90. Lee H, Sohn SI, Cho YW, et al. Cerebellar infarction presenting isolated vertigo: frequency and vascular topographical patterns. Neurology. 2006;67:1178–83.

91. Moon IS, Kim JS, Choi KD, et al. Isolated nodular infarction. Stroke. 2009;40:487–91.

92. Kim HA, Lee H. Isolated vestibular nucleus infarction mimicking acute peripheral vestibulopathy. Stroke. 2010;41:1558–60.

93. Newman-Toker DE, Kattah JC, Alvernia JE, Wang DZ. Normal head impulse test differentiates acute cerebellar strokes from vestibular neuritis. Neurology. 2008;70:2378–85.

94. Halmagyi GM, Curthoys IS. A clinical sign of canal paresis. Arch Neurol. 1988;245:737–9.

95. Kattah JC, Talkad AV, Wang DZ et al. HINTS to diagnose stroke in Acute Vestibular Syndrome. Stroke. 2009 (Nov); 40 (11):3504–10.

# TINNITUS SYMPTOMATOLOGY: DIAGNOSIS AND MANAGEMENT

# 9 Tinnitus Symptomatology: Diagnosis and Management

*Abha Kumari and Uma Patnaik*

## CONTENTS

## INTRODUCTION

The word tinnitus is derived from Latin word *tinnire*, meaning 'to ring'. The first recorded use of the word was in 1693 in Blanchard's physician dictionary. Since then, many attempts have been made for a scientific description and classification by various scientists (1). Tinnitus can be defined as the perception of sound in the absence of external or internal acoustic source or electric stimulation, and is a common reason for an Ear, Nose and Throat (ENT) consultation (2). It can be acute, lasting from minutes to weeks or chronic lasting for more than 3 months. Severity can range from mild to severe, with potential for disruption of daily activity. The prevalence of tinnitus is around 30% in the general population and 1–5% of individuals with tinnitus have severe or disabling tinnitus impairing their daily activities (3–5). It can occur in isolation or as a part of other diseases. The effects of tinnitus depend on the aetiology and vary from person to person. Despite being a debilitating illness with an adverse effect on the quality of life, no well-established single treatment is available. A comprehensive history, complete ENT and systemic examination and multidisciplinary approach is required for appropriate management. We will discuss the various forms of tinnitus, approach to diagnosis and available management options.

## HISTORY

The earliest attempts to understand tinnitus began in ancient Egypt and first attempt to treat tinnitus was made in 2500 BC by instillation of medicine into the ear (6). After that, the need to understand and treat tinnitus was felt in many civilizations like the Roman and Byzantine.

## EPIDEMIOLOGY

Various studies have shown that the prevalence of tinnitus is affected by age, race, socioeconomic status, noise exposure and hearing status (7). The prevalence of tinnitus is more in men and increases with age. It is seen to be more in Caucasians than Afro-Americans and in lower socio-economic status. Studies showed no significant difference in the laterality of tinnitus (8).

Cole et al. showed that the tinnitus was more severe in patients with hearing loss (9). Various risk factors have been identified like genetic predisposition, type D personality, food low in carbohydrates, high in fruits and caffeine, smoking and alcohol consumption, low socio-economic class etc. (10–12). Other risk factors are hypertension, cardiovascular diseases, head injury and use of ototoxic drugs like salicylates, aminoglycosides and quinine.

## CLASSIFICATION

Historically, various attempts have been made to classify tinnitus based on aetiology or symptoms. Tinnitus can be unilateral or bilateral, within the ear or outside. The character can vary from hissing, sizzling or buzzing to more than one sound. Tinnitus can be acute or recent onset if it is present for less than 6 months and thereafter it is classified aschronic (13). Tinnitus can be continuous when present throughout the day or intermittent.

Shulman in 1980 classified tinnitus into two main varieties: otological and neurotological (14).

Otological causes are due to diseases of the external ear, middle ear, ossicles or middle ear muscle abnormality. This can be differentiated based on history and physical examination.

Under neurotological classification, most of the patients have subjective idiopathic tinnitus diagnosed after complete cochleovestibular evaluation, including radiology and audiology evaluation. Nodar, in 1996, gave another classification which can be used to describe almost any type of tinnitus. It can be remembered with use of mnemonic ABC-CLAP (15):

A – aurium (one ear)

B – both ear

C – centred in head

c  cause

C – composition: buzz, roar, hissing

L – loudness

A – annoyance due to tinnitus

P – pitch

The most commonly used and simplest classification divides tinnitus into subjective and objective type (Table 9.1) (16, 17). Subjective tinnitus is perceived only by the patient and not by the observer. The prevalence ranges from 8% to 30% based on definition, severity and diagnostic methods (3, 5, 18). Objective tinnitus can be perceived by both the patient and examiner. It can be heard by means of stethoscope or ear-level microphones. Tinnitus can be pulsatile or non-pulsatile. Pulsatile tinnitus is further classified as synchronous or non-synchronous in relation to the heartbeat.

## PATHOPHYSIOLOGY

The understanding of pathophysiological mechanism of tinnitus is a major challenge as it is complex, involving both auditory and non-auditory systems. Recent theories assume the involvement of extra-auditory brain regions, which engage multiple active dynamic and

## Table 9.1: Classification of Tinnitus

| Objective tinnitus | Pulsatile | • Synchronous<br>  – *Arterial causes:* AV fistula, carotid artery stenosis, persistent stapedial artery, paraganglioma – glomus tympanicum/ Jugulare<br>  – *Venous:* Venous hum, sigmoid sinus or Jugular bulb anomaly<br><br>• Asynchronous<br>  – Palatal myoclonus, tensor tympani or stapedial myoclonus |
|---|---|---|
| | Non-pulsatile | • Eustachian tube dysfunction, spontaneous otoacoustic emission |
| | Tinnitus associated with hearing loss – presbycusis, NIHL, Ménière's disease, acoustic trauma | |
| Subjective tinnitus | *Somatic tinnitus:* The loudness, tone and laterality of tinnitus can be modulated by somatic modulation like TM joint dysfunction, cervical dysfunction, gaze /cutaneous evoked | |
| | *Typewriter tinnitus:* It is an intermittent, staccato tinnitus similar to typewriter's tapping. It is often triggered by physiological stimulus appropriate for that cranial nerve. It is mostly seen in elderly, chronic in nature and shows good response to carbmazepine (16). Vascular compression of auditory nerve on the side of the tinnitus may be seen (17) | |
| | Musical/complex | |
| | Intrusive | |

overlapping networks for tinnitus to reach conscious perception.

Jastreboff stated that the origin of tinnitus is related to aberrant neural activity in the auditory system (19). This auditory perception that results from aberrant neural activity at cochlear level and perceived through auditory pathways is referred to as peripheral tinnitus (19, 20). Many pathological processes which damage the auditory pathway like cochlear OHC damage due to noise, aminoglycosides, calcium channel dysfunction and neurotransmitters like glutamate have been proposed in generation of tinnitus (19, 21).

Initially, cochlear origin of tinnitus was favoured as a link between high-frequency hearing loss and tinnitus. However, current research appears to indicate the importance of central auditory pathways (22–24). Central tinnitus refers to origin of tinnitus at auditory brain centres by aberrant neural activity (25–28). Damage to the auditory system can also lead to central mechanisms like increased spontaneous firing, reorganization of neurons and spontaneous synchronized activity in auditory cortex, in response to damage to peripheral auditory system leading to generation of tinnitus (29–31).

The psychological theory given by Hallem et al. works on bio-psycho-social model wherein moderating and mediating factors like psychological and social factors impact the individual's response to tinnitus (32). Relaxation therapy and cognitive behaviour therapy to reduce the impact of tinnitus are based on this principle (33).

## DIFFERENT FORMS OF TINNITUS

The presentation of tinnitus can be clinically heterogenous according to aetiology, perceptual characteristics, accompanying symptoms and its modulating factors. Different subtypes can be tinnitus associated with hearing loss, post-traumatic tinnitus, tinnitus with temporo-mandibular disorder and tinnitus with hyperacusis. These different forms vary in pathophysiology and response to therapeutic intervention. However, clear-cut differentiating criteria for subtypes are still missing and research may be required for this (34).

The management of tinnitus is multidisciplinary and must be individualized based on the subtype. A stepwise approach is advised to reach a conclusion and treat the condition accordingly. Some of the rare subtypes may benefit from specific treatment of the underlying pathology like cochlear implantation in unilateral deafness, microvascular

decompression in tinnitus arising from microvascular conflict and carbamazepine in typewriters tinnitus (35–37).

## APPROACH TO A PATIENT WITH TINNITUS

A stepwise approach, including detailed history, clinical examination, assessment of tinnitus and its severity based on self-administered questionnaires, hearing status, audiological measurements of tinnitus, imaging if necessary, is required in all cases. Further diagnostic tests like metabolic workup for catecholamine secreting tumours are indicated based on case subtypes.

### Audiological Tests

Pure tone audiometry is the basic investigation done in all cases of tinnitus. Hearing loss is present in conditions like presbycusis, NIHL etc. Other tests which can be done are speech reception threshold, speech discrimination score, otoacoustic emissions, and auditory brainstem response.

### Tinnitus: Clinical Tests

These include several tests like tinnitus localization tests, tinnitus pitch matching, loudness matching and determining the minimum masking level. Though the reliability of these tests is variable, these tests are helpful in optimal management (34).

- *Tinnitus loudness measure:* Here a pure tone auditory stimulus is presented to the patient, and he is asked which matches best with his tinnitus loudness. This has therapeutic benefit as the tinnitus loudness measure is often used to ascertain the outcome of drug treatment and surgery (35, 36).

- *Pitch matching:* Here the patient is presented multiple pure tones, and he is directed to select the tone that best matches the pitch of his tinnitus.

- *Minimum masking level (MML):* It is the minimum level of broadband noise required to make the tinnitus inaudible for the patient.

### Tinnitus Questionnaires

Several self-assessment tests to grade tinnitus are available, which form an important tool for research (37). These are used in clinical practice to determine functional, physical and psychological effects of tinnitus and what measures the patient is using to cope with it. Some of the scales commonly in use are tinnitus handicap

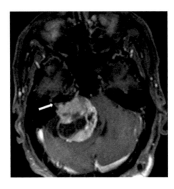

**Figure 9.1** Vestibular schwannoma (right). Axial CEMRI image shows heterogeneously enhancing well-defined right cerebellopontine angle mass, extends into and expands the adjacent portion of the internal acoustic meatus (arrow), with lesion's morphology imparting ice-cream cone-like appearance. The presence of canalicular extension and non-enhancing areas within the mass is consistent with diagnosis of vestibular schwannoma.

questionnaire, the tinnitus handicap inventory, the mini tinnitus questionnaire, tinnitus functional index and tinnitus coping style questionnaire (38–42).

### Imaging

MRI is considered useful in cases of asymmetrical sensorineural hearing loss, unilateral tinnitus, when there is suspicion of vestibular schwannoma, sudden sensorineural hearing loss or to rule out a retrocochlear pathology. Figure 9.1 illustrates a case of vestibular schwannoma who presented with unilateral tinnitus.

### Comorbidities Associated with Tinnitus

Psychological conditions like anxiety, depression and mood disorders are often associated with severe debilitating tinnitus (43, 44). It may be accompanied with insomnia and other emotional disturbances. Their identification and proper treatment are important as they interfere with clinical improvement. Some of the tests which can be done in clinic are beck depression inventory, hospital anxiety depression scale, insomnia severity index (45, 46).

### TREATMENT

The treatment of tinnitus is multipronged and the results are variable. They vary from a good outcome in cases where the pathology is treatable, such as cholesteatoma and sudden sensorineural hearing loss, to poor outcomes in idiopathic chronic tinnitus sufferers.

Various treatment options are available and are discussed here:

- Counselling and reassurance
- Hearing aids
- Tinnitus Retraining Therapy (TRT)
- Other sound therapy
- Cognitive behavioural therapy
- Other psychological treatment
- Laser
- Surgery
- Pharmacological treatment
- Alternative treatment

### Counselling and Reassurance

This forms the initial step in the management. The patient is educated about the condition, its causes and effects. Patients are counselled by practitioners that the perceived loudness of tinnitus and its emotional impact will improve with time. Various RCTs have supported its role (47–49). A systematic review with meta-analysis done by Phillips et al. showed that there is improvement in global severity of tinnitus over time in patients taking no intervention or waiting list controls, but the effect is highly variable across individuals (50).

### Hearing Aids

As hearing loss and tinnitus are often linked, use of hearing aids helps in ameliorating symptoms in patients with audiometrically proven hearing loss and tinnitus (51). The results are good if supported with proper counselling and education along with hearing amplification (52).

### Tinnitus Retraining Therapy

The aim of TRT is to make the patient habituated for tinnitus with combination of sound enrichment and appropriate counselling. This consists of combining counselling with sound therapy based on neurophysiological model of tinnitus. The aim of this approach is to break the functional connection between auditory and limbic and autonomic nervous system so that patient becomes habituated to tinnitus perception and its reactions. The main goal is to reclassify tinnitus into one of the neural stimuli and to decrease the strength of tinnitus-related neuronal activity. It works to delink the connection between auditory and other systems in the brain, so any aetiology of tinnitus including somatosounds can be treated via this modality (53). Studies

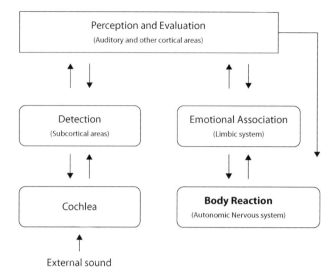

**Figure 9.2** Tinnitus retraining therapy model.

have compared TRT with waiting list controls and found a significant reduction in TQ score (54, 55). TRT model is depicted in Figure 9.2.

#### Other Sound Therapies

Sound therapy is given either as a part of TRT or separate treatment to suppress or mask tinnitus in 95% of cases of tinnitus (56). The principle behind this sound is that externally generated sound is less disturbing than the tinnitus and it masks the tinnitus.

This sound can be delivered by various methods like hearing aids which produce masking by amplifying ambient sound, tinnitus maskers or sound generators which generate wide band noise, white noise generators and external sound generators to modify environmental sound. Such devices can deliver a masking or sound therapy at a mixing point and that depends on the output level set on the device. Another method is use of non-wearable devices like electric fans, water features, wind chimes and electronic external sound generators that produce sound in the external environment of the patient. Sound therapy is supposed to facilitate the habituation process.

*New sound therapy:* Various devices are available which deliver sound therapy that specifically targets tinnitus instead of simply masking it.

*Neuromonics tinnitus therapy (NTT):* It is an acoustic desensitization protocol which combines features of sound therapy, systematic desensitization and directive counselling along with coping strategies, stress and sleep management. Here the neuromonics sound processor device

delivers music in a dynamic range with peaks and troughs in it through a set of earphones with the idea to compensate for any hearing loss. The tinnitus is audible in troughs with intention that slowly patient gets habituated to tinnitus. Initially the patient listens to intermittent tinnitus with perception of tinnitus alternating with tinnitus masking through music. Gradually therapeutic music is given in the treatment programme. The patient gets gradually habituated to the tinnitus and it is accompanied along with education and counselling. An RCT done showed promising results similar to ear-level sound generators (57).

*Serenade:* Serenade delivers sound therapy in dubbed "S" tones and uses temporally altered sound in range of patient's tinnitus and his hearing loss. It has shown benefit as compared to wide band sound (58).

*Noise cancellation:* Here the therapeutic sound is delivered which cancels out the tinnitus for one third of the total time. Limited data has been available for its use (59).

*Ultrasound:* Ultrasound delivers high-frequency sound through bone conduction directly to cochlea without hindering with sound transmission in the normal auditory system.

*Transcranial magnetic stimulation (TMS):* It is a method based on stimulation of neuronal tissue by application of brief, intense electric current to the scalp. Magnetic stimulation leads to changes in neuronal activity in different regions of the cortex. The depth of penetration is less than 2 cm (60). TMS is used to treat tinnitus by inhibiting abnormal cortical activities in the affected area. Repetitive TMS refers to regularly repeated TMS delivered to a single scalp site to attenuate the tinnitus-associated hyperactivity in the primary auditory cortex and other associated areas. Repetitive TMS is given with aim to suppress tinnitus for a longer duration of time. It can induce alterations in neuronal activity which outlast the actual stimulation period for a longer duration of time. Many studies have suggested the use of radiological findings to assist in positioning of the coil to increase efficacy. Studies have been done with use of PET, EEG, and functional MRI to determine the hyperactive auditory cortex area. Mennemeir et al. showed no evidence for use of PET in guiding effective treatment, nor was any advantage gained in stimulating one hemisphere or the other (61). Khedr et al. in their studies found a decrease in the mean score of tinnitus in patients of chronic tinnitus with the use of rTMS (62). Other studies have, however, failed to show improvement in tinnitus with rTMS (63, 64).

### Cognitive Behaviour Therapy (CBT)

This is the main psychological treatment for tinnitus. CBT is a form of psychotherapy aimed to reduce the reactivity associated with tinnitus. It does not reduce the loudness of tinnitus but with help of behavioural therapies, it helps the patient to overcome the association between tinnitus and counterproductive responses (avoiding tinnitus-increasing activities). Cognitive therapies modify the relationship between thoughts and emotions associated with experience of tinnitus (65, 66). Behaviour is also modified as the actions taken by person in response to tinnitus make them stressful and deteriorate their quality of life. The patient avoids the opportunity to disprove or question the negative cognition. This avoidance behaviour inhibits habituation to tinnitus. So, during therapy, these unhelpful behaviours are identified and change is supported. Cognitive and behavioural therapy helps to modify the behavioural responses and dysfunctional thought process that maintain adverse reaction.

When a person hears tinnitus or experiences negatively biased interpretations or thoughts, it produces a dysfunctional emotional or behavioural response. Cognitive and behavioural therapy identifies this biased or irrational thinking style and replaces it with a more adaptive alternative helpful thought/response. The person learns that tinnitus is no longer related to being in distress. It overall reduces generalized anxiety and depression associated with tinnitus and improves self-reported quality of life.

A meta-analysis revealed clear evidence that CBT is effective in reducing tinnitus-related distress and has a significant positive effect on mood (67). A Cochrane review also showed improvement in tinnitus-related distress after CBT but no effect on tinnitus loudness (68). The evidence in meta-analytic reviews recommend CBT for the treatment of tinnitus. However, the result depends on willingness of patient to undergo CBT.

### Other Psychological Treatment

Mindfulness meditation and acceptance and commitment therapy are also used in the treatment of tinnitus and have been shown to reduce stress (69, 70). Here emphasis is given on accepting unwanted thoughts, sufferings or feelings as the attempts to resist these can lead to more stress. These psychological approaches do not make tinnitus to disappear, but enable the person to lead a more normal and meaningful life by reducing distress.

### Laser

Some theories have proposed increased cell proliferation, increased blood flow to inner ear and growth factor secretion as probable mechanisms of low-power laser irradiation in treatment of tinnitus (58, 70, 71).

The role of low-power lasers has been studied in chronic tinnitus and has shown good results (72, 73). A study done by Mirvakilli et al. on 120 patients of SNHL with tinnitus showed a statistically significant difference between the group treated by LLR than control group in tinnitus severity at the end of 3 months (74). However, two more trials showed no benefit of LLR over placebo in tinnitus severity (75, 76).

### Surgery

- *Cochlear implant:* A significant suppression of tinnitus has been reported in patients of bilateral profound hearing loss with tinnitus after restoration of hearing with cochlear implant surgery.

- *Otosclerosis:* Surgery has shown definite improvement in suppression of tinnitus in patients of otosclerosis when stapedectomy is done (77, 78).

- *Ménière's disease:* Endolymphatic sac decompression has been used to control vertigo; few studies have been done to see effect on tinnitus but has showed no advantage over other treatment (79).

- Cochlear neurectomy has also been tried, but there is no good evidence for its use.

## Pharmacological Treatment

Many causes, pathways and triggers have been associated with tinnitus and hence various pharmacological treatments have been tried for the treatment of tinnitus. Non-classical pathway of auditory system, somatosensory system and limbic system have a role in the activation of some forms of tinnitus. Pharmacological treatment can modulate the neural activity and can improve some forms of tinnitus. Most of the pharmacological studies in humans are based on clinical or theoretical underpinnings. Several clinical, pathophysiological and surgical treatment similarities exist between pain and tinnitus, and depression is common comorbidity associated with tinnitus (80–83). The pharmacological treatment is commonly directed towards the comorbid or the associated condition:

- *Antidepressants:* Antidepressants like trimipramine, nortriptyline, amitriptyline and selective serotonin reuptake inhibitors (SSRIs) have been used to combat mood disorders associated with tinnitus. Many antidepressants have been studied, they do not have direct effects on tinnitus but help in patients of tinnitus deal with comorbid depression or anxiety (84–89).

- *Benzodiazepines:* Benzodiazepines like alprazolam and clonazepam have been used widely in management of tinnitus and have shown good results in control of tinnitus with associated anxiety (35, 90, 91).

- *Anticonvulsants and other drugs:* Antiepileptics, vasodilators, anti-spasmodics and betahistine have been used in the treatment of tinnitus, but the results are not very promising (92–96).

- *Vitamins and micronutrients:* Birkiten et al. studied the role of vitamin B12 in tinnitus and hearing loss, the subjects were treated with vitamin B12 but there was no significant difference between pre- and post-treatment in tinnitus (97). Zinc sulfate has also been studied but did not result in any improvement in tinnitus patients (98).

- *Intratympanic treatment:* Intratympanic steroids have been used in the treatment of idiopathic refractory tinnitus. The anti-inflammatory effect of steroids on inner ear hair cells and immune-mediated effect on neuroepithelium of hair cells have been explored to treat tinnitus. A placebo-controlled study done by Seong Jun et al. in patients of refractory tinnitus with intratympanic dexamethasone and saline for control showed no statistical difference in two groups in tinnitus relief (99).

## Alternative Therapy

Yoga, tai chi, herbal medicine and meditation are also mentioned to help in non-specific ways in patients with tinnitus.

## PREVENTION

Ototoxicity and NIHL are some of the preventable causes of tinnitus. Adequate precautions should be taken during exposure to these agents. Multivitamins with antioxidants are thought to help by delaying apoptosis and to delay inner ear damage. The role of stem cell and gene therapy is being investigated.

## PULSATILE TINNITUS

Pulsatile tinnitus is a specific subtype of tinnitus which merits special mention. It is the perception of a rhythmic sound which is most commonly, but not exclusively, due to an underlying vascular pathology. The sound can be clicking, pulsating or fluttering in nature. In subjective pulsatile tinnitus, patients perceive the pulsating sound as rushing, humming or flowing with a few describing accentuations of these with physical activity or in recumbent position (100). Objective pulsatile tinnitus can be observed by clinician on auscultation (mastoid or neck region).

### Synchronous Pulsatile Tinnitus

It is generally seen in the presence of vascular anomalies adjacent to the peripheral auditory system. It can also be seen in conditions with hyperdynamic circulation, benign intracranial hypertension or pseudotumor cerebri. It can be further classified based on pathology: arterial, venous or microvascular conditions of middle ear.

### Nonsynchronous Pulsatile Tinnitus

It occurs due to repetitive myoclonic contractions of middle ear muscles like tensor tympani and stapedius. It mostly occurs in young age but can be seen in elderly too. It can be buzzing, fluttering or clicking in nature.

Differentiation between arterial and venous causes of tinnitus may be possible clinically, with significant reduction or resolution of noise noted on strong manual compression of ipsilateral carotid artery in case of former. Performing the Valsalva manoeuvre and rotation of head to the side of tinnitus results in reduction of venous tinnitus with no effect observed in tinnitus of arterial origin. Similarly, increase in tinnitus is

## Table 9.2: Causes of Pulsatile Tinnitus

| Arterial | Venous | Arterio-venous Transition | Hypervascular Tumours | Non-vascular |
|---|---|---|---|---|
| ICA narrowing<br>• Atherosclerotic<br>• Dissection<br>• - Fibro-muscular dysplasia | Idiopathic intracranial hypertension† | DAVF | Paraganglioma | Palatal myoclonus |
| Variant/anomalous vessel within temporal bone<br>• Aberrant ICA<br>• Lateralized ICA<br>• - Persistent Stapedial artery | Variant /anomalous vessel within temporal bone<br>• Sigmoid sinus diverticulum‡<br>• Laterally placed sigmoid sinus‡<br>• Jugular bulb diverticulum‡‡<br>• High-riding Jugular bulb‡‡ | AVM | Haemangioma | Middle ear myoclonus |
| Aneurysm<br>• ICA<br>• Vertebral<br>• - AICA | Abnormal mastoid emissary veins | | Meningioma | |
| | | | Langerhans cell histiocytosis | |
| | | | Metastases | |

*Abbreviations:* ICA: Internal Carotid Artery; AICA: Anterior Inferior Cerebellar Artery; †: with or without associated transverse sinus stenosis; ‡: with or without sigmoid plate dehiscence; ‡‡ with or without Jugular plate dehiscence; DAVF: Dural Arteriovenous Fistula; AVM: arteriovenous malformation.

observed during Muller manoeuvre and with rotation of head towards opposing side in cases with venous aetiology of tinnitus. The various causes of pulsatile tinnitus can be grouped into arterial, venous, arterio-venous transition and non-vascular (Table 9.2) (100–103).

### Approach to a Patient with Pulsatile Tinnitus

Table 9.3 summarizes clinical characteristics, the presence of which suggest a particular diagnostic consideration. Other tests which can aid in diagnosis are audiology and electrophysiologic examination.

## Table 9.3: Clinical Characteristics as Pointers to a Specific Diagnosis

| Clinical Characteristics | Diagnosis to Consider |
|---|---|
| **History** | |
| Rhythmic noise, synchronous with patient's heartbeat | Pulsatile tinnitus |
| Change in intensity of tinnitus with various manoeuvre (Mueller's, Valsalva and head rotation) | Venous aetiology<br>Pseudotumor cerebri |
| Young, obese women with pulsatile tinnitus | DAVF |
| Diplopia, proptosis, visual disturbances and tinnitus | Carotid artery dissection |
| Young patient with sudden onset of pulsatile tinnitus, headache, dizzy spells and syncope | ACAD |
| Recurrent TIA or stroke, old age, smoker, hypertension, diabetes mellitus and hyperlipidaemia | |
| **Head and neck examination findings** | |
| • Soft palate contractions | Palatal myoclonus |
| • Palpable thrill | AVM, AVF, DAVF |
| • Bruit in orbital and mastoid region | DAVF |
| • - Bruit in neck region | Carotid stenosis |
| **Ear Examination/ Otoscopy** | |
| • Rhythmic movement of tympanic membrane | Tensor tympani myoclonus |
| • Retro-tympanic pulsatile mass | High Jugular bulb, glomus tumour and aberrant ICA |

*Abbreviations:* DAVF: dural arteriovenous fistula; ACAD: atherosclerotic carotid artery disease; AVM: arteriovenous malformation; AVF: arteriovenous fistula; ICA: internal carotid artery.

### Imaging in Pulsatile Tinnitus

CT, MRI and digital subtraction angiography (DSA) provide complementary information in the evaluation of pulsatile tinnitus. The characteristic imaging findings and the usual standard treatment for common diseases leading to pulsatile tinnitus, such as sigmoid sinus dehiscence (104, 105), Jugular bulb diverticulum (106), high-riding Jugular bulb (107, 108), dehiscent Jugular bulb, aberrant ICA (109), DAVF and paraganglioma (110) are summarized in Table 9.4.

## Table 9.4: Imaging Features and Treatment Modalities of Various Causes Leading to Pulsatile Tinnitus

| Disease | Imaging Appearances | Treatment /Key Points |
|---|---|---|
| Sigmoid sinus diverticulum | *CTV/MRV*: Outpouching from sigmoid sinus → intrude into the mastoid bone<br>*CT*: Remodelling or erosion of sigmoid plate | *Endovascular:* Stenting of sigmoid sinus and coil embolization of the diverticulum<br>*Surgical:* Resurfacing of sigmoid plate, bone wax packing or electrocoagulation of diverticulum |
| Sigmoid sinus dehiscence | *CT* : "air-on-sinus" sign (no bony separation between lateral portion of sigmoid sinus and mastoid air cells) | Sigmoid sinus wall reconstruction or resurfacing, using hydroxyl apatite cement, soft tissue graft and/or autologous bone |
| Jugular bulb diverticulum | *CTV/MRV*: Outpouching from Jugular bulb<br>*CT*: Smooth remodelling of Jugular foramen and adjacent temporal bone by diverticulum | *Endovascular:* Stenting of Jugular bulb and coil embolization of the diverticulum<br>*Surgical:* Mastoidectomy and bone wax packing of diverticulum |
| High-riding Jugular bulb (HRJB) | Varying definitions of axial level above which HRJB terminology is used:<br><br>• Floor of IAC<br>• 2 mm below floor of IAC<br>• Inferior rim of round window niche<br>• Basal turn of cochlea<br>• Inferior rim of the tympanic annulus or floor of the external auditory canal | |
| Dehiscent Jugular bulb | *CTA and HRCT*: Absent sigmoid plate (normally present between a high-riding Jugular bulb and middle ear) → wall of Jugular bulb bulges into middle ear cavity | This retro-tympanic vascular mass if mistaken for a middle ear tumour and biopsied → disastrous consequences<br>*DD:* High-riding Jugular bulb (shows intact sigmoid plate) |
| Carotid (ICA) stenosis | *Doppler study*: Assess plaque morphology and degree of stenosis<br>*CTA*: Important for detailed assessment prior to revascularization procedure | Carotid stenting or carotid endarterectomy |
| Aberrant ICA | *CT and CTA*: Enlarged inferior tympanic canaliculus, enhancing vessel across the inferior cochlear promontory, absent carotid plate and absent or hypoplastic vertical segment of the carotid canal<br>*DSA*: Enlarged inferior tympanic branch of ascending pharyngeal artery, lateral extension of ICA with pinched contour of the vessel | This retro-tympanic vascular mass if mistaken for a middle ear tumour and biopsied → disastrous consequences<br>*DD:* Lateralized ICA (protrudes into the anterior mesotympanum, does not course across cochlear promontory, no enlargement of inferior tympanic canaliculus) |
| DAVF | *DSA*: Gold standard in both diagnosis and accurate classification | *Most common site of DAVF:* Transverse/ sigmoid sinus<br>*Conservative:* Low-grade DAVF<br>*Endovascular:* Presence of retrograde venous reflux or persistent symptoms |
| Paragangliomas | *HRCT (glomus tympanicum):*<br>Enhancing soft tissue mass lateral to cochlear promontory (if large, may fill middle ear cavity, invade eustachian tube or mastoid)<br>Intact Jugular bulb | *DD:* Glomus Jugulare paraganglioma ( dehiscent Jugular bulb)<br>Surgical resection is the treatment of choice |

*Abbreviations:* CTV: CT Venography; MRV: MR Venography; DSA: Digital Subtraction Angiography; ICA: Internal Carotid Artery; DAVF: Dural Arterio-Venous Fistula; DD: Differential Diagnosis.

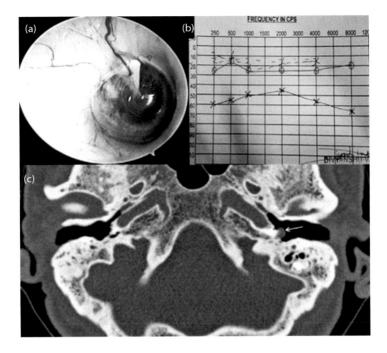

**Figure 9.3** Glomus tympanicum (left). Forty-year-old female with left-sided pulsatile tinnitus. (a) Otoendoscopy examination shows a pulsating vascular mass in middle ear. (b) Pure tone audiogram shows conductive hearing loss pattern. (c) HRCT image shows a small soft tissue attenuation mass overlying the cochlear promontory (arrow in part c), consistent with glomus tympanicum.

Figures 9.3 and 9.4 illustrate cases of glomus tympanicum and carotid-cavernous fistula, respectively.

## CONCLUSION

- Tinnitus is a common symptom and can be a manifestation of other diseases.

- The pathophysiology and management are not completely clear in many cases.

- Subjective idiopathic tinnitus is the most common, and patients get habituated with time and it is never an alarming condition, so reassurance helps.

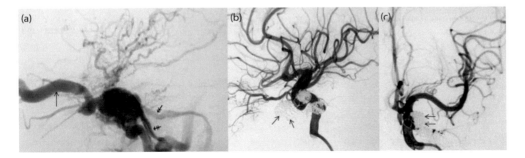

**Figure 9.4** Direct carotid-cavernous fistula (left). Twenty-eight-year-old male with history of diplopia and tinnitus on left side for 1 week, following history of trauma. (a) Pre-embolization digital subtraction angiogram demonstrates a dilated superior ophthalmic vein (arrow in part a), superior petrosal sinus (two-headed arrow in part a) and inferior petrosal sinus (arrow with double stroke in part a) during the arterial phase, consistent with a direct CCF. (b and c) Post-procedure angiograms show complete obliteration of the fistula with coils (arrow in parts b and c).

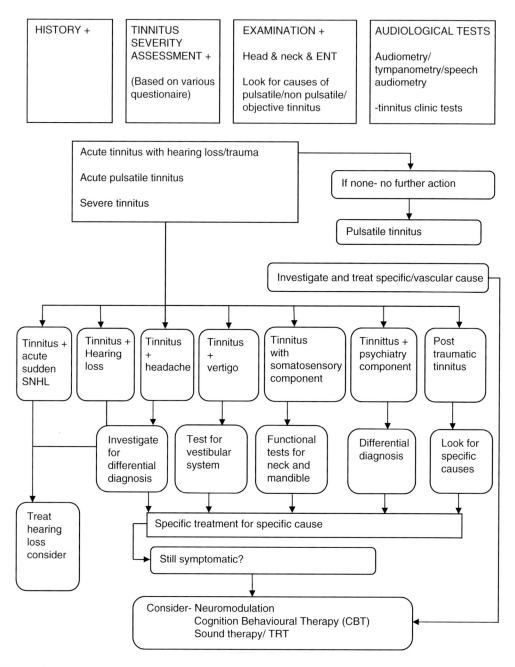

**Figure 9.5** Suggested algorithm for management of tinnitus.

- It is often associated with comorbid conditions like anxiety and depression. Hence, psychological management need to be considered

- A detailed history, complete physical examination and essential investigations help in management of the patient. If associated with hearing loss, intervention may help.

- A suggested algorithm for management is as depicted in Figure 9.5.

### REFERENCES

1. Baguley D, Anderson G, Ferran DM, et al. Tinnitus: A Multidisciplinary Approach, 2nd ed. UK: John Wiley & Sons, Inc., 2013.

2. Holgers KM, Hakansson BE. Sound stimulation via bone conduction for tinnitus relief: a pilot study. Int J Audiol. 2002;41:293–300.

3. National Center for Health Statistics. Hearing status among adults, United States, 1960–1962. Washington, DC: US Department of Health, Education and Welfare, 1968.

4. Nondahl DM, Cruickshanks KJ, Wiley TL, et al. Prevalence and 5-year incidence of tinnitus among older adults: the epidemiology of hearing loss study. J Am Acad Audiol. 2002;13(6):323–31.

5. Cooper JC, Jr. Health and nutrition examination survey of 1971–75: Part II. Tinnitus, subjective hearing loss, and well-being. J Am Acad Audiol. 1994;5(1): 37–43.

6. Stephens SDG. Historical aspects of tinnitus. In: Hazell JWP, editor. Tinnitus. New York: Churchill Livingstone, 1987, p. 1–19.

7. Adams PF, Hendersot GE, Marano MA. Current estimates from the National Health Interview Survey, 1996. Vital and Health Statistics: Series 10, National Center for Health Statistics, 1999, p. 81–103.

8. Chung DY, Gannon RP, Mason K. Factors affecting the prevalence of tinnitus. Audiology. 1984;23:441–52.

9. Coles RR. Epidemiology of tinnitus: demographic and clinical features. J Laryngol Otol Suppl. 1984; 9:195–202.

10. Kvestad E, Czajkowski N, Engdahl B, et al. Low heritability of tinnitus: results from the second Nord-Trondelag health study. Arch Otolaryngol Head Neck Surg. 2010;136:178–82.

11. Bartels H, Middel B, Pedersen SS, et al. The distressed (type D) personality is independently associated with tinnitus: a case-control study. Psychosomatics. 2010;51:29–38.

12. Davis A, El Rafaie A. Epidemiology oftinnitus. In: Tyler RS, editors. Tinnitus Handbook. San Diego: Singular, 2000, p. 1–23.

13. Tunkel DE, Bauer CA, Sun GH, et al. Clinical practice guideline: Tinnitus. Otolaryngol Head Neck Surg. 2014;151:S1–40.

14. Shulman A. Classification of tinnitus. In: Shulman A, Aran J, Tonndorf J, et al. Tinnitus: Diagnosis/ Treatment. Philadelphia: Lea & Febiger, 1991, p. 248–52.

15. Nodar RH. Tinnitus reclassified: new oil in an old lamp. Otolaryngol Head Neck Surg. 1996;114:582–5.

16. Mardini MK. Ear-clicking "tinnitus" responding to carbamazepine. N Engl J Med. 1987;317(24):1542.

17. Levine RA. Typewriter tinnitus: a carbamazepine-responsive syndrome related to auditory nerve vascular compression. ORL J Otorhinolaryngol Relat Spec. 2006;68(1):43–6.

18. Sindhusake D, Golding M, Newall P, et al. Risk factors for tinnitus in a population of older adults: the Blue Mountains hearing study. Ear Hear. 2003;24(6):501–7.

19. Jastreboff PJ. Phantom auditory perception (tinnitus): mechanisms of generation and perception. Neurosci Res. 1990;8(4):8221–54.

20. Guitton MJ, Caston J, Ruel J, et al. Salicylate induces tinnitus through activation of cochlear NMDA receptors. J. Neurosci. 2003;23:3944–52.

21. Puel JL. Chemical synaptic transmission in the cochlea. Prog Neurobiol. 1995;47(6):449–76.

22. Baguley DM. Mechanisms of tinnitus. Br Med Bull. 2002;63:195–212.

23. Eggermont JJ, Roberts LE. The neuroscience of tinnitus. Trends Neurosci. 2004;27:676–82.

24. Salvi RJ, Lockwood AH, Burkard R. Neural plasticity and tinnitus. In: Tyler RS, editors. Tinnitus Handbook. San Diego: Singular, 2000, p. 123–48.

25. Eggermont JJ. Pathophysiology of tinnitus. Prog Brain Res. 2007;166:19–35.

26. Kaltenbach JA. Summary of evidence pointing to a role of the dorsal cochlear nucleus in the etiology of tinnitus. Acta Otolaryngol. 2006;556:20–6.

27. Eggermont JJ. Tinnitus: neurobiological substrates. Drug Discov Today. 2005;10:1283–90.

28. Mulders WH, Robertson D. Hyperactivity in the auditory midbrain after acoustic trauma: dependence on cochlear activity. J Neurosci. 2009;164:733–46.

29. Norena AJ, Eggermont JJ. Changes in spontaneous neural activity immediately after an acoustic trauma: implications for neural correlates of tinnitus. Hear Res. 2003;183:137–53.

30. Seki S, Eggermont JJ. Changes in spontaneous firing rate and neural synchrony in cat primary auditory cortex after localized tone-induced hearing loss. Hear Res. 2003;180:28–38.

31. Eggermont JJ, Komiya H. Moderate noise trauma in juvenile cats results in profound cortical topographic map changes in adulthood. Hear Res. 2000;142:89–101.

32. Hallam RS, Rachman S, Hinchcliffe R. Psychological aspects of tinnitus. Contributions to Medical Psychology, 3rd ed. Oxford: Pergamon Press, 1984, p. 31–53.

33. Andersson G. A cognitive-affective theory for tinnitus: experiments and theoretical implications. In: Patuzzi R, editor. Proceedings of the Seventh International Tinnitus Seminar. Fremantle: University of Western Australia, 2002, p. 197–200.

34. Hoare DJ, Edmondson-Jones M, Gander PE, et al. Agreement and reliability of tinnitus loudness matching and pitch likeness rating. PLOS ONE. 2014;9(11):4553.

35. Johnson RM, Brummett R, Schleuning A. Use of alprazolam for relief of tinnitus. Arch Otolaryngol Head Neck Surg. 1993;119:842–5.

36. Cope TE, Baguley DM, Moore BC. Tinnitus loudness in quiet and noise after resection of vestibular schwannoma. Otol Neurotol. 2011;32:488–96.

37. Landgrebe M, Azevedo A, Baguley D, et al. Methodological aspects of clinical trials in tinnitus: a proposal for an international standard. J Psychosom Res. 2012;73:112–21.

38. Kuk FK, Tyler RS, Russell D, et al. The psychometric properties of a tinnitus handicap questionnaire. Ear Hear. 1990;11:434–45.

39. Newman CW, Jacobson GP, Spitzer JB. Development of the tinnitus handicap inventory. Arch Otolaryngol Head Neck Surg. 1996;122:143–8.

40. Hiller W, Goebel G. Rapid assessment of tinnitus-related psychological distress using the mini-TQ. Int J Audiol. 2004;43:600–4.

41. Meikle MB, Henry JA, Griest SE, et al. The tinnitus functional index: development of a new clinical measure for chronic, intrusive tinnitus. Ear Hear. 2012;33:153–76.

42. Budd RJ, Pugh R. Tinnitus coping style and its relationship to tinnitus severity and emotional distress. J Psychosom Res. 1996;41:327–35.

43. Halford JB, Anderson SD: Anxiety and depression in tinnitus sufferers. J Psychosom Res. 1991;35(4):383–90.

44. Henry JL, Wilson PH: Coping with tinnitus: two studies of psychological and audiological characteristics of patients with high and low tinnitus-related distress. Int Tinnitus J. 1995;1(2):85–92.

45. Zigmond AS, Snaith RP. The hospital anxiety and depression scale. Acta Psychiatr Scand. 1983;67:361–70.

46. Bastien CH, Vallieres A, Morin CM. Validation of the insomnia severity index as an outcome measure for insomnia research. Sleep Med. 2001;2:297–307.

47. Henry JA, Loovis C, Montero M, et al. Randomized clinical trial: group counseling based on tinnitus retraining therapy. J Rehabil Res Dev. 2007;44:21–32.

48. Kaldo V, Cars S, Rahnert M, et al. Use of a self-help book with weekly therapist contact to reduce tinnitus distress: a randomized controlled trial. J Psychosom Res. 2007;63:195–202.

49. Malouff JM, Noble W, Schutte NS, et al. The effectiveness of bibliotherapy in alleviating tinnitus-related distress. J Psychosom Res. 2010;68:245–51.

50. Phillips JS, McFerran DJ, Hall DA, et al. The natural history of subjective tinnitus in adults: systematic review and meta-analysis of no-intervention periods in controlled trials. Laryngoscope. 2018;128(1):217–27.

51. Trotter MI, Donaldson I. Hearing aids and tinnitus therapy: a 25-year experience. J Laryngol Otol. 2008;122:1052–6.

52. Searchfield GD, Kaur M, Martin WH. Hearing aids as an adjunct to counseling: tinnitus patients who choose amplification do better than those that don't. Int J Audiol. 2010;49:574–9.

53. Jastreboff PJ. 25 years of tinnitus retraining therapy. HNO. 2015;63(4):307–11.

54. Caffier PP, Haupt H, Scherer H, et al. Outcomes of long-term outpatient tinnitus-coping therapy: psychometric changes and value of tinnitus-control instruments. Ear Hear. 2006;27:619–27.

55. Seydel C, Haupt H, Szczepek AJ, et al. Long-term improvement in tinnitus after modified tinnitus retraining therapy enhanced by a variety of psychological approaches. Audiol Neurootol. 2010;15:69–80.

56. Vernon JA, Meikle MB. Masking devices and alprazolam treatment for tinnitus. Otolaryngol Clin North Am. 2003;36:307–20.

57. Newman CW, Sandridge SA. A comparison of benefit and economic value between two sound therapy tinnitus management options. J Am Acad Audiol. 2012;23:126–38.

58. Tyler R, Stocking C, Secor C, et al. Amplitude modulated S-tones can be superior to noise for tinnitus reduction. Am J Audiol. 2014;23:303–8.

59. Vermeire K, Heyndrickx K, De Ridder D, et al. Phase-shift tinnitus treatment: an open prospective clinical trial. B-ENT. 2007;3(Suppl 7):65–9.

60. Wagner T, Gangitano M, Romero R, et al. Intracranial measurement of current densities induced by transcranial magnetic stimulation in the human brain. Neurosci Lett. 2004;354(2):91–4.

61. Mennemeier M, Chelette KC, Allen S, et al. Variable changes in PET activity before and after rTMS treatment for tinnitus. Laryngoscope. 2011;121(4):815–22.

62. Khedr EM, Rothwell JC, Ahmed MA, et al. Effect of daily repetitive transcranial magnetic stimulation for treatment of tinnitus: comparison of different stimulus frequencies. J Neurol Neurosurg Psychiatr. 2008;79(2):212–5.

63. Piccirillo JF, Garcia KS, Nicklaus J, et al. Low-frequency repetitive transcranial magnetic stimulation to the temporoparietal junction for tinnitus. Arch Otolaryngol Head Neck Surg. 2011;137(3):221–8.

64. Anders M, Dvorakova J, Rathova L, et al. Efficacy of repetitive transcranial magnetic stimulation for the treatment of refractory chronic tinnitus: a randomized, placebo-controlled study. Neuro Endocrinol Lett. 2010;31(2):238–49.

65. Ellis A, Grieger R, editors. Handbook of Rational-Emotive Therapy, Vol. 1, New York: Springer, 1977.

66. Beck AT. Cognitive Therapy and the Emotional Disorders. New York: International Universities Press, 1979.

67. Hesser H, Weise C, Westin VZ, et al. A systematic review and meta-analysis of randomized controlled trials of cognitive behavioural therapy for tinnitus distress. Clin Psychol Rev. 2011;31(4):545–53.

68. Martinez-Devesa P, Perera R, Theodoulou M, et al. Cognitive behavioural therapy for tinnitus. Cochrane Database Syst Rev. 2010;(9):CD005233.

69. Kreuzer PM, Goetz M, Holl M, et al. Mindfulness- and body-psychotherapy-based group treatment of chronic tinnitus: a randomized controlled pilot study. BMC Complement Altern Med. 2012;12:235.

70. Westin VZ, Schulin M, Hesser H, et al. Acceptance and commitment therapy versus tinnitus retraining therapy in the treatment of tinnitus: a randomized controlled trial. Behav Res Ther. 2011;49:737–47.

71. Neri G, De Stefano A, Baffa C, et al. Treatment of central and sensorineural tinnitus with orally administered melatonin and sulodexide personal experience from a randomized controlled study. Acta Otorhinolaryngol Ital. 2009;29:86–91.

72. Shiomi Y, Takahashi H, Honjo I, et al. Efficacy of transmeatal low power laser irradiation on tinnitus: a preliminary report. Auris Nasus Larynx. 1997;4:39–42.

73. Walger M, Von Wedel H, Hoenen S, et al. Effectiveness of the low power laser and ginko extract i.v. therapy in patients with chronic tinnitus. In: Vernon JA, editor. Tinnitus: Treatment and Relief. Boston: Allyn and Bacon, 1998, p. 68–73.

74. Mirvakili A, Mehrparvar A, Mostaghaci M, et al. Low level laser effect in treatment of patients with intractable tinnitus due to sensorineural hearing loss. J Lasers Med Sci. 2014;5(2):71–4.

75. Mirz F, Zachariae R, Andersen SE, et al. The low-power laser in the treatment of tinnitus. Clin Otolaryngol Allied Sci. 1999;24:346–54.

76. Nakashima T, Ueda H, Misawa H, et al. Transmeatal low-power laser irradiation for tinnitus. Otol Neurotol. 2002;23:296–300.

77. Gersdorff M, Nouwen J, Gilain C, et al. Tinnitus and otosclerosis. Eur Arch Otorhinolaryngol. 2000;257:314–6.

78. Ayache D, Earally F, Elbaz P. Characteristics and postoperative course of tinnitus in otosclerosis. Otol Neurotol. 2003;24:48–51.

79. Pullens B, Verschuur HP, van Benthem PP. Surgery for Meniere's disease. Cochrane Database Syst Rev. 2013;(2): CD005395.

80. Moller AR. Similarities between chronic pain and tinnitus. Am J Otol. 1997;18:577–85.

81. Moller AR. Similarities between severe tinnitus and chronic pain. J Am Acad Audiol. 2000;11:115–24.

82. Tonndorf J. The analogy between tinnitus and pain: a suggestion for a physiological basis of chronic tinnitus. Hear Res. 1987;28:271–5.

83. De Ridder D, Elgoyhen AB, Romo R, et al. Phantom percepts: tinnitus and pain as persisting aversive memory networks. Proc Natl Acad. 2011;108(20): 8075–80.

84. Langguth B, Elgoyhen AB. Current pharmacological treatments for tinnitus. Expert Opin Pharmacother. 2012;13:2495–509.

85. Trellakis S, Lautermann J, Lehnerdt G. Lidocaine: neurobiological targets and effects on the auditory system. Prog Brain Res. 2007;166:303–22.

86. Baldo P, Doree C, Molin P, et al. Antidepressants for patients with tinnitus. Cochrane Database Syst Rev. 2012;9:CD003853.

87. Bayar N, Boke B, Turan E, et al. Efficacy of amitriptyline in the treatment of subjective tinnitus. J Otolaryngol. 2001;30:300–3.

88. Podoshin L, Ben-David Y, Fradis M, et al. Idiopathic subjective tinnitus treated by amitriptyline hydrochloride/biofeedback. Int Tinnitus J. 1995;1:54–60.

89. Sullivan M, Katon W, Russo J, et al. A randomized trial of nortriptyline for severe chronic tinnitus. Arch Intern Med. 1993;153:2251–9.

90. Jalali MM, Kousha A, Naghavi SE, et al. The effects of alprazolam on tinnitus: a cross-over randomized clinical trial. Med Sci Monit. 2009;15:155–60.

91. Han SS, Nam EC, Won JY, et al. Clonazepam quiets tinnitus: a randomised crossover study with ginkgo biloba. J Neurol Neurosurg Psychiatry. 2012; 83:821–7.

92. Donaldson I. Tegretol: a double blind trial in tinnitus. J Laryngol Otol. 1981;95:947–51.

93. Simpson JJ, Gilbert AM, Weiner GM, et al. The assessment of lamotrigine, an antiepileptic drug in the treatment of tinnitus. Am J Otol. 1999;20:627–31.

94. Westerberg BD, Roberson JB, Stach BA. A double-blind placebo-controlled trial of baclofen in the treatment of tinnitus. Am J Otol. 1996;17:896–903.

95. Davies WE, Knox E, Donaldson K. The usefulness of nipodipine, an L-calcium channel antagonist, in the treatment of tinnitus. Br J Audiol. 1994;28:125–9.

96. Jayarajan V, Coles R. Treatment of tinnitus with frusemide. J Audiol Med. 1993;2:114–9.

97. Berkiten G, Yildirim G, Topaloglu I, et al. Vitamin B12 levels in patients with tinnitus and effectiveness of vitamin B12 treatment on hearing threshold and tinnitus. BENT. 2013;9:111–6.

98. Coelho C, Witt SA, Hansen MR, et al. Zinc to treat tinnitus in the elderly: a randomized placebo-controlled crossover trial. Otol. Neurotol. 2013;34:1146–54.

99. Seong JC, Jong BL, Hye JL. Intratympanic dexamethasone injection for refractory tinnitus: prospective placebo-controlled study. Laryngoscope. 2013,123:2817–22.

100. Grierson KE, Grierson BHP, Grierson DJ, Grierson FPA. The assessment of pulsatile tinnitus: a systematic review of underlying pathologies and modern diagnostic approaches. Aust J Otolaryngol 2016;8(3):e11.

101. Hofmann E, Behr R, Neumann-Haefelin T, Schwager K. Pulsatile tinnitus: imaging and differential diagnosis. Deutsches Arzteblatt Int. 2013;110 (26):451–8.

102. Miller TR, Serulle Y, Gandhi D. Arterial abnormalities leading to tinnitus. Neuroimaging Clin N Am. 2016;26 (2):227–36.

103. Sismanis A. Pulsatile tinnitus: contemporary assessment and management. Curr Opin Otolaryngol Head Neck Surg. 2011;19 (5):348–57.

104. Lansley JA, Tucker W, Eriksen MR, Riordan-Eva P, Connor SEJ. Sigmoid sinus diverticulum, dehiscence, and venous sinus stenosis: potential causes of pulsatile tinnitus in patients with idiopathic intracranial hypertension? Am J Neuroradiol. 2017;38 (9):1783–8.

105. Zeng R, Wang GP, Liu ZH, et al. Sigmoid sinus wall reconstruction for pulsatile tinnitus caused by sigmoid sinus wall dehiscence: a single-center experience. PLOS ONE. 2016;11(10): e0164728.

106. Mortimer AM, Harrington T, Steinfort B, Faulder K. Endovascular treatment of Jugular bulb diverticula causing debilitating pulsatile tinnitus. BMJ Case Rep. 2017;38(9):1783–8.

107. Park JJ, Shen A, Loberg C, Westhofen M. The relationship between Jugular bulb position and Jugular bulb related inner ear dehiscence: a retrospective analysis. Am J Otolaryngol. 2015;36(3):347–51.

108. Overton SB, Ritter FN. A high placed Jugular bulb in the middle ear: a clinical and temporal bone study. Laryngoscope. 1973;83(12):1986–91.

109. Glastonbury CM, Harnsberger HR, Hudgins PA, Salzman KL. Lateralized petrous internal carotid artery: imaging features and distinction from the aberrant internal carotid artery. Neuroradiology. 2012;54(9):1007–13.

110. Gary Jackson C, Glasscock ME, Harris PF. Glomus tumors: diagnosis, classification, and management of large lesions. Arch Otolaryngol. 2012;54(9):1007–13.

# SECTION VI

# FACIAL PALSY IN OTOLOGY: APPROACH TO A PATIENT

# 10 Facial Palsy in Otology: Approach to a Patient

*SK Singh, Sunil Goyal and Roohie Singh*

## CONTENTS

"You're never fully dressed without a smile."

–**Martin Charnin for the Broadway musical** *Annie*

## INTRODUCTION

The human face has an important role in social interaction by providing non-verbal clues regarding a person's identity, race, sexual dimorphism, emotion and overall health. Facial deformity secondary to facial palsy results in functional, communicative and social impairment along with a negative impact on the quality of life and emotional well-being of a person.

Acute Flaccid Facial Paralysis (FFP) results from Facial nerve (VII N) insults and can have a spectrum of recovery, ranging from complete recovery of facial function to persistence of complete paralysis. Today, we have many therapeutic options available to restore facial function and to reduce long-term sequelae. An algorithm-based treatment approach based on Evidence-Based Medicine (EBM) can help us cut through the haze of multiple treatment options available and provide best possible outcomes. This chapter aims to present a systematic approach to a patient presenting with acute Flaccid Facial palsy of otologic origin.

## SURGICAL ANATOMY

While an understanding of VII N anatomy is a prerequisite in the management of Facial palsy, however, we shall be concentrating only on its applied aspects.

The VII N consists of about 10,000 fibres of which approximately 7000 are myelinated branchial motor fibres which innervate the muscles of facial expression. The rest of the fibres are somatosensory and secretomotor which constitute the nervus-intermedius.

The VII N has four components (Figure 10.1):

1. Special Visceral Efferent (SVE) – motor nucleus

2. General Visceral Efferent (GVE) – superior salivatory nucleus

3. Special Visceral Afferent (SVA) – nucleus tractus solitarius

4. General Somatic Afferent (GSA) – spinal nucleus of Trigeminal

The upper part of face gets bilateral supranuclear innervation and is hence spared in Upper Motor Neuron (UMN) lesions. Better topographic organization of the nerve at the level of the Central Nervous System (CNS) than at the peripheral end explains the existence of dissociated volitional and emotional Facial palsy and the phenomenon of synkinesis.

While exiting the brainstem at the pontomedullary junction, the VII N has an intimate relationship with the abducens nerve in the floor of fourth ventricle. Hence, brainstem lesions usually involve the VI and VII nerves simultaneously. The relative location of the VII N, Trigeminal nerve (V N), Vestibulocochlear nerve (VIII N) and the relative diameter of VII N to VIII N (1.8 mm vs. 3 mm) are of great importance in lateral skull base surgery involving

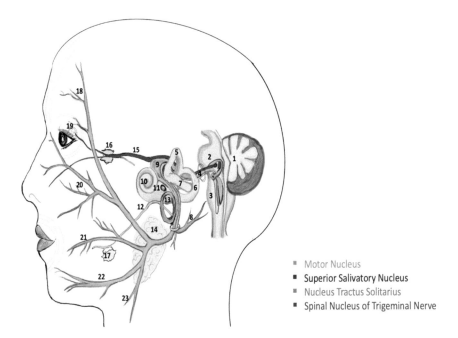

- Motor Nucleus
- Superior Salivatory Nucleus
- Nucleus Tractus Solitarius
- Spinal Nucleus of Trigeminal Nerve

**Figure 10.1** Schematic diagram of Facial nerve anatomy showing Facial nerve nucleus, pathway and terminal branches: [1] cerebellum; [2] pons; [3] medulla; [4] iac; [5] superior SCC; [6] posterior SCC; [7] lateral SCC; [8] Posterior Auricular nerve; [9] geniculate ganglion; [10] cochlea; [11] oval window; [12] Chorda tympani; [13] nerve to stapedius; [14] parotid gland; [15] Greater Superficial Petrosal nerve (GSPN); [16] Pterygopalatine ganglion; [17] submandibular gland; [18] temporal branch; [19] lacrimal gland; [20] zygomatic branch; [21] buccal branch; [22] marginal mandibular branch; [23] cervical branch.

cerebellopontine angle (CP Angle) lesions. The sensory roots of V N and the nervus-intermedius are prone to distortion, which explains loss of corneal reflex and presence of Hitzelberger's sign in CP Angle lesions. The intracranial VII N with VIII N and nervus intermedius enter the porus of the Internal Auditory Canal (IAC). Here it is covered only with pia mater (perineurium is absent) which makes it vulnerable to injury in CP Angle surgeries.

The intrameatal part of the VII N shares dural investment with the nervus intermedius and VIII N, making it vulnerable during surgical manipulation. The motor component merges with nervus intermedius at the fundus of the IAC. Here, the crista falciformis and Bill's bar are important landmarks in identifying the nerves, as depicted in Figure 10.2.

The labyrinthine segment, with the geniculate ganglion forming the first genu, is the narrowest and shortest segment with an anatomic "bottleneck" of dense arachnoid band around it, is prone to trauma in temporal bone fractures and ischaemia caused by oedema, secondary to inflammation, as in Bell's palsy. The Greater

Superficial Petrosal nerve (GSPN) arises onto the floor of the Middle Cranial Fossa (MCF).

The tympanic segment of the VII N lies above the oval window and its proximal end passes just above cochleariform process. It then makes the second genu hugging the antero-inferomedial aspect of the lateral semicircular canal. The pyramidal eminence is another landmark for the second genu, marking the beginning of mastoid or vertical segment of the VII N. The Chorda tympani, a landmark for posterior tympanotomy, emerges just 3–5 mm proximal to the exit of the VII N from the stylomastoid foramen (SMF). The ampulla of the posterior semicircular canal lies medial to the vertical segment of the VII N. This holds importance during labyrinthectomy done as a part of translabyrinthine approach to IAC.

The tympanomastoid suture is the most reliable landmark to identify VII N after it exits the Stylomastoid foramen. Here, it is encircled by the fibrous tendon of the digastric muscle which requires sharp dissection while following the extracranial VII N into the parotid gland. The nerve here is superficial in children <2 years of

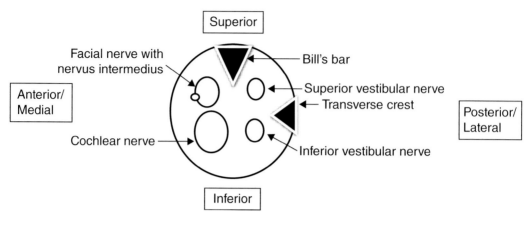

**Figure 10.2** Schematic representation of fundus of IAC with Facial nerve, Cochlear nerve, Superior and Inferior Vestibular nerves.

age due to a poorly developed mastoid process and hence susceptible to trauma during forceps delivery and mastoid surgery.

The relative position of the VII N in the IAC and the temporal bone with contiguous critical structures is important in mastoid surgery and lateral skull base surgery, as depicted in Figures 10.3 and 10.4.

## REVIEW OF LITERATURE

The summary of certain relevant definitions pertaining to Facial palsy used in the text is provided in Table 10.1.

Facial palsy is a devastating experience for a patient with functional and aesthetic sequelae resulting in profound Quality of Life (QOL) impairment (1, 2). Depending on the degree of neural injury in acute Flaccid Facial palsy,

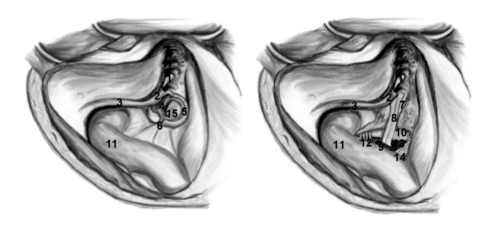

**Figure 10.3** Surgical landmarks and relationship of Facial nerve during translabyrinthine approach (R) ear: [1] incus; [2] second genu of Facial nerve; [3] vertical or mastoid segment of Facial nerve; [4] vestibule; [5] superior SCC; [6] vestibular aqueduct; [7] Facial nerve at fundus of IAC (anterosuperior quadrant); [8] Superior and Inferior Vestibular nerve at IAC (posterior part of IAC); [9] anteroinferior cerebellar artery (AICA); [10] brainstem; [11] sigmoid Jugular complex; [12] cranial nerve IX, X, XI (lower cranial nerves); [13] Basilar artery; [14] Trigeminal nerve at superior part of Cerebellopontine angle; [15] subarcuate artery through subarcuate fossa.

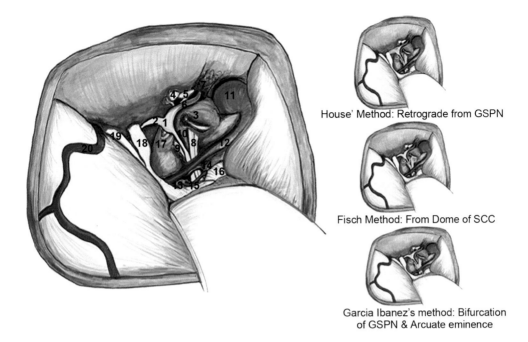

House' Method: Retrograde from GSPN

Fisch Method: From Dome of SCC

Garcia Ibanez's method: Bifurcation
of GSPN & Arcuate eminence

**Figure 10.4**  Surgical landmarks and relationship of Facial nerve during middle cranial fossa approach (R) ear [1] geniculate ganglion; [2] GSPN; [3] superior SCC; [4] malleus; [5] incus stapes complex; [6] tympanic segment of Facial nerve; [7] aditus and mastoid; [8] superior and inferior Vestibular nerve; [9] Cochlear nerve at modiolus of cochlea; [10] Bill's bar at fundus of IAC; [11] sigmoid sinus; [12] superior petrosal sinus draining into sigmoid sinus; [13] Basilar artery; [14] porus of IAC; [15] AICA arising from Basilar artery; [16] cerebellum; [17] cochlea; [18 and 19] Trigeminal nerve V3 and V2; [20] Middle Meningeal artery.

outcomes can range from persistent and complete Flaccid Facial palsy to a full return of normal function. In between these extremes exist zonal permutations of hypoactivity and hyperactivity and synkinesis, often with symptomatic gustatory epiphora and facial discomfort, a condition known as post-paralytic Facial nerve syndrome (PFNS) which is postulated to result from aberrant regeneration of the VII N (3–6).

Bell's palsy is the commonest cause of acute Flaccid Facial palsy and accounts for up to 70% of cases. The second most common aetiology is congenital Facial palsy followed by Ramsay Hunt Syndrome (7). Bell's palsy is the commonest cause in paediatric population followed by infections (otitis media [OM], zoster) and trauma (8). The incidence of Bell's palsy has been reported to be between 18 and 40 cases per 100,000 persons annually (7, 9–11). Aetiology is thought to be reactivation of latent Herpes simplex virus (HSV) or Varicella zoster virus (VZV) or human Herpes virus 6 (12–14). However, Bell's

## Table 10.1:  Relevant Definitions in Facial Palsy

| | |
|---|---|
| Facial palsy | Entire spectrum of facial movement disorders, including flaccid facial palsy, facial paresis and post-paralytic palsy |
| Flaccid facial palsy (FFP) | Complete or near complete absence of facial movement and tone without synkinesis or hyperactivity |
| Facial synkinesis | Involuntary and abnormal facial muscle activation accompanying volitional or spontaneous expression |
| Post-paralytic Facial nerve syndrome (PFNS) | Syndrome comprising facial synkinesis, facial muscle rigidity, spasm, contracture or pain. Gustatory epiphora (crocodile tears or Bogorad syndrome) is often present. Result of aberrant regeneration or ephaptic transmission following VII N insult |
| Post-paralytic facial palsy (PFP) | Facial movement disorder or PFNS comprising of varying degrees of zonal synkinesis, hypoactivity and hyperactivity |

## Table 10.2: **Aetiology of Facial Palsy**

| Category | Disease |
|---|---|
| Infections | Bell's palsy (BP) |
| | Ramsay Hunt syndrome (RHS) |
| | Lyme disease |
| | HIV |
| Congenital | Birth trauma |
| | Geniculate ganglion vascular malformation (GGVM) |
| | Pontine vascular malformation |
| | Pontine developmental venous anomaly |
| | Hemifacial macrosomia |
| Iatrogenic | Otological and lateral skull base surgery |
| | Parotid surgery |
| | Head and neck surgery |
| Trauma | Temporal bone fracture |
| | Penetrating trauma |
| | Birth trauma |
| Otologic | Acute otitis media (AOM) |
| | Chronic otitis media (COM) |
| | Cholesteatoma |
| | Malignant otitis externa (MOE) or lateral skull base osteomyelitis (LSBO) |
| Tumour | Temporal bone carcinoma |
| | VII and VIII CN schwannoma |
| | Leptomeningeal carcinomatosis |
| Systemic autoimmune | Melkersson-Rosenthal syndrome (MRS) |
| | Sarcoidosis |
| | Guillain-Barre syndrome (GBS) |
| | Multiple sclerosis |
| | Amyloidosis |
| | Wegener granulomatosis |
| | Sjogren's syndrome |
| | Systemic lupus erythematosus |
| | Behçet's disease |
| Metabolical | Hyperthyroidism |
| | Pregnancy |
| | Diabetes mellitus |
| Vascular | Brainstem cerebrovascular accident |
| | Central CVA |
| | Hemifacial spasm |

palsy is a diagnosis of exclusion and should be given only after all other diagnoses have been ruled out. The aetiology of Facial palsy is listed in Table 10.2.

Recurrent Bell's palsy (ipsilateral or contra-lateral) is the commonest cause for recurrent facial palsy (RFP). However, it is pertinent to rule out VII N tumours in recurrent ipsilateral Facial palsy. Alternating recurrent Facial palsy can be seen in some rare disorders of which Melkersson-Rosenthal syndrome (MRS) is the next commonest cause, after recurrent Bell's palsy (15, 16).

Bilateral facial palsy, which may occur simultaneously (within 30 days of first side) or asynchronously, represents 0.2–3% of all cases of Facial palsy (17, 18). Overall, the commonest cause of Bilateral Facial palsy is Bell's palsy followed by Lyme disease. The most common cause of simultaneous Bilateral Facial palsy is Lyme disease, followed by posterior fossa tumours, trauma, immune-mediated Guillain-Barre syndrome (GBS), CNS lymphoma and HIV infection. Among asynchronous cases of Bilateral Facial palsy, Bell's palsy is the commonest cause followed by neurofibromatosis type 2 (NF-2)-associated vestibular schwannoma (VS) and MRS (18, 19). Endocrine, metabolic, autoimmune and systemic causes of Facial palsy should always be considered in Recurrent Facial palsy or Bilateral Facial palsy. Imaging and relevant diagnostic laboratory investigations should be carried out where indicated.

### APPROACH TO A PATIENT WITH FACIAL PALSY
#### History

It is incumbent upon the treating clinician to establish a diagnosis for underlying cause of facial movement disorder. History taking is the key to making a correct diagnosis and effective management. A particular diagnosis can almost always be ascertained 80–90% of time by taking an accurate history.

*Onset and Course:* Enquiry should begin with the onset of Facial palsy and any associated prodrome. Idiopathic or viral acute Flaccid Facial palsy has a sudden onset and is usually associated with a prodrome. Bell's palsy generally evolves over 3 days with varying degree of Flaccid Facial palsy. Recovery of facial tone and movement usually occurs within 4 months. However, there may be continued recovery of facial function up to a period of 12–18 months.

Approximately 70% of Bell's palsy will show complete recovery, while the remainder will show varying degrees of aberrant regeneration and facial synkinesis (7). Ramsay Hunt Syndrome or zoster-associated Facial palsy usually presents as complete palsy and takes longer to recover with higher chances of having PFP and post-herpetic neuralgia.

History of head injury preceding onset of acute Flaccid Facial palsy would suggest a temporal bone fracture, while a recent history of otological surgery would suggest an iatrogenic cause. Post-traumatic sudden onset complete palsy makes VII N transection a strong possibility, while delayed onset palsy would be indicative of palsy secondary to oedema. Temporal bone fractures generally occur due to Road Traffic Accidents (RTA) and are usually associated with head injury. Most of these patients are admitted in the Intensive Care Unit (ICU) and the presence of Facial palsy gets overlooked because of life-saving measures and ventilatory support taking priority. It would be difficult to determine whether Facial palsy had been of immediate onset or a delayed onset in such a scenario.

An insidious onset slowly progressive Facial palsy may indicate a benign lesion (e.g. VII N schwannoma), while a rapidly progressive Facial palsy may indicate a malignant lesion (e.g. carcinoma temporal bone).

*Age:* Age at onset is an important clue in reaching a diagnosis. Facial palsy present since birth could be either developmental or traumatic in origin. Birth trauma (e.g. forceps delivery) can affect one or more branches of VII N and is evident with the first cry or grimace and usually improves with time. History of prolonged labour, forceps use during delivery, facial and periauricular ecchymoses at delivery or shortly thereafter would suggest birth trauma. Presence of other congenital anomalies and lack of improvement in facial function would point to a developmental cause (e.g. hemifacial macrosomia).

Ramsay Hunt Syndrome generally presents with complete palsy in patients older than 45 years or immunocompromised individuals, while Bell's palsy presents with varying severity of Facial palsy at any age, including immunocompetent patients.

*Duration:* The duration of palsy has a very important role in deciding the treatment. Given the plethora of therapeutic options available in the management of Facial palsy, it is useful to determine the domains of treatment plan to which individual patient belong, as mentioned in Table 10.3. The five management domains are based on timing of presentation, status of VII N and facial musculature.

*History of Travel to Lyme Disease Endemic Area:* A high index of suspicion is required as patient

## Table 10.3: Management Domains Based on Duration of Facial Nerve Palsy

| Time Frame | Facial Nerve Anatomically Intact | Facial Nerve Not Intact |
|---|---|---|
| Onset to first 2 weeks | Acute flaccid facial palsy (FFP) | Flaccid Facial palsy |
| 2 weeks to 6 months | Flaccid Facial palsy with potential for spontaneous recovery | Flaccid Facial palsy with potential for spontaneous recovery |
| | | Flaccid Facial palsy with viable facial musculature with low potential for spontaneous recovery |
| 6–12 months | Flaccid Facial palsy with potential for spontaneous recovery | Flaccid Facial palsy with viable facial musculature with low potential for spontaneous recovery |
| | Flaccid Facial palsy with viable facial musculature with low potential for spontaneous recovery | |
| | Post-paralytic facial palsy (PFP) | |
| 1–2 years | Flaccid Facial palsy with viable facial musculature with low potential for spontaneous recovery | Flaccid Facial palsy with viable facial musculature with low potential for spontaneous recovery |
| | PFP | PFP |
| | Flaccid Facial palsy without viable facial musculature | Flaccid Facial palsy without viable facial musculature |
| >2 years | Flaccid Facial palsy without viable facial musculature | Flaccid Facial palsy without viable facial musculature |
| | PFP | PFP |

*Note:* The five domains of treatment plan includes: (a) acute Flaccid Facial palsy; (b) Flaccid Facial palsy with potential for spontaneous recovery; (c) Flaccid Facial palsy with viable facial musculature with low potential for spontaneous recovery; (d) Flaccid Facial palsy without viable facial musculature; and (e) PFP.

often do not recall a tick bite or a rash. Any history of recent travel to endemic areas (e.g. the United States) or tick exposure should be obtained. Differentiation is imperative as steroids, which are the mainstay of medical management in acute Flaccid Facial palsy, may be associated with worse prognosis and post-paralytic synkinesis here.

*Recurrent or Bilateral:* Although Bell's palsy is the commonest cause for recurrent and bilateral Facial palsy, a history of recurrent or bilateral Facial palsy would warrant an investigation into other diagnoses. Appropriate radiological imaging should be considered to rule out a tumour and diagnostic laboratory studies are required to rule out endocrine, metabolic, autoimmune and other systemic causes.

*Associated Otological Symptoms:* These symptoms have an important role in reaching a diagnosis in patients of Facial palsy. Otalgia may be an associated symptom in up to 50% of patients with Bell's palsy and almost all with Herpes zoster oticus (Ramsay Hunt Syndrome), but rarely in tumours. The character of pain is typical of post-herpetic neuralgia in Ramsay Hunt Syndrome, while malignant otitis externa (MOE) has a deep-seated aural pain which is worse at night.

Mastoiditis requires to be ruled out if Facial palsy is associated with otalgia and hearing loss. Acute Facial palsy seen in chronic OM usually presents with otalgia, otorrhoea and hearing loss, while in AOM fever usually coexists.

Gradually progressive Facial palsy with hearing loss may be indicative of a mass lesion in the middle ear cleft or a lesion involving the IAC. Acute Flaccid Facial palsy with hearing loss and dizziness could be the presentation following temporal bone trauma and Ramsay Hunt Syndrome, which also has vesicles in a segmental pattern. Facial palsy with hearing loss and pulsatile tinnitus may be a presentation of vascular lesion like a jugulo tympanic paraganglioma (JTP).

*Other Cranial Nerve Involvement:* Jugular fossa tumours can present with Facial palsy along with involvement of lower cranial nerves (LCNs). A very large vestibular schwannoma can also cause Facial palsy, although less likely acute Facial palsy. It can present with loss of corneal sensation and LCNs involvement. Facial Nerve Schwannomas (FNS) may also cause Facial palsy, as they slowly grow and expand, and may rarely present with acute Facial palsy. However, acute Flaccid Facial palsy is more likely secondary to treatment of these tumours.

*Associated Symptoms:* Associated symptoms help in reaching a diagnosis and also help in determining the treatment plan. Photophobia with an irregular pupil can be present in Facial palsy caused by sarcoidosis, while Facial palsy with ophthalmoplegia with a normal pupil can be seen in diabetic neuropathy. Rarely Facial palsy may be the presenting feature of metastatic cancers of breast, lung, thyroid, kidney, ovary or prostate along with headache and seizures. Cerebrovascular Accidents (CVAs) can involve multiple cranial nerves, including VII N along with unilateral weakness of limbs, headache, vomiting and seizures.

Associated symptoms can vary according to the timing of presentation and degree of recovery. Patients with acute Flaccid Facial palsy would complain of ocular irritation (secondary to paralytic lagophthalmos), facial asymmetry and oral incompetence. However, patients presenting at a later stage of PFP may complain of facial synkinesis and epiphora. Platysmal synkinesis results in neck discomfort and facial fatigue while periocular synkinesis results in a narrowed palpebral fissure. Lack of meaningful smile occurs in severe cases.

*Past Medical History:* Peripheral neuropathies such as Facial palsy have been associated with conditions such as Diabetes mellitus (DM), alcoholism, collagen vascular disorders and hypertension (20). DM is a risk factor for MOE and also associated with a worse outcome in Bell's palsy. In patients presenting with Recurrent Facial palsy or Bilateral Facial palsy, enquiry into known medical or family history of autoimmune disease should be made.

It is not clear whether pregnancy increases the risk of Facial palsy over the general population; however, it occurs more frequently during the third trimester. Bell's palsy during the third trimester carries a worse prognosis compared with a cohort of non-pregnant women of the same age (21).

*Family History:* Enquiry may reveal a family history of Facial palsy. An association with paralysis of multiple VII N branches and specific alleles 3q21 and 3q22 with an autosomal dominant transmission has been found. However, no gene has yet been identified (22). MRS is an inherited disorder that presents with Recurrent Facial palsy, fissured tongue and facial swelling.

*Treatment History:* Enquiry into treatment history may reveal possible iatrogenic causes of Facial palsy or details about previous attempts at surgical correction of Facial palsy. In tumours involving the middle ear cleft and vestibular schwannoma, Facial palsy is typically caused or aggravated by treatment of these lesions either by resection or irradiation, or both. Middle ear and mastoid surgery can also result in iatrogenic Facial palsy in less than 1% of individuals, more so during revision surgery.

Toxicity due to certain medications like isoniazid has been reported to be accompanied by Facial palsy. Acute porphyrias characterized by abdominal pain and photosensitivity may be precipitated by medication, such as sulfonamides and barbiturates, and may also present with Bilateral Facial palsy. Similarly, vaccinations against polio, rabies and influenza have been noted to be followed by neuropathies including Facial palsy.

### Examination

The primary aim of examination is to determine whether it is a Lower Motor Neuron (LMN) lesion or an Upper Motor Neuron (UMN) lesion and its severity. A meticulous examination is required to determine any associated synkinesis, contractures and other cranial nerve involvement and to look for causes of Facial palsy. The following aspects of examination of patients with Flaccid Facial palsy are mandatory:

*Physical Examination:* Examination of skin to look for rash or nodule suggestive of a systemic disease (like SLE, sarcoidosis), Lyme disease or skin cancer. Dermatomal distribution of vesicles along cranial nerve V, VII, IX or X or cervical nerves with Facial palsy would be diagnostic of Herpes zoster oticus or Ramsay Hunt Syndrome. Scars on face may be suggestive of head injury or road traffic accident with associated temporal bone fracture or surgical scars which patient may not have revealed in history.

Paediatric patients should also be examined for other stigmata of syndromes, including craniofacial dysmorphism (e.g. hemifacial microsomia), and features of birth trauma (periauricular ecchymosis). The neck should be examined for any mastoid-related abscess or regional lymph nodes. Inspection and palpation of the parotid area and tonsillar fossa may reveal a parotid mass with Facial palsy suggestive of parotid malignancy. A fissured tongue (lingua plicata) in a patient with Recurrent Facial palsy may suggest a diagnosis of MRS.

*Examination of Ears:* Pre- and post-auricular regions are inspected and palpated for features of acute mastoiditis or mastoid abscess or previous surgery scar. Vesicles over the concha, external auditory canal (EAC) and tympanic membrane (TM) would clinch a diagnosis of Ramsay Hunt Syndrome. Granulations in the EAC in an immunocompromised patient not responding to treatment would most likely be MOE; however, a biopsy from the granulations is a must to rule out malignancy.

Examination of the TM would confirm the presence of AOM and COM with or without cholesteatoma. A traumatic perforation of the TM with blood in the EAC or hemotympanum would be indicative of temporal bone fracture. Facial palsy with a reddish mass behind an intact TM, CHL and pulsatile tinnitus would make a clinical diagnosis of a vascular lesion like a JTP (Figure 10.2). A mass behind an intact TM would warrant appropriate radiological investigation, which shall be discussed later in chapter.

*Hearing Evaluation:* Tuning fork tests (TFTs) would help determine the type of hearing loss and the side affected. Gradually progressive Facial palsy with conductive hearing loss (CHL) may be indicative of a mass lesion in the middle ear cleft, whereas sensorineural hearing loss (SNHL) would be suggestive of a pathology involving the inner ear.

*Otoneurological Examination:* Facial palsy with vertigo may be peripheral, because of involvement of the inner ear or central in origin. A simple bedside HINTS examination (head impulse test, nystagmus and test of skew) would help in differentiating a peripheral from central cause of vertigo.

Head impulse test (HIT) addresses the question of a unilateral or bilateral vestibular Ocular Reflex (VOR) deficit. Brief, high acceleration horizontal head thrusts are applied at random intervals and order, while keeping the patient's eyes in primary gaze position. The slow phase of nystagmus will be evoked towards the lesioned labyrinth (positive HIT).

It is important to use Frenzel's glasses (+16 diopters), in particular to differentiate between a peripheral vestibular spontaneous nystagmus (suppressed by visual fixation) and a central nystagmus (also present during fixation or even intensified by it). In unilateral vestibular hypofunction, the horizontal component beats towards the intact ear and the torsional component involves beating of superior poles of the eyes towards the intact ear. Direction changing horizontal nystagmus or any vertical or rotatory nystagmus indicates a central lesion.

Test of skew is performed by examining the eye in straight ahead gaze to look for vertical divergence (one eye is higher than the other), cover test is used to detect skew deviation. Test of skew has principally been identified as a central sign in those with posterior fossa pathology. The test is specific but not sensitive for central pathology.

*Examination of Facial Palsy:* One should make note of the type of paralysis (UMN or LMN), complete flaccid or partial flaccid and any synkinesis or contractures. This is important in not only determining the cause but will also aid in deciding the treatment plan.

In the analysis of VII N function, it is crucial to have a zonal assessment (horizontal thirds) of facial function at rest and in motion and compared with normal side in unilateral palsy. Examination for facial function begins with the upper third of the face, making note of the presence or absence of forehead wrinkles and the position of the eyebrows. Symmetry of the upper third of face may indicate a central cause of Facial palsy, warranting further evaluation including imaging.

In Flaccid Facial palsy, middle third of the face will show a flaccid ptosis of mid cheek and fat pad. The nasal alae may also be displaced inferomedially with the philtrum pulled to the opposite side. Obstruction of the external nasal valve is often present. The Nasolabial Fold (NLF) on affected side is effaced.

In the lower third, the oral commissure may be inferiorly displaced along with weakening of the lower lip and oral incompetence.

The presence and degree of brow, ocular, midfacial, depressor, mentalis and platysmal synkinesis are also evaluated. Attention should also be paid to the contralateral hemiface with regard to whether weakening of a given paired muscle group, such as hemibrow or depressor labii inferioris, is likely to result in improved symmetry.

Several clinician-graded scoring systems have been described and validated for documentation of Facial palsy, but no one system has gained universal acceptance. The House Brackmann system (Table 10.4) was the first widely accepted outcome measure in Facial palsy and it continues to be used by clinicians because of its familiarity despite its limitations (23). The Sunnybrook facial grading scale (24) and Facial nerve grading system 2.0 (Table 10.5) (25) are also used.

Alternatively, documentation of severity of Facial palsy and outcome measures can be done with photography and videography at the first and follow-up visits. Photography and videography to document the appearance of the face at rest and with volitional facial movements (brow elevation, light and full effort eye closure, and smile, lip pucker, lower lip depression) on presentation and follow-up are essential. This allows for ongoing evaluation as the patient recovers or as interventions are performed.

*Assessment of Eye and Periocular Complex:* This includes eye closure, corneal reflex and presence of Bell's phenomenon (protective superior rotation of globe on eye closure). Schirmer test may be done to evaluate the viability of tear film and its ability to keep the eye moist. It is vital to note that the vertical height of the median palpebral fissure will be increased in Flaccid Facial palsy.

The position of the lower eyelid relative to the iris and snap test of the lower eyelid is done to evaluate elasticity of the lower eyelid skin and compared with the normal side as it is indicative of the tone of the orbicularis oculi muscle.

*Cranial Nerve Examination:* A quick cranial nerve examination is necessary to rule out diagnoses other than Bell's palsy. Multiple cranial nerves involvement may be seen in tumours involving the CP Angle and Jugular fossa but are more commonly secondary to treatment of such tumours. Inflammatory diseases and autoimmune conditions can also involve multiple cranial nerves.

## DIFFERENTIAL DIAGNOSIS

At the end of an astute history taking and clinical examination, an otologist would be able to reach at a diagnosis in 90% of cases and only the remaining 10% would require further evaluation to determine the aetiology, as depicted in

## Table 10.4: House Brackmann Facial Nerve Grading System (23)

| Grades | Gross | At Rest | On Motion (Forehead, Eye and Mouth) |
|---|---|---|---|
| I Normal | Normal | Normal | Normal |
| II Mild dysfunction | Slight weakness noticeable on close inspection (slight synkinesis) | Normal symmetry and tone | *Forehead:* moderate to good function; *eye:* complete closure with minimal effort; *mouth:* slight asymmetry |
| III Moderate dysfunction | Obvious weakness but not disfiguring | Normal symmetry and tone | *Forehead:* slight to moderate to function; *eye:* complete closure with effort; *mouth:* slightly weak with maximal effort |
| IV Moderately severe dysfunction | Obvious weakness with disfiguring asymmetry (severe synkinesis) | Normal symmetry and tone | *Forehead:* none; *eye:* incomplete closure with maximal effort; *mouth:* asymmetry with maximal effort |
| V Severe dysfunction | Only barely perceptible motion | Asymmetry | *Forehead:* none; *eye:* incomplete closure; *mouth:* slight movement |
| VI Total palsy | No movement | Loss of tone | No movement |

## Table 10.5: Facial Nerve Grading Scale 2.0 (FNGS 2.0)

| Score | Evaluation of Eye | | Evaluation of Eyebrow, Nasolabial Fold and Oral Region | | Synkinesis | |
|---|---|---|---|---|---|---|
| 0 | Not applicable | | Not applicable | | No synkinesis | |
| 1 | Normal | | Normal | | Slight synkinesis | |
| 2 | >75% movement, complete eye closure | | >75% movement | | Obvious synkinesis | |
| 3 | >50% movement, resting symmetry | | >50% movement, resting symmetry | | Disfiguring synkinesis | |
| 4 | <50% movement, resting asymmetry | | <50% movement, asymmetry | | Not applicable | |
| 5 | Trace movement | | Trace movement | | Not applicable | |
| 6 | No movement | | No movement | | Not applicable | |
| Total = 27 | 6 | | 6 x 3 =18 | | 3 | |
| FNGS 2.0 | I | II | III | IV | V | VI |
| Score | 4 | 5–9 | 10–14 | 15–19 | 20–23 | 24–27 |

*Source:* Adaptation of Vrabec (25).

Figure 10.5. In this section, we would be discussing the differential diagnosis of important otological causes of Facial palsy, which would help in deciding the management.

*Idiopathic Facial Palsy (Bell's Palsy):* It is the diagnosis in a majority of patients who have acute Flaccid Facial palsy. However, it is always a diagnosis of exclusion and should be given only after all other diagnoses have been excluded. Bell's palsy is diagnosed clinically based on Taverner's criteria (26).

A typical Bell's palsy will progress over 3 days, is self-limiting with spontaneous recovery in up to 70% of patients even without treatment (7). Prognosis is better in cases with incomplete paralysis at onset, paediatric patients, intact taste, intact stapedius reflex, absence of postauricular pain and in those with signs of recovery within 3 weeks (7, 27, 28). Poor prognostic indicators include diabetes, pregnancy, advanced age (>60), hypertension and complete Flaccid Facial palsy at onset (26). Management protocol in Bell's palsy is depicted in Figures 10.6 and 10.7.

When the history and physical examination are consistent with Bell's palsy, further investigation is not required except in Lyme endemic areas, where serology is always prudent. Lyme disease patients may also report fatigue and severe headache.

Herpes zoster oticus or Ramsay Hunt Syndrome is characterized by unilateral Facial palsy, pain, cochleovestibular symptoms and vesicles in a segmental pattern (8). Vesicles may not appear simultaneously with the palsy. Zoster sine herpete occurs with an absence of vesicles and may make diagnosis more difficult. Treatment includes corticosteroid and antiviral medications. Ramsay Hunt Syndrome has a poorer prognosis with delayed recovery compared with Bell's palsy. Without treatment, only about 20% will fully recover (7).

In the setting of acute Flaccid Facial palsy, red flags suggesting a diagnosis other than Bell's palsy include the following:

1. Recurrent Facial palsy or Bilateral Facial palsy

2. Slow onset of facial weakness

3. Asymmetric weakness across facial zones at onset

4. Constitutional symptoms (fever, lethargy, malaise, myalgias)

5. Headache

6. Presence of other focal neurological deficits

7. Absence of recovery of facial tone within 4 months of onset

*Otitis Media:* In the modern era, only about 0.005% of patients with OM develop Facial palsy, as compared with 0.7% in the pre-antibiotic era (29).The pathogenesis of Facial palsy associated with OM is unclear, but several hypotheses exist. OM may cause retrograde infection, ascending along the chorda tympani or FNC, causing reactivation of latent viral infection; or peripheral demyelination of VII N may occur due to presence of inflammatory bacterial toxins. Inflammatory process of OM in later stages may spread into FNC leading to inflammation

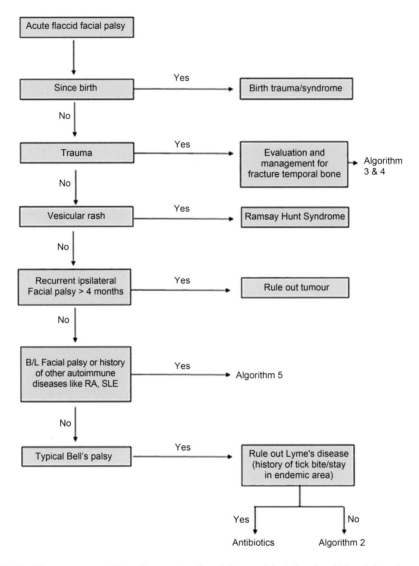

**Figure 10.5**  History as an aid to diagnosis of aetiology of facial palsy (Algorithm 1).

and compression of VII N. Lastly, an inflammatory polyp or a cholesteatoma may cause direct erosion into FNC (30).

COM causing Facial palsy is most likely due to cholesteatoma in 60–80% of cases (31, 32). Three percent of patients with cholesteatoma may present with sudden or gradual Facial palsy. The treatment of cholesteatoma is surgical.

*Malignant Otitis Externa:* MOE usually begins as an otitis externa, progresses to an osteomyelitis of temporal bone and skull base with risk to adjacent neural and cranial structures. Levenson's criteria are most commonly used for clinical diagnosis of MOE. Risk factors include diabetes, previous radiation therapy, advanced

age and an immunocompromised state. VII N is the earliest cranial nerve to get affected. As the disease progresses, other cranial nerves (IX, X, XI, XII) can also get affected.

Erythrocyte sedimentation rate (ESR) and C-reactive protein (CRP), though non-specific, are found to be raised in MOE. Serial ESR and CRP rates are also used to assess response to treatment. Biopsy from granulation tissues should be obtained which helps in differentiating from tumours of the temporal bone. Imaging includes a high-resolution computed tomography (HRCT) scan of temporal bone and an MRI. If results are equivocal, technetium or gallium scans may also aid diagnosis.

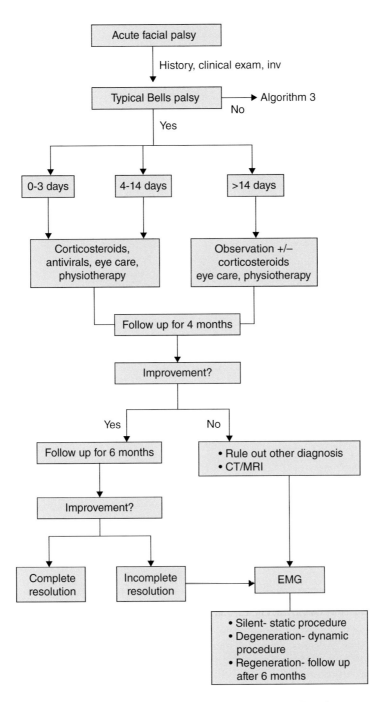

**Figure 10.6**  Management algorithm for typical Bell's palsy (Algorithm 2).

*Temporal Bone Fracture:* Trauma to the face or skull can produce acute Flaccid Facial palsy. Approximately 20% of cases of peripheral Facial palsy are attributed to trauma. Most cases of blunt trauma-induced Facial palsy show complete recovery (33). In suspected fracture of temporal bone, HRCT of temporal bone may demonstrate a fracture line. Otic capsule involving fractures are less common but have a higher risk of VII N injury compared to otic capsule sparing fractures (34). Facial palsy may be secondary to bony impingement or perineural inflammation

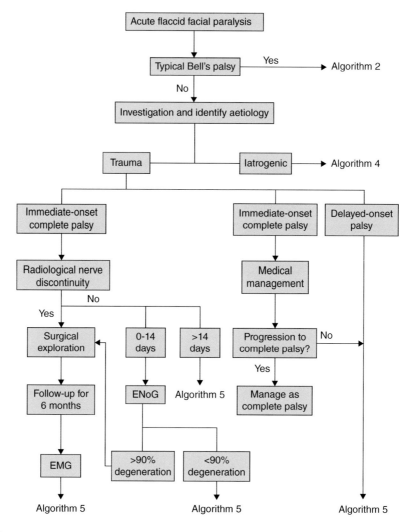

**Figure 10.7** Management algorithm for traumatic facial palsy (Algorithm 3).

and subsequent neural ischaemia. Typical management protocol for traumatic Facial palsy is depicted in Figures 10.7 and 10.9.

*Iatrogenic Facial Palsy:* Iatrogenic injury of intratemporal VII N presents a special problem for an otologist and neuro-otologist. Certain otological procedures like lateral skull base surgery carry an increased risk of VII N injury. Middle ear and mastoid surgery can be associated with VII N injury and the risk increases in revision surgery. The most common site of inadvertent injury in middle ear surgery is second genu and vertical segment of VII N. Figures 10.8 and 10.9 depict the management protocol for iatrogenic Facial palsy.

*Temporal Bone Tumours:* FNS is a rare tumour which most commonly presents in the 5th decade of life with Facial palsy being the most common presentation. Facial twitching and spasms are also commonly reported in about 25% of patients. Persistent or progressive hemifacial twitching suggests an ongoing degenerative process and increases the suspicion of a VII N tumour. A VII N examination showing elements of both weakness and hypertonicity or synkinesis in different zones of face is also highly suggestive of VII N tumours. Hearing loss (CHL/SNHL) is common at presentation with FNS.

Congenital intraosseous venous malformations (VII N hemangioma) of temporal bone adjacent to geniculate ganglion or intraosseous VII N characteristically enlarge throughout patient's life and can exert direct pressure on VII N to present as acute Facial palsy or Recurrent Facial palsy later in life (35). Because

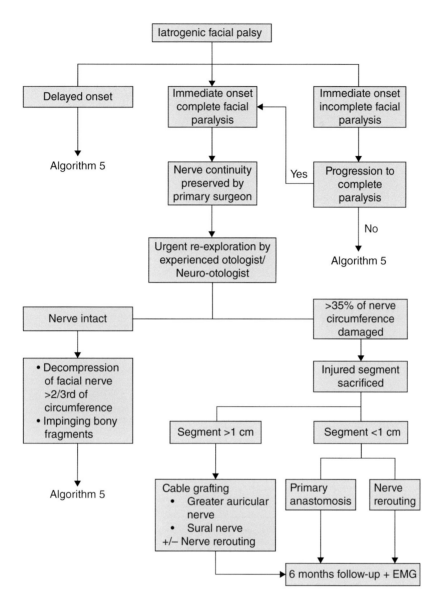

**Figure 10.8**  Management algorithm for iatrogenic facial palsy (Algorithm 4).

the natural history is to expand over time, surgical exploration is warranted in the presence of Facial palsy.

Treatment option is driven by desire to preserve facial function for longest period of time and at best possible level (7). Treatment and approach have to be individualized and stringent selection criteria in deciding on appropriate surgical management are crucial.

Head and neck tumours, such as temporal bone carcinoma and parotid malignancies, can present with acute or slowly progressive Facial palsy. CEMRI of temporal bone and neck will delineate tumour and any VII N involvement.

Treatment of tumour will depend on the clinical and pathological stage. Planned surgical extirpation with VII N reconstruction will depend on the extent of tumour as well as patient factors. In a retrospective study by Grundfast et al. (36), 12% of patients admitted to a children's hospital in 1990 with idiopathic Facial palsy were found to have malignancies. Clinical features such as gradual progression of paralysis lasting more than 3 weeks, no return of function in 6 months, ipsilateral recurrence, hemifacial spasm, other associated cranial neuropathies, and pain and single branch involvement should raise suspicion of a neoplastic aetiology.

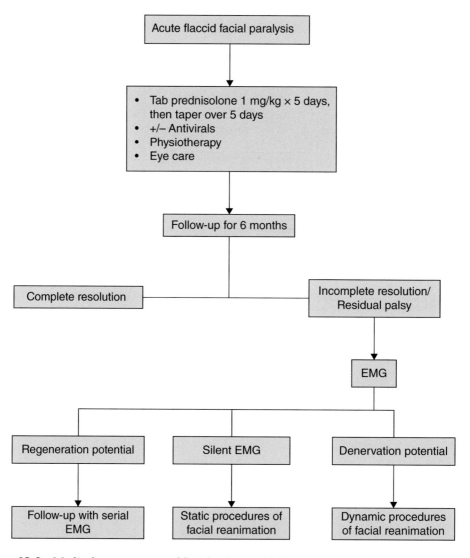

**Figure 10.9** Medical management of facial palsy and follow-up (Algorithm 5).

## INVESTIGATIONS

In presence of red flag signs suggestive of diagnosis other than Bell's palsy, appropriate further investigations should be done to reach a diagnosis and plan treatment strategy.

*Pure Tone Audiometry (PTA):* PTA helps determine the type and severity of hearing loss and also the hearing status of the normal side. It also helps in deciding the surgical approach, as in case the hearing is unserviceable, then a more radical translabyrinthine approach may be preferable with complete excision of temporal bone disease or tumour.

*Impedance Audiometry:* In Bell's palsy, ipsilateral stapedial reflex may be diminished or absent in up to 90% of cases. It is interesting to note that patients with intact stapedial reflex

have been shown to have better prognosis in Bell's palsy.

*Imaging:* Imaging studies (such as a HRCT of temporal bone with/without contrast, and/ or CEMRI of brain and neck; PET scan; Tc99m scan, Gallium scan, DOTANAC scan etc.) are indicated to rule out tumours in relation to the temporal bone, MOE, COM, fracture temporal bone etc. Clinical evaluation warranting imaging would include the following:

1. Red flag signs of Facial palsy suggesting diagnosis other than Bell's palsy

2. Setting of abnormal otoscopy

3. Palpable parotid or neck mass

4. Abnormal audiological evaluation

Imaging aims to determine site and type of lesion, extent, radiological characteristics, any additional tumours (e.g. NF2) and is required for preoperative surgical planning.

*Laboratory/Serological Tests:* Laboratory investigations have a limited role in setting of Facial palsy. In Lyme endemic area and serology (ELISA and Western blot test) should be sent for spirochete Borrelia burgdorferi. In Bilateral Facial palsy or Recurrent Facial palsy with a suspicion of an autoimmune aetiology, targeted laboratory investigations would include rheumatoid factor (RF), antinuclear antibody (ANA), antiphospholipid antibody and angiotensin-converting enzyme (ACE). Investigations like complete blood count (CBC), ESR, CRP, blood sugar level (BSL) and HIV ELISA may be indicated on case-to-case basis. Role of lumbar puncture for CSF studies to rule out meningitis and neuroborreliosis in Facial palsy is controversial (37, 38).

*Electrodiagnostic Tests:* Electrophysiological testing provides an objective means of assessing nerve function and is indicated for patients with complete paralysis. Those with incomplete paralysis carry a favourable prognosis and electrophysiological testing is not indicated. Electrophysiological testing also offers prognostic value for recovery in patients with complete paralysis, thereby identifying those who may be candidates for surgical intervention.

*Electroneuronography (ENoG) and Electromyography (EMG):* ENoG and EMG are the two most accurate and reliable electrophysiological tests currently in use. ENoG estimates relative proportion of nerve fibres that have undergone Wallerian degeneration and is most useful between day 4 and 14 of complete Facial palsy (39, 40). ENoG uses an evoked, supramaximal electrical stimulus to activate VII N as it exits the skull at Stylomastoid foramen. Maximum amplitude of CMAP correlates with number of remaining nerve fibres that are responsive (41), which is then compared with CMAP of normal side and a percentage of degenerated nerve fibres is calculated (42).

Voluntary EMG measures motor activity with needle electrodes placed in orbicularis oris and orbicularis oculi muscle while patient is asked to make forceful facial contractions. It is conducted after 3 weeks of onset of Facial palsy. In acute phase of Facial palsy, it is used when ENoG shows more than 90% degeneration (43), to confirm absence of muscle function. Presence of active motor units on EMG in a setting of severe degeneration on ENoG indicates a phenomenon termed deblocking (43), which is a sign of nerve regeneration and portends a favourable prognosis and does not warrant surgical intervention.

*Histopathological Examination (HPE):* Any mass or granulation in EAC should be subjected to HPE unless suspected to be of a vascular nature.

## TREATMENT

At the end of the clinical evaluation and investigations, one should be able to place the patient into one of five management domains of Facial palsy (44), as given in **Table 10.3**. A brief elaboration on the management domains is elucidated below:

*Acute Flaccid Facial Palsy:* This domain encompasses the first 2 weeks following onset of acute Flaccid Facial palsy. Once the diagnosis and severity of Facial palsy is established, it is imperative to initiate medical therapy as indicated, manage exposure keratopathy and determine candidacy for surgical intervention.

In Bell's palsy, administration of corticosteroids within 72 hours of symptom onset has been shown to shorten recovery time (45). Combined use of antivirals and corticosteroids may be of additional clinical benefit, especially for those with severe to complete paralysis (46–48). All delayed onset Facial palsy or incomplete Facial palsy secondary to trauma or iatrogenic warrants corticosteroids and observation.

Typical prednisolone dosing in most studies has been 60 mg orally once daily for 5 days followed by a 5-day taper (45, 49). Recent American Academy of Otolaryngology Head and Neck Surgery (AAO-HNS) clinical practice guidelines for Bell's palsy recommend a 10-day course of oral corticosteroids with at least 5 days at a high dose (prednisolone 50 mg for 10 days or prednisone 60 mg for 5 days) and tapering over 5 days. In paediatric patients, dosing is weight based, such as prednisolone 1–2 mg/kg per day for 10 days with a 3–5-day taper (50) or prednisolone 0.5–1.0 mg/kg per day (51). Alternatively, intravenous delivery is an option, though not commonly used (52).

Lyme-disease-associated Facial palsy is treated with a prolonged course (10–21 day course) of oral antibiotics, such as doxycycline, cefuroxime, amoxicillin or intravenous ceftriaxone (53). Although adjuvant corticosteroid therapy is commonly prescribed, its role in Lyme disease is controversial (54, 55, 56).

AOM associated with Facial palsy warrants a wide myringotomy (with or without mastoidectomy), steroids and antibiotics (57).

Facial palsy noticed immediately after surgical intervention warrants urgent re-exploration unless the primary surgeon documents having identified VII N and preserved it intact. Patients with complete idiopathic or posttraumatic paralysis with an ENoG response demonstrating greater than 90% degeneration, and absent voluntary motor units on EMG are considered for surgical intervention, ideally within 14 days of symptom onset (45). Treatment protocol for surgical intervention is provided in Figure 10.7 and 10.8.

Eye lubrication with night-time taping to close the affected eye is indicated to prevent exposure keratopathy. Physiotherapy and education on upper eyelid stretching to aid passive closure may be of benefit. Role of surgery in acute setting of Bell's palsy is controversial in contemporary literature.

*Flaccid Facial Palsy with Potential for Spontaneous Recovery:* In the setting of Flaccid Facial palsy of less than 6 months duration where VII N continuity is thought to be intact (VII N continuity either preserved or repaired intraoperatively), a potential for spontaneous recovery exists. Complete or partial return of facial tone and movement are expected within 6–12 months. Patients may benefit from physiotherapy, corneal protective measures, static periocular reanimation and temporary chemodenervation (e.g. Botox injection) of the healthy side depressor labii inferioris muscle to improve oral competence and articulation during this period. Close follow-up (every 3 months) is warranted to monitor recovery of function.

*Flaccid Facial Palsy with Viable Facial Musculature and Low Potential of Spontaneous Recovery:* When there exists a documented discontinuity of VII N or absent recovery of facial function (on electrophysiological studies) noted within 6–12 months of onset of Facial palsy with intact facial musculature, the potential for spontaneous recovery is low (58). VII N repair and transfers are indicated within 24 months from onset of Facial palsy as facial musculature remains receptive to reinnervation for periods up to 24 months following denervation (59, 60). Interposition graft repair (sural nerve or greater auricular nerve) should be considered in the setting of neural discontinuity. Alternatively, split hypoglossal nerve transfer to main trunk of VII N is an option.

The goal of VII N repairs and transfers is to restore facial tone and some form of blink; meaningful reanimation of expression is rarely achieved. Volitional expressions may be restored through targeted nerve transfers during this period. Static periocular reanimation (such as upper-lid weighting and lateral tarsal strip procedure) may be offered early in course of palsy onset where recovery is likely to take several months.

*Flaccid Facial Palsy Without Viable Facial Musculature:* Flaccid Facial palsy without viable facial musculature can occur either because facial musculature is absent or facial musculature is unreceptive to reinnervation (silent EMG). In such a scenario, nerve repair or transfers are no longer indicated.

Conservative approaches would include physiotherapy and targeted chemodenervation of the healthy side, while more aggressive options would include surgical interventions, including static facial suspensions, static periocular reanimation, and muscle transfers.

*Post-paralytic Facial Palsy (PFP):* PFP is a result of spontaneous aberrant regeneration or following grafting of VII N trunk, 6–18 months following severe VII N insult. It is always permanent in nature. Rarely, lagophthalmos may occur. Physiotherapy is the first-line treatment. A comprehensive program should include patient education, soft tissue mobilization, mirror and EMG biofeedback and neuromuscular retraining (61). In cases with severe restriction of oral commissure, regional (e.g. temporalis) or free (e.g. gracilis) muscle transfer may be considered for dynamic smile reanimation. Targeted nerve transfers, such as nerve to masseter transfer to the diseased side zygomatic branches for smile reanimation, are largely ineffective in the setting of PFP.

## OUTCOME TRACKING IN FACIAL PALSY

Systematic tracking of therapeutic outcomes is a prerequisite to clinical excellence. No single outcome measure can capture all of the complex domains of Facial palsy. An optimal panel of outcome measures should be objective, sensitive to change and easy to implement and compare results. An optimal outcome measure panel in Facial palsy includes (62) (1) patient reported outcome measures; (2) automated and clinician graded Facial palsy grading systems; (3) layperson assessment equivalent; and (4) spontaneous smile analysis.

QOL impact may be assessed using generalized patient-graded scales such as Facial Disability Index (63), Facial Clinimetric Evaluation (1) and Synkinesis Assessment Questionnaire (64). A computer-vision-based facial landmark recognition algorithm has recently been used within a novel freeware application (Emotrics, Massachusetts Eye and Ear Infirmary) for objective measurement of various facial displacements (e.g. smile excursion) from clinical photographs (65).

## KEY LEARNING POINTS

1. Facial deformity secondary to Facial palsy results in functional, communicative and social impairment along with a negative impact on quality of life and emotional well-being of a person.

2. History taking is the key to making a correct diagnosis and effective management. Diagnosis can almost always be ascertained 80–90% of time by obtaining an accurate history and conducting a thorough clinical examination.

3. Bell's palsy or idiopathic Facial palsy is the commonest cause of Facial palsy. However, in the presence of red flag signs suggestive of diagnosis other than Bell's palsy, appropriate further investigations (including imaging) should be done to reach a diagnosis and plan the treatment strategy.

4. A plethora of therapeutic options are available in the management of Facial palsy. Treatment is individualized depending on the primary aetiology and severity of Facial palsy and timing of presentation.

## ACKNOWLEDGEMENT

Surg Lt Cdr (Dr) Mahesh Ravunnikutty (Postgraduate trainee – MS ENT) for making the anatomical diagrams and algorithms.

## REFERENCES

1. Kahn JB, Gliklich RE, Boyev KP, et al. Validation of a patient-graded instrument for Facial nerve paralysis: the FaCE scale. Laryngoscope. 2001;111(3):387–98.

2. Ishii LE, Godoy A, Encarnacion CO, et al. What faces reveal: impaired affect display in facial paralysis. Laryngoscope. 2011;121(6):1138–43.

3. Valls-Sole J, Tolosa ES, Pujol M. Myokymic discharges and enhanced Facial nerve reflex responses after recovery from idiopathic facial palsy. Muscle Nerve. 1992;15(1):37–42.

4. Montserrat L, Benito M. Facial synkinesis and aberrant regeneration of Facial nerve. Adv Neurol. 1988; 49:211–24.

5. Kimura J, Rodnitzky RL, Okawara SH. Electrophysiologic analysis of aberrant regeneration after Facial nerve paralysis. Neurology. 1975;25(10):989–93.

6. Wetzig P. Aberrant regeneration of oculomotor and Facial nerves. Rocky Mt Med J. 1957;54(4):347–8.

7. Peitersen E. Bell's palsy: the spontaneous course of 2,500 peripheral Facial nerve palsies of different etiologies. Acta Otolaryngol Suppl. 2002;(549):4–30.

8. Cha CI, Hong CK, Park MS, et al. Comparison of Facial nerve paralysis in adults and children. Yonsei Med J. 2008;49(5):725–34.

9. Vrabec JT. The Facial nerve. In: Slattery WH, Azizzadeh B, editors. Medical Treatment of Bell Palsy. New York: Thieme; 2014.

10. De Diego JI, Prim MP, Madero R, et al. Seasonal patterns of idiopathic facial paralysis: a 16-year study. Otolaryngol Head Neck Surg. 1999;120(2):269–71.

11. Yanagihara N. Incidence of Bell's palsy. Ann Otol Rhinol Laryngol Suppl. 1988; 137:3–4.

12. Murakami S, Mizobuchi M, Nakashiro Y, et al. Bell palsy and Herpes simplex virus: identification of viral DNA in endoneurial fluid and muscle. Ann Intern Med. 1996;124(1 Pt 1):27–30.

13. Furuta Y, Fukuda S, Suzuki S, et al. Detection of Varicella-zoster virus DNA in patients with acute peripheral facial palsy by the polymerase chain reaction, and its use for early diagnosis of zoster sine herpete. J Med Virol. 1997;52(3):316–9.

14. McCormick DP. Herpes-simplex virus as a cause of Bell's palsy. Lancet. 1972;1(7757):937–9.

15. Rivera-Serrano CM, Man LX, Klein S, et al. Melkersson-Rosenthal syndrome: a Facial nerve center perspective. J Plast Reconstr Aesthet Surg. 2014;67(8): 1050–4.

16. Liu R, Yu S. Melkersson-Rosenthal syndrome: a review of seven patients. J Clin Neurosci. 2013; 20(7):993–5.

17. Sathirapanya P. Isolated and bilateral simultaneous facial palsy disclosing early human immunodeficiency virus infection. Singapore Med J. 2015;56(6):e105–6.

18. Gaudin RA, Jowett N, Banks CA, et al. Bilateral facial paralysis: a 13-year experience. Plast Reconstr Surg. 2016;138(4):879–87.

19. Oosterveer DM, Benit CP, de Schryver EL. Differential diagnosis of recurrent or bilateral peripheral facial palsy. J Laryngol Otol. 2012;126(8):833–6.

20. Yanagihara N, Hyodo M. Association of diabetes mellitus and hypertension with Bell's palsy and Ramsay Hunt syndrome. Ann Otol Rhinol Laryngol Suppl. 1988;137:5–7.

21. Phillips KM, Heiser A, Gaudin R, et al. Onset of Bell's palsy in late pregnancy and early puerperium is associated with worse long-term outcomes. Laryngoscope. 2017;127(12):2854–9.

22. Alrashdi IS, Rich P, Patton MA. A family with hereditary congenital facial paresis and a brief review of the literature. Clin Dysmorphol. 2010;19(4):198–201.

23. House JW, Brackmann DE. Facial nerve grading system. Otolaryngol Head Neck Surg. 1985;93(2):146–7.

24. Ross BG, Fradet G, Nedzelski JM. Development of a sensitive clinical facial grading system. Otolaryngol Head Neck Surg. 1996;114(3):380–6.

25. Vrabec JT, Backous DD, Djalilian HR, et al. Facial nerve grading system 2.0. Otolaryngol Head Neck Surg. 2009;140(4):445–50.

26. Taverner D. Surgery versus conservative treatment in peripheral facial palsies: round table discussion. (Jongkees LBW, moderator). Arch Otolaryngol. 1965;81:532–46.

27. Takemoto N, Horii A, Sakata Y, et al. Prognostic factors of peripheral facial palsy: multivariate analysis followed by receiver operating characteristic and Kaplan-Meier analyses. Otol Neurotol. 2011;32(6):1031–6.

28. Byun H, Cho YS, Jang JY, et al. Value of electroneurography as a prognostic indicator for recovery in acute severe inflammatory facial paralysis: a prospective study of Bell's palsy and Ramsay Hunt syndrome. Laryngoscope. 2013;123(10):2526–32.

29. Ellefsen B, Bonding P. Facial palsy in acute otitis media. Clin Otolaryngol Allied Sci. 1996;21:393Y395.

30. Gaio E, Marioni G, de Filippis C, et al. Facial nerve paralysis secondary to acute otitis media in infants and children. J Paediatr Child Health. 2004;40:483Y486.

31. Ikeda M, Nakazato H, Onoda K, et al. Facial nerve paralysis caused by middle ear cholesteatoma and effects of surgical intervention. Acta Otolaryngol. 2006;126(1):95–100.

32. Savic DL, Djeric DR. Facial paralysis in chronic suppurative otitis media. Clin Otolaryngol Allied Sci. 1989;14(6):515–7.

33. Guerrissi JO. Facial nerve paralysis after intratemporal and extratemporal blunt trauma. J Craniofac Surg. 1997;8:431Y437.

34. Patel A, Groppo E. Management of temporal bone trauma. Craniomaxillofac Trauma Reconstr. 2010; 3(2):105–13.

35. Benoit MM, North PE, McKenna MJ, et al. Facial nerve hemangiomas: vascular tumors or malformations? Otolaryngol Head Neck Surg. 2010;142(1):108–14.

36. Grundfast KM, Guarisco JL, Thomsen JR, et al. Diverse etiologies of facial paralysis in children. IJPORL. 1990;19:223Y239.

37. Sandstedt P, Hyden D, Odkvist LM, et al. Peripheral facial palsy in children: a cerebrospinal fluid study. Acta Paediatr Scand. 1985;74:281Y285.

38. Albisetti M, Schaer G, Good M, et al. Diagnostic value of cerebrospinal fluid examination in children with peripheral facial palsy and suspected Lyme borreliosis. Neurology. 1997;49:817Y824.

39. Gantz BJ. Traumatic facial paralysis. In: Current Therapy in Otolaryngology Head and Neck Surgery. Hamilton (ON): BC Decker, 1987, p. 112–5.

40. Fisch U. Facial nerve grafting. Otolaryngol Clin North Am. 1974;7(2):517–29.

41. Krarup C. Compound sensory action potential in normal and pathological human nerves. Muscle Nerve. 2004;29(4):465–83.

42. Gantz BJ, Gmuer AA, Holliday M, et al. Electroneurographic evaluation of the Facial nerve: method and technical problems. Ann Otol Rhinol Laryngol. 1984;93(4 Pt 1):394–8.

43. Fisch U. Maximal nerve excitability testing vs. electroneuronography. Arch Otolaryngol. 1980;106(6): 352–7.

44. Jowett N. A general approach to facial palsy. OCNA. 2018;51(6):1019–31.

45. Engstrom M, Berg T, Stjernquist-Desatnik A, et al. Prednisolone and valaciclovir in Bell's palsy: a randomised, double-blind, placebo-controlled, multicentre trial. Lancet Neurol. 2008;7(11):993–1000.

46. McAllister K, Walker D, Donnan PT, et al. Surgical interventions for the early management of Bell's palsy. Cochrane Database Syst Rev. 2013;(10):CD007468.

47. de Almeida JR, Al Khabori M, Guyatt GH, et al. Combined corticosteroid and antiviral treatment for Bell palsy: a systematic review and meta-analysis. JAMA. 2009;302(9):985–93.

48. Murakami S, Hato N, Horiuchi J, et al. Treatment of Ramsay Hunt syndrome with acyclovir-prednisone: significance of early diagnosis and treatment. Ann Neurol. 1997;41(3):353–7.

49. Austin JR, Peskind SP, Austin SG, et al. Idiopathic Facial nerve paralysis: a randomized double blind controlled study of placebo versus prednisone. Laryngoscope. 1993;103(12):1326–33.

50. Unuvar E, Oguz F, Sidal M, et al. Corticosteroid treatment of childhood Bell's palsy. Pediatr Neurol. 1999;21(5):814–6.

51. Pitaro J, Waissbluth S, Daniel SJ. Do children with Bell's palsy benefit from steroid treatment? A systematic review. Int J Pediatr Otorhinolaryngol. 2012;76(7):921–6.

52. Lagalla G, Logullo F, Di Bella P, et al. Influence of early high-dose steroid treatment on Bell's palsy evolution. Neurol Sci. 2002;23(3):107–12.

53. Wormser GP, Dattwyler RJ, Shapiro ED, et al. The clinical assessment, treatment, and prevention of Lyme disease, human granulocytic anaplasmosis, and babesiosis: clinical practice guidelines by the Infectious Diseases Society of America. Clin Infect Dis. 2006;43(9):1089–134.

54. Jowett N, Gaudin RA, Banks CA, et al. Steroid use in Lyme disease associated facial palsy is associated with worse long-term outcomes. Laryngoscope. 2017;127(6):1451–8.

55. Clark JR, Carlson RD, Sasaki CT, et al. Facial paralysis in Lyme disease. Laryngoscope. 1985;95(11):1341–5.

56. Halperin JJ, Shapiro ED, Logigian E, et al. Practice parameter: treatment of nervous system Lyme disease (an evidence-based review): report of the Quality Standards Subcommittee of the American Academy of Neurology. Neurology. 2007;69(1):91–102.

57. Redaelli de Zinis LO, Gamba P, Balzanelli C. Acute otitis media and Facial nerve paralysis in adults. Otol Neurotol. 2003;24(1):113–7.

58. Rivas A, Boahene KD, Bravo HC, et al. A model for early prediction of Facial nerve recovery after vestibular schwannoma surgery. Otol Neurotol. 2011; 32(5):826–33.

59. Wu P, Chawla A, Spinner RJ, et al. Key changes in denervated muscles and their impact on regeneration and reinnervation. Neural Regen Res. 2014; 9(20):1796–809.

60. Conley J. Hypoglossal crossover–122 cases. Trans Sect Otolaryngol Am Acad Ophthalmol Otolaryngol. 1977;84(4 Pt 1):Orl-763–8.

61. Wernick Robinson M, Baiungo J, Hohman M, et al. Facial rehabilitation. Oper Tech Otolaryngol Head Neck Surg. 2012;23(4):288–96.

62. Dusseldorp JR, Van Veen MM, Mohan S, Hadlock TA. Outcome tracking in facial palsy. Otolaryngol Clin N Am. 2018;51(6):1033–50.

63. Van Swearingen JM, Brach JS. The Facial Disability Index: reliability and validity of a disability assessment instrument for disorders of the facial neuromuscular system. Phys Ther. 1996;76(12): 1288–98 [discussion: 1298–300].

64. Mehta RP, Wernick Robinson M, Hadlock TA. Validation of the synkinesis assessment questionnaire. Laryngoscope. 2007;117(5):923–6.

65. Guarin DL, Dusseldorp JR, Hadlock TA, et al. A machine learning approach for automated facial measurements in facial palsy. JAMA Facial Plast Surg. 2018; 20(4):335–7.

# NEOPLASMS IN OTOLOGY: GUIDE TO DIAGNOSIS AND MANAGEMENT

# 11 Malignant Neoplasms in Otology

*Smriti Panda, Chirom Amit Singh and Uma Patnaik*

## CONTENTS

## INTRODUCTION

Temporal bone malignancies (TBM) constitute 0.2% of all head and neck malignancies with an annual incidence of 6 per million people (1–3). Demographic studies have shown that primary TBM have a predilection for males in the 5th to 7th decades (4). A practitioner of otology will encounter malignant tumours in this region arising either from the external ear or from the temporal bone (Figure 11.1) (5). The temporal bone is more frequently involved by neoplastic process arising in the parotid, temporo-mandibular joint or the skull base (paranasal sinus and nasopharynx). The prime focus of this chapter shall remain malignancies arising from the external ear and the temporal bone.

Given the architectural and histological complexity of the temporal region, a wide variety of neoplasms have been reported (Table 11.1). Broadly, neoplasms can be of epithelial, mesenchymal or minor salivary gland origin. The most commonly encountered histology is squamous cell carcinoma (60–80%) followed by basal cell carcinoma and adenoid cystic carcinoma (6).

### Aetiology

1. *Ultraviolet radiation:* Ultraviolet radiation and fair skin are the prime aetiological factors to be taken into account for cutaneous squamous cell carcinoma, basal cell carcinoma or malignant melanoma (7). External auditory canal tumours and carcinoma arising from the pinna are often associated with actinic changes (8, 9).

2. *Chronic otitis media:* A history of chronic otitis media is frequently encountered prior to the development of temporal bone squamous cell carcinoma (10). Older literature implicated cholesteatoma to be a causative factor in 85% of all TBM (11).

3. *Prior radiotherapy:* The first report of radiation-induced TBM was by Ruben et al. in 1977 (11). Criteria for labelling a tumour as radiation induced were laid out by Cahan et al. (12):

    a. The tumour should arise in the field of prior radiotherapy.

    b. There should be a latent period of at least 5 years.

    c. There should be histologically documented evidence of the irradiated and present tumour to be different.

In a cohort of nasopharyngeal carcinoma patients who were irradiated, follow-up revealed

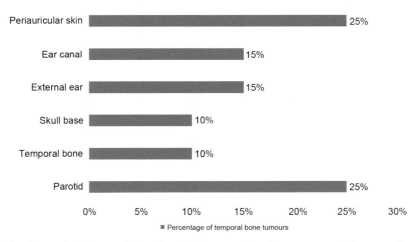

**Figure 11.1** Chart depicting subsite distribution contributing to temporal bone malignancy.

a radiation-induced TBM in 0.13%, which is much higher than the general population (13).

1. *Human papilloma virus:* The association of HPV with cholesteatoma to the tune of 36% has led many investigators to question its aetiological role in TBM (14–16).

2. Other postulated aetiological factors include trauma (17), immunosuppression and systemic lupus erythematosus (18).

### Clinical Presentation

The clinical features of a TBM overlap with those of inflammatory conditions of the temporal bone. This results in significant delay in diagnosis at an early stage. Some studies have reported a treatment delay of an average of 13 months (19). Based on the demographic details and aetiological factors enumerated, a high index of suspicion needs to be maintained

### Table 11.1: Histological Differential Diagnosis for a Temporal Bone Neoplasm

| Tissue of Origin | Tumour |
|---|---|
| 1. Epithelial | Squamous cell carcinoma<br>Basal cell carcinoma<br>Adenoid cystic carcinoma<br>Basosquamous carcinoma<br>Hidradenocarcinoma<br>Melanoma<br>Sebaceous cell carcinoma<br>Sarcomatoid carcinoma<br>Endolymphatic sac tumour |
| 2. Mesenchymal | Rhabdomyosarcoma<br>Chondrosarcoma<br>Synovial sarcoma<br>Osteosarcoma<br>Malignant peripheral nerve sheath tumour<br>Fibrous dysplasia<br>Ossifying fibroma<br>Aneurysmal bone cyst |
| 3. Salivary gland | Adenoid cystic carcinoma<br>Mucoepidermoid carcinoma<br>Acinic cell carcinoma |
| 4. Intermediate-grade tumours | Chordoma<br>Chondroblastoma<br>Solitary fibrous tumour<br>Glomangiopericytoma<br>Langerhans cell histiocytosis |
| 5. Metastasis | Solid organ malignancy: kidney, lung, breast, thyroid<br>Hematolymphoid: granulocytic sarcoma/chloroma |

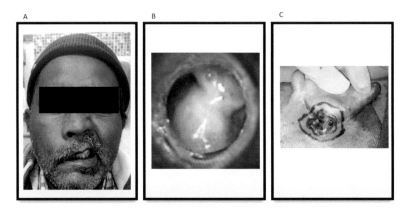

**Figure 11.2**   Clinical presentation in temporal bone malignancy. (a) Right-sided House-Brackman grade 6 facial palsy. (b) Examination under microscope of the same patient revealing a proliferative growth filling the external auditory canal. Histology in this case was squamous cell carcinoma. (c) Cutaneous malignancy arising from the pinna (conchal cartilage and postauricular sulcus). Proliferative, well-defined, pigmented lesion is seen. Histopathology in this case was basal cell carcinoma.

for inflammatory conditions refractory to conservative management.

Tumours arising from the external auditory canal or the pinna present with a visible proliferative lesion with ulceration and bleeding (Figure 11.2). Those located in the bony canal and middle ear initially manifest with otorrhea, hearing loss and otalgia, thereby delaying diagnosis. Skin involvement, sensorineural hearing loss, facial palsy and trismus are late features. The latter is a pointer towards infratemporal fossa extension or temporomandibular joint involvement. Locally extensive tumours with intracranial extension can present with VI nerve palsy and anaesthesia in the V nerve's distribution due to petrous apex involvement, followed by cavernous sinus extension (Figure 11.3).

### DIAGNOSTIC WORKUP

*Cross-Sectional Imaging:* Computed tomography and magnetic resonance imaging provide complementary information pertaining to bone erosion and soft tissue extension, respectively. Computed tomography of the temporal bone should be of high resolution (HRCT) with a slice thickness of 1 mm or less (Figure 11.4). While

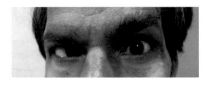

**Figure 11.3**   Left-sided lateral rectus palsy due to petrous apex extension of temporal bone lesion.

interpreting the disease extent on an HRCT temporal bone, it is essential to remember its shortcomings. Leonetti et al. studied the pattern of spread in case of TBM and found that HRCT was accurate for staging only in cases of anterior and inferior growth patterns. HRCT underestimated disease spread for tumours with posterior, superior and medial extensions (20). To identify bone erosions in the anterior wall of external auditory canal, minimum of 2-mm erosion is required to be accurately identified by HRCT (21). Considerable artefacts have been identified in HRCT temporal bone from dental implants and ossified cartilage (22).

Contrast-enhanced MRI of the temporal region and brain provides excellent soft tissue delineation (Figure 11.5). It also helps to differentiate tumour involvement from fluid collection in the mastoid air cells. It is the currently the gold standard for defining the extent of intracranial extension and perineural neural invasion on fat-suppressed sequence. The character of the lesion on various sequences of MRI can also provide a clue to its histological variant (**Table 11.2**) (23). Sigmoid sinus obstruction and encasement of petrous internal carotid artery are informative to assess the operability of the tumour (24).

*Cerebral Cross-circulation:* The neurotologist is often faced with the situation of tumour closely abutting the internal carotid artery or the sigmoid sinus. Cerebral cross-circulation for the arterial and venous phases will determine the future course of action in these cases (Figure 11.6). Indiscriminate ligation of the carotid system is associated with a 40%

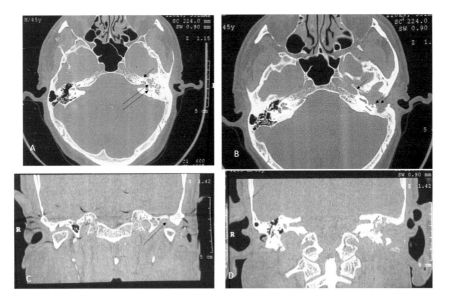

**Figure 11.4** HRCT temporal bone of a patient with squamous cell carcinoma of temporal bone. (a) Axial cut showing homogeneous, destructive soft tissue density filling mastoid air cells and middle ear. There is surrounding sclerosis of mastoid air cells. Ossicles are partly destroyed. Osseous destruction is seen over the dome of the lateral semicircular canal (double arrow). Dehiscence possibly disease related is seen in the region of the second genu of the Facial nerve (single arrow). (b) Disease extending to petrous apex abutting petrous ICA (single arrow), mastoid segment of Facial nerve eroded (double arrow). (c and d) Corresponding coronal section showing disease extension into temporomandibular joint space (arrow).

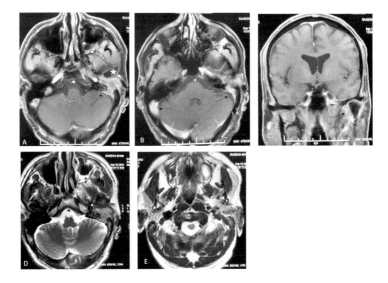

**Figure 11.5** Contrast MRI of the same patient showing better soft tissue delineation. (a) T1 contrast-enhanced sequence showing enhancing infiltrative mass lesion of the mastoid air cells and middle ear. Extension to petrous apex is seen. Dural enhancement is seen along the posterior fossa dura (arrow). Tumour infiltration noted into the temporomandibular joint space (star). (b) Dural venous sinus is noted to be less prominent on the left side, suggesting the possibility of sigmoid sinus thrombosis. (c) Coronal section showing soft tissue infiltration along temporomandibular joint space. (d) Outline of petrous carotid artery is seen to be preserved. (e) Extensive soft tissue infiltration is seen into the infratemporal fossa.

## Table 11.2: Radiological Features of Common Temporal Bone Pathologies

| | T1 | T1+Gad | T2 | CT | Additional Findings |
|---|---|---|---|---|---|
| Squamous cell carcinoma | Isointense | Enhancing | Hyperintense | Destructive infiltrative | |
| Salivary gland tumour | Hypointense | Focal enhancement | Hypointense/ isointense | Cystic, poorly defined spaces | |
| Lymphoma | Hypointense | Variable, enhancement in higher grade | Hypointense | Smooth borders | |
| Chordoma | Hypointense | Intense enhancement | Hyperintense | Lobulated, bone destruction, calcific spicules | |
| Granulocytic sarcoma | Hypointense | Enhancement | Isointense | Expansile homogeneous | Involves middle ear cleft, enhancement along Facial nerve due to direct tumour infiltration in paediatric patients and dehiscent nerves |
| Rhabdomyosarcoma | Hypointense | Enhancement | Hyperintense | Destructive/ infiltrative | |
| Osteosarcoma | Irregular | Irregular enhancement | Mixed | Radiolucent | Sun-burst appearance |
| Langerhans cell histiocytosis | Variable | Enhancing | Hyperintense | Well-defined osseous destruction centred over the mastoid tip | Relative sparing of ossicles, petrous apex and middle ear |
| Metastasis from solid organ | Hypointense | Variable | Isointense | Irregular with smooth margin | Involves temporal squama, petrous apex, Facial nerve. Middle ear cleft involvement is rare |

incidence of cerebrovascular accident with mortality in 50% of these patients. Long-term excess mortality rates have been found to be 17% with a yearly stroke rate of 0.5% (25). Venous insufficiency in the absence of venous cross-circulation with an incidence of 1.5 per 1000 skull base procedures similarly predisposes to venous infarct and obstructing hydrocephalus (26). A multimodality testing protocol for cerebral cross-circulation consisting of endovascular balloon test occlusion with monitoring of neurological status, electrocardiography (ECG), electroencephalography (EEG), single-photon emission computed tomography (SPECT) imaging of regional cerebral blood flow with Tc-99-HMPAO, transcranial Doppler of ipsilateral middle cerebral artery was used and testing was repeated following acetazolamide administration. Despite such a rigorous testing, 2 out of 45 developed cerebrovascular accident following carotid occlusion (27). Revascularization procedure is recommended in patients failing these tests, in younger individuals and patients with bilateral tumours.

*Histopathology:* Tissue diagnosis is essential to identify the histological type of TBM. Squamous cell carcinoma, for example, requires 1-cm gross

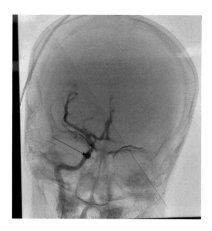

**Figure 11.6** Cerebral cross-circulation study by balloon test occlusion of the right ICA system. Flow is seen to be established on the ipsilateral side through anterior communicating collateral.

margin with elective lymph nodal treatment in the parotid and cervical nodal basin. Basal cell carcinoma is only locally infiltrative with no predilection for lymph nodal metastasis requiring 4-mm margins. In case of adenoid cystic carcinoma, perineural invasion needs to be addressed surgically and with adjuvant treatment. Biopsy also helps to identify tumours which do not require upfront surgery, for example: lymphoma, Langerhans cell histiocytosis (LCH), rhabdomyosarcoma (RMS) etc. Biopsy should be performed under microscopic magnification; the procedure can be performed under local anaesthesia in adults but requires general anaesthesia in children.

*Metastatic Screening:* Temporal bone squamous cell carcinoma is locally aggressive with a tendency to fail locoregionally (28). Therefore, there is limited role for routine whole-body PET-CT for distant metastasis screening (Figure 11.7). Instead of HRCT of the chest, chest X-ray is a more cost-effective option. PET-CT in TBM is indicated when a metastatic skull base lesion is suspected from an unknown primary like kidney, breast and prostate (29).

*Pre-anaesthetic Workup:* Poor general condition of the patient precludes the extensive skull base approaches which form a part of temporal bone resection. Baseline investigations and screening for comorbid illnesses should be performed prior to embarking on surgery. If lower cranial nerve weakness is expected postoperatively, preoperative incentive spirometry may ameliorate aspiration risk (30).

*Staging and Patterns of Spread of TBM:* One of the challenges encountered in the management of TBM is the lack of a cogent staging system by AJCC/UICC. External ear (pinna) squamous cell carcinoma is staged according to head and neck

cutaneous squamous cell carcinoma (Table 11.3) (31). Over the years, many staging systems and their modifications have been suggested for temporal bone carcinoma (Table 11.4) (32).

Stell and McCormick et al. proposed a staging system for TBM in 1985; however, this staging system did not distinguish patients with extracranial soft tissue extension from patients with intracranial disease. This drawback was noted by Clark et al. in their observation of ten patients staged as T3 according to the Stell and McCormick classification. Patients with extracranial soft tissue extension had better outcomes than those with intracranial disease. This was subsequently incorporated in the staging modification (32, 33).

The staging system more popularly followed is the Pittsburgh System proposed by Arriaga et al. modified by Moody et al. (34, 35). This modification was a result of an analysis which demonstrated significant difference in survival in patients with preoperative Facial nerve palsy and other patients staged T3 according to the original Pittsburgh Classification (36). Since the outcome of patients with Facial nerve palsy paralleled the T4 patients, this important prognostic marker was incorporated into the staging system.

*Pathways of Spread of TBM:* TBM spread in an orderly fashion along various preformed pathways (Figure 11.8). Knowledge of the pathways of spread will help us in appreciating the "compartmentalized resection" strategies that form the basis for various types of temporal bone resection (20).

1. *Anterior spread:* For a tumour located in the external auditory canal, discontinuity in the cartilaginous canal (fissures of Santorini)

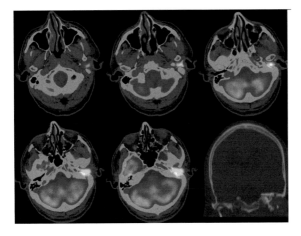

**Figure 11.7** Whole body 18F-FDG PET-CT of the same patient showing no uptake suggestive of distant metastasis.

## Table 11.3: AJCC 8th Edition Staging for Cutaneous Squamous Cell Carcinoma of the Pinna

**Definition of Primary Tumour (T)**

| T category | T criteria |
| --- | --- |
| Tx | Primary tumour not identified |
| Tis | Carcinoma in situ |
| T1 | Tumour smaller than 2 cm in greatest dimension |
| T2 | Tumour 2 cm or larger, but smaller than 4 cm in greatest dimension |
| T3 | Tumour 4cm or larger in maximum dimension or minor bone invasion or perineural invasion or deep invasion (invasion beyond subcutaneous fat, >6 mm as measured from the granular cell layer of the adjacent normal epidermis. PNI defined as tumour cells within nerve sheath of a nerve lying deeper than the dermis or measuring 0.1 mm or larger in calibre, or presenting with clinical or radiographic involvement of named nerves without skull base invasion or transgression) |
| T4 | Tumour with cortical bone/marrow, skull base invasion and or skull base foramen invasion |
| T4a | Tumour with gross cortical bone/marrow invasion |
| T4b | Tumour with skull base invasion and or skull base foramen involvement |

**Clinical N**

| | |
| --- | --- |
| Nx | Regional lymph node cannot be assessed |
| N0 | No regional lymph nodal metastasis |
| N1 | Metastasis in single ipsilateral lymph nodes 3 cm or smaller in greatest dimension and ENE– |
| N2a | Metastasis in a single ipsilateral node greater than 3 cm but not larger than 6 cm in greatest dimension and ENE– |
| N2b | Metastasis in multiple ipsilateral nodes, none larger than 6 cm in greatest dimension and ENE– |
| N2c | Metastasis in bilateral or contralateral nodes, none larger than 6 cm in greatest dimension and ENE– |
| N3a | Metastasis in a lymph node larger than 6 cm in greatest dimension and ENE– |
| N3b | Metastasis in any node and ENE+ |

*Abbreviations:* ENE: Extranodal Extension; PNI: Perineural Invasion.

facilitates spread towards the superficial lobe of parotid. The foramen of Huschke is a defect in the bony canal which can help track tumour cells into the infratemporal fossa and deep lobe of parotid. Once the parotid is involved, Facial nerve weakness can result from spread along extratemporal course of Facial nerve.

2. *Posterior spread:* Erosion of the posterior canal wall will provide access to the mastoid air cell system. Depending on the extent of pneumatization, these cells provide a pathway of least resistance causing the tumour to grow unimpeded along the cell tracts. Another feature of posterior spread is the involvement of Facial nerve either in the mastoid segment or at the stylomastoid foramen.

3. *Medial spread:* The tympanic membrane acts as a barrier for spread. Some authors have also coined the term "Ohngren's line for temporal bone" for the tympanic membrane (37). Tumours restricted to the external auditory canal are therefore amenable to lateral temporal bone resection (LTBR). Breach of the annulus and tympanic membrane result in involvement of middle ear mucosa.

4. Once in the middle ear, medial spread results in inner ear involvement. Anterior spread occurs along eustachian tube, peritubal cells and petrous apex, Gasserian ganglion, cavernous sinus and nasopharynx. The tumour can encase the petrous carotid in this region. Superior spread can result in involvement of tympanic segment of Facial nerve. Posterior spread results in involvement of the mastoid air cell, vertical segment of the Facial nerve and the vestibule. Continued disease extension medially and posteriorly will cause posterior fossa extension and sigmoid sinus involvement, respectively.

## Table 11.4: Staging Systems for Temporal Bone Carcinoma

| T | Arriaga et al. Original Pittsburgh 1990 (34) | Moody's Modification of Pittsburgh Staging (2000) (35) | Stell and McCormick's Staging 1985 (33) | Clark's Modification of Stell's Staging 2018 (32) |
|---|---|---|---|---|
| T1 | Tumour limited to EAC without bone erosion or soft tissue involvement | No change | Tumour limited to the site of origin, i.e., no bone erosion or facial palsy | No change |
| T2 | Tumour with limited EAC bone involvement (not full thickness) and <0.5 cm soft tissue involvement | No change | Tumour extending beyond the site of origin as indicated by facial palsy or radiological evidence of bone erosion but does not extend beyond the organ of origin | No change |
| T3 | Tumour involving full thickness osseous destruction of EAC with <0.5 cm soft tissue involvement or tumour involving middle ear, mastoid and Facial nerve | Tumour involving full thickness osseous destruction of EAC with <0.5 cm soft tissue involvement or tumour involving middle ear, mastoid air cells | Clinical or radiological evidence of extension beyond the organ of origin (TMJ, dura, skull base, parotid gland, etc.) | Clinical or radiological evidence of extension to extracranial structures – TMJ, parotid gland, skin |
| T4 | Tumour eroding the cochlea, petrous apex, carotid canal, Jugular foramen, dura, extensive soft tissue involvement (>0.5 cm), such as involvement of TMJ/styloid process | Tumour eroding the cochlea, petrous apex, carotid canal, Jugular foramen, dura, extensive soft tissue involvement (>0.5 cm), such as involvement of TMJ/ styloid process and Facial nerve involvement | | Clinical or radiological evidence of extension to cranial structures like skull base and dura |

*Abbreviations:* TMJ: Temporomandibular Joint; EAC: External Auditory Canal.

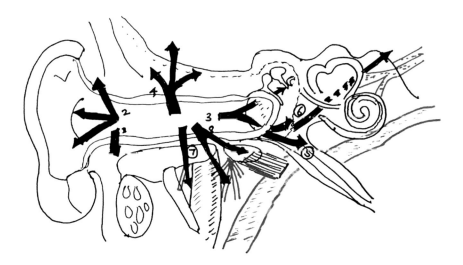

**Figure 11.8** Pathways of spread of temporal bone malignancy. 1: Anterior spread through cartilaginous canal. 2: Through concha into posterior auricular sulcus. 3: Through tympanic membrane into middle ear. 4: posteriorly into mastoid. 5: Through anterior mesotympanum into eustachian tube and carotid artery. 6: Into inner ear through round window and otic capsule. 7: Into infratemporal fossa through Facial nerve. 8: Inferomedially into Jugular fossa, carotid space and lower cranial nerves. (Adapted from Moody SA, Hirsch BE, Myers EN. Squamous cell carcinoma of the external auditory canal: an evaluation of a staging system. *Am J Otol* 2000;21:582–8.)

5. *Superior spread:* Perpetuation of disease process superiorly will result in intracranial extension following erosion of tegmen tympani or tegmen antri.

6. *Inferior spread:* This is a late event during a TBM. Sequential involvement of the hypotympanum is followed by Jugular foramen extension. The latter brings on the symptoms of lower cranial nerve palsy.

The frequency of these pathways encountered was studied by Gidley et al. (38). Anterior extension through the external auditory canal was the most common route of spread as seen in 63%, Jugular foramen extension in 23%, carotid artery and infratemporal fossa involvement in 11% and temporomandibular joint involvement in 4%.

## REVIEW OF LITERATURE

An extensive literature search revealed the following limitations at present:

1. Most studies are limited to retrospective, single-institution experience.

2. There is heterogenicity in the histologies considered for inclusion. There is often an overlap with cutaneous squamous cell carcinoma.

3. Lack of a universal staging system makes it difficult to compare treatment outcomes.

4. Evaluation of non-surgical treatment modalities is difficult owing to a large number of studies from pre-conformal radiotherapy era.

*Evaluation of Prognostic Factors and Outcomes:* In Tables 11.5 and 11.6, we have summarized the prognostic factors, their significance and oncological outcomes in various notable series (39–42). Higgins et al. performed a systematic review and pooled survival analysis of 21 studies involving 348 cases of temporal bone squamous cell carcinoma (36). The overall and disease-specific survival was found to be worse for patients with Facial nerve involvement. There are studies which do not show significant difference in terms of local control following dural resection, as in the study by Dean et al. (76.9% vs. 71.7%) (43).

Margin positivity directly translates to poor local control. Margin positivity rates in various series are in the range of 20–33% (28, 44). Morris et al. have shown disease-specific survival dropping from 81.7% to 50% with positive margins (28). As evident by the staging systems in practice, middle ear involvement is associated with worse outcome. Middle ear involvement brings down survival from 60% to 20% irrespective of treatment modality (19).

*Role of Parotidectomy and Neck Dissection:* The next important prognostic factor is lymph node positivity. As a dictum in head and neck oncology, lymph node positivity reduces long-term survival outcomes by 50% (45). However, unlike mucosal head and neck subsites, the incidence of lymph nodal positivity in neck dissection specimens from temporal bone squamous cell carcinoma patients is less than 20% (13). Interesting findings from the study by McRackan et al. were that 50% of those who were N+ recurred more commonly at distant sites, while N0 patients failed at the primary site. The pattern of lymph nodal spread from the temporal bone is as follows: level II (20.4%), level III (13.3%), periparotid (11.2%), level IV (6.1%), perifacial (4.1%) and level V (4.1%) (4). Contrary to these findings, there is tendency towards addressing the neck nodes electively in temporal bone squamous cell carcinoma with neck dissection rates of 88.5–93.3% in literature (46). McRackan et al. study also revealed that the risk of recurrence was higher with cervical nodal positivity than periparotid nodal involvement (13).

The parotid gland can get involved either through direct infiltration through the external auditory canal or via intraparotid lymph nodes. The reported incidence of parotid gland involvement range between 10% and 62% (47). There are currently no clear-cut guidelines for incorporating parotidectomy in every case of temporal bone resection. Though some authors routinely perform a superficial parotidectomy, few forego this step in T1 and T2 tumours if anterior wall is free of disease (48).

*En-Bloc vs. Piecemeal Excision:* Halstedian principles governing oncology have always insisted on en-bloc resection of malignancy with tumour-free margin. In the temporal bone, this would entail resection of the petrous carotid artery, Facial nerve and Jugular foramen structures (49). Though many surgeons practice en-bloc resection for early stage TBM, the same principles for locally advanced tumours would result in unnecessary morbidity (48). To strike a balance between morbidity and oncology, following a LTBR, disease is cleared under microscopic guidance from vital neurovascular structures and confirmed with frozen section. The surrounding bone is drilled till bleeding edges are seen (44).

*Need for Mastoid Obliteration:* The incidence of osteoradionecrosis following tympanomastoid exenteration and radiation have been

## Table 11.5: Summary of the Results from Studies Evaluating Prognostic Factors in Temporal Bone Malignancies

| Study (Year) | n | Histology | Treatment Modality | Study Duration | Staging System | Prognostic Factors | Univariate Analysis | Multivariate Analysis |
|---|---|---|---|---|---|---|---|---|
| Sinha (2017)[39] | 56 | SCC – 54% Salivary gland – 18% BCC – 9% | LTBR-56 Preop RT-21 PORT-56 PO CT-15 | 2008–2015 | UP | Age, T, RT, parotidectomy, neck dissection, Facial nerve sacrifice Residual disease, positive nodes, PNI | Positive nodes and PNI | Not done |
| Gandhi (2015)[40] | 43 | SCC | SBTR-4 LTBR-12 Rad RT-14 PORT-11 Pal RT-11 CRT-5 PO CRT-2 NACT-1 | 2001–2012 | SM | T, Facial nerve, lymph node, surgery vs. RT, age, RT technique, margin, intracranial extension | T, Facial nerve | None significant |
| Gidley (2012)[4] | 157 | SCC – 38% BCC – 14% Adcc – 7.6% Others – 40% | Mastoidectomy – 28% LTBR – 59.2% SBTR – 2.5% TTBR – 3.2% Others – 15% PORT – 50.3% POCRT – 17% NACT – 2.5% | 1999–2009 | UP | Positive nodes, facial palsy, extratemporal site, positive margin, post-op RT | — | All sig for OS |
| Zanoletti (2013)[42] | 41 | SCC | LTBR-30 STBR-11 PORT-23 | 1980–2008 | UP | T, N, grade, neck dissection, parotidectomy, Facial nerve, PORT, dura mater | Dura and Facial nerve, pattern of spread, LN, grade, T | Dura, LN |

*Abbreviations:* SCC: Squamous Cell Carcinoma; BCC: Basal Cell Carcinoma; Adcc: Adenoid Cystic Carcinoma; LTBR: Lateral Temporal Bone Resection; STBR: Subtotal Temporal Bone Resection; TTBR; Total Temporal Bone Resection; PORT: Postoperative Radiotherapy; NACT: Neoadjuvant Chemotherapy; POCRT: Postoperative Chemoradiation; Preop RT: Preoperative Radiotherapy; Pal RT: Palliative Radiotherapy; Rad RT: Radical Radiotherapy; UP: University of Pittsburgh Staging; SM: Stell and McCormick Staging; LN: Lymph Node; PNI: Perineural Invasion; OS: Overall Survival.

## Table 11.6: Oncological Outcomes in Various Series of Temporal Bone Malignancy

| Study (year) | n | | | | | Survival Outcome | | | | |
|---|---|---|---|---|---|---|---|---|---|---|
| | Total | T1 | T2 | T3 | T4 | Full Cohort | T1 | T2 | T3 | T4 |
| Sinha (2017)[39] | 56 | 10.7% | 12.5% | 10.7% | 62.5% | Mean OS 4.6+/-4 years | 5 Year: 82% | | 5 year: 40% | |
| Gandhi (2015)[40] | 43 | 4.6% | 39.5% | 41.8% | Unknown 13.9 | 2 year OS 50.7% | 2 year PFS 28.6% | | 15.5% | |
| Gidley (2012)[4] | 157 | 7% | 5% | 3% | 21%, unknown 36.3% Recurrent-32% | 5 Year OS 58% 5 Year DFS 54.9% | — | | | |
| Yin (2005)[41] | 95 | — | — | — | — | 5 Year OS 66.8% | Stage I and II 100% | | Stage III 67.2% Stage IV 29.5% | |
| Zanoletti (2013)[42] | 41 | 17% | 14.6% | 36.5% | 31.7% | — | pT 5 Year DFS 95% | | pT 5 Year DFS 47% | |

*Abbreviations:* OS: Overall Survival; DFS: Disease Free Survival.

reported, varying from 19 to 52% (50, 51). In the study by Nadol et al., osteoradionecrosis was avoided in the subgroup of patients that underwent mastoid obliteration (51). The same study describes an open and closed technique, depending upon whether cul-de-sac closure of external auditory canal is performed. Mastoid obliteration can be performed by rotating surrounding muscles like temporalis and sternomastoid. More extensive defects would require pedicled flaps like pectoralis major myocutaneous flap or trapezius flap and free flaps like radial artery forearm flap or anterolateral thigh flap.

## DIFFERENTIAL DIAGNOSIS AND MANAGEMENT

### Cutaneous Malignancy of the Pinna

Figure 11.9 shows cutaneous squamous cell carcinoma of the pinna. The principles of excision are the same as cutaneous malignancies elsewhere. For basal cell carcinoma, 4-mm margins are considered for tumours <2 cm (52, 53). For squamous cell carcinoma, 4–6-mm margins are taken (54). Management of melanoma is a bit more complex. Here the depth of the tumour is of prime concern along with necrosis to guide the margin of resection and lymph nodal sampling (55).

### Squamous Cell Carcinoma of the Temporal Bone

Surgery offers the best chance of cure for temporal bone squamous cell carcinoma. The following are the various surgical options (Figure 11.10):

a. Sleeve Resection: This procedure involves excision of the cartilaginous canal and excision of a cuff of the skin of the osseous canal.

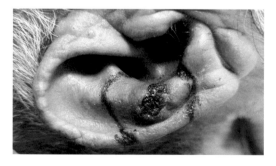

**Figure 11.9** Cutaneous squamous cell carcinoma located over the anti-helix. Violet marking depicts the required 4–6-mm margin for these cases.

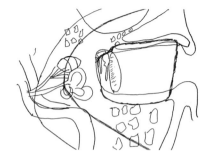

**Figure 11.10** Sagittal cross section of temporal bone depicting the limits of temporal bone resection. Red: lateral temporal bone resection; green: subtotal temporal bone resection; blue: total temporal bone resection.

The indication at present for such a procedure would be verrucous hyperplasia and premalignant lesions of the external auditory canal. Sleeve resection is discouraged as the external auditory canal skin is very thin and is not considered as a barrier for tumour spread. Austin et al. identified a local failure rate of 60% when sleeve resection alone was used to manage T1 tumours (56). Similarly, Zhang et al. noted margin positivity of 54% and local control of 46% with sleeve resection (47).

b. Lateral Temporal Bone Resection: It is the minimum oncologically accepted procedure for temporal bone squamous cell carcinoma. It is indicated in tumours restricted to external auditory canal. The disease-free status of the middle ear needs to be ascertained prior to surgery with a combination of HRCT and MRI. This surgery involves resection of the external auditory canal, mastoid air cells, middle ear mucosa and ossicles till the incudostapedial joint. In case the Facial nerve is intact, the procedure can be performed under Facial nerve monitoring. The incisions for LTBR and surgical resection are shown in Figures 11.11 and 11.12, respectively. Depending on the tumour extent, resection may include the part of the pinna and the underlying muscle and periosteum of the temporal region. A modification of LTBR has been described by Ghavami et al. which involves preservation of the tympanic membrane and ossicles resulting in better post-op hearing (57).

c. Subtotal Temporal Bone Resection (STBR): Tumours with middle ear involvement require a STBR. The initial steps include a LTBR, beyond this tumour resection occurs

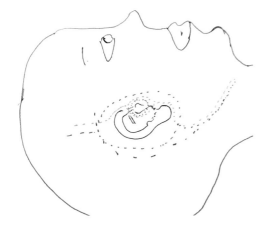

**Figure 11.11** Incisions for temporal bone resection. Red: postauricular incision; blue: auriculectomy incision; green: preauricular incision.

in a piecemeal fashion guided by radiological tumour extent and frozen section. On a sagittal plane, the medial most limit of SBTR is at the internal auditory canal (Figure 11.13). This procedure includes labyrinthectomy and/or a cochleotomy tailored to the tumour extent. The tumour may require clearance from the middle fossa or posterior fossa dura. In the presence of Facial nerve involvement, proximal segment can be traced up to internal auditory canal followed by labyrinthectomy. Dural repair needs to be meticulous and can be performed in a multilayered fashion using fascia lata and abdominal fat augmented with fibrin glue.

d. Total Temporal Bone Resection (TTBR): This is the most morbid of all temporal bone resection. This involves resection of petrous apex: petrous ICA, cavernous sinus and associated

dura. In view of the anticipated morbidity, possible mortality and negligible survival advantage, the present recommendation is piecemeal excision following STBR (48).

e. Fisch Partial Mastoidotympanectomy: Though this procedure is not indicated for temporal bone neoplasms, it has been mentioned since it is a form of temporal bone resection for malignant neoplasms. It is mainly described by Fisch and Mattox for malignant tumours of the parotid or upper cervical lymph nodes, which by the virtue of their location in the retromandibular fossa involve the inferior aspect of the temporal ring (58) (Figure 11.14).

### Indication for Adjuvant Treatment

The absolute indications for adjuvant radiotherapy are positive margins, positive lymph nodes, perineural invasion, recurrent tumour and bone erosion (37). T2 tumours according to Modified Pittsburgh staging have bone erosion, many studies have found better survival outcomes in patients who have received adjuvant radiotherapy (38, 59). On the other hand, no advantage was gained on subjecting patients with T1 tumours to adjuvant radiotherapy (60).

### Non-surgical Treatment Options

Radiotherapy has also been used in the definitive setting to a dose of 70 Gy as a function preservation alternative for T1 tumours (61). Definitive chemoradiation with cisplatin has been shown by Morita et al. to have similar outcomes in unresectable T4 tumours (60). The criteria for unresectability were petrous apex involvement, dural invasion and encasement of petrous ICA. Another strategy for tumours with extension to petrous apex and ICA encasement is preoperative chemoradiation (62). Nakagawa et al.

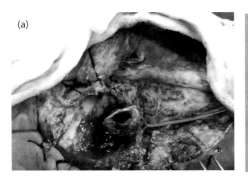
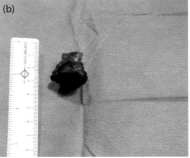

**Figure 11.12** Lateral temporal bone resection. (a) Completed cortical mastoidectomy and extended facial recess. Extratemporal Facial nerve seen under the blue sling. (b) En-bloc resected specimen.

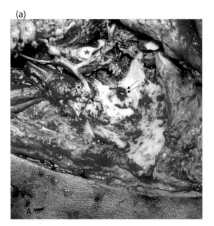
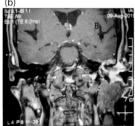
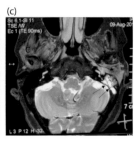

**Figure 11.13** Subtotal temporal bone resection for adenoid cystic carcinoma of the temporal bone. (a) Intraoperative picture showing proximal end of Facial nerve at the stylomastoid foramen (single arrow). The intratemporal segment of Facial nerve had to be sacrificed. Total conservative parotidectomy was performed. Mastoid air cell system and the vestibule have been completely exenterated till the internal auditory canal (double arrows). Condylectomy has been performed, ascending ramus is visualized (star). (b and c) CE-MRI of the same patient, showing tumour in the EAC and middle ear (star), infiltrating TMJ capsule (single arrow). Mastoid air cell system is filled with effusion (double arrow).

used preoperative chemoradiation in 8 out of 12 patients with extensive temporal bone squamous cell carcinoma (62). The regime consisted of 40 Gy in 20 fractions preoperative radiation with intralesional bleomycin used as radiosensitizer with 250 mg of intravenous 5-fluorouracil. Negative surgical margins could be obtained in five out of six patients. Patients with no shrinkage of disease from petrous apex went on to receive definitive chemoradiation. Intra-arterial chemotherapy by the RADPLAT (intra-arterial supradose cisplatin with intravenous sodium thiosulfate) has shown promise in phase II trials of head and neck squamous cell carcinoma (63). Though this trial which also included temporal bone tumours resulted in four complete responders, the same effect could not be replicated in a phase III setting (64).

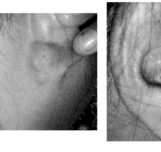
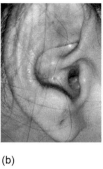
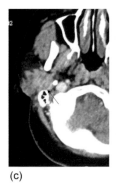
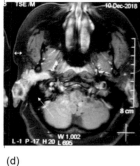

(a)        (b)        (c)        (d)

**Figure 11.14** Candidacy for partial mastoidotympanectomy. (a) A 55-year-old female with postauricular mass with central discharging sinus. (b) Examination of the ear canal revealed skin-covered mass arising from the floor and anterior wall of external auditory canal. (c) Contrast CT revealed heterogeneously enhancing mass arising from the parotid and extending to the region of the stylomastoid foramen (arrow). (d) CEMRI was performed to evaluate the accurate soft tissue extension. MRI reveals involvement of the temporal bone to be restricted to the external auditory canal and the mastoid air cells being free (arrow). Histopathology in this case was high-grade mucoepidermoid carcinoma. This patient requires a partial mastoidotympanectomy as described by Fisch and Mattox.

*Summarizing Treatment Options*

Systematic review of 26 studies involving 141 patients by Prasad and Janecka led to the following conclusions (65):

1. Outcome of patients with tumour in the external auditory canal did not depend on the type of surgical resection (mastoidectomy/LTBR/STBR), with no additional benefit of radiotherapy.

2. With disease extending to middle ear, STBR offered better cure rates than LTBR. However, conclusive evidence on the role of adjuvant radiotherapy is elusive.

3. The value of surgical resection when tumour extended to petrous apex is doubtful.

4. Resection of dura failed to improve survival across all studies, though data is confounded on the way margin status was reported.

5. Data was considered insufficient at the time of the publication to recommend resection of brain parenchyma or ICA.

Though there has not been much change in the surgical principles since the publication of this systematic review (1994), there has been revolutionary change in the field of conformal radiation. A meta-analysis published in 2014 showed 5-year survival rates of patients undergoing surgery +/-radiation, preoperative chemoradiation, definitive chemoradiation and postoperative chemoradiation were: 53.5%, 85.7%, 43.6% and 0%, respectively (66). Results are skewed in favour of preoperative chemoradiation due to a single study.

Taking into consideration the evidence from all the available literature, our suggested treatment algorithm is shown in Figure 11.15.

## Rhabdomyosarcoma

Presence of rapidly progressing, ulcerated mass with facial palsy, postauricular swelling with or without cervical lymphadenopathy in a paediatric age group should raise the suspicion of a soft tissue sarcoma. The most common soft tissue sarcoma in that age group is RMS accounting for 60% of all soft tissue sarcoma (23). Diagnosis requires biopsy from the tumour either through the ear canal or from the mastoid antrum (representative areas). On contrast-enhanced MRI, RMS appears hypointense on T1-weighted images, enhancing with gadolinium, and hyperintense on T2-weighted images. Tumour is locally destructive with infiltrative margins. Treatment is primarily by chemoradiation. The role for the surgeon in majority of the cases is for obtaining a biopsy. Temporal bone resection is rarely reserved for residual tumour (67). Temporal bone RMS is staged as

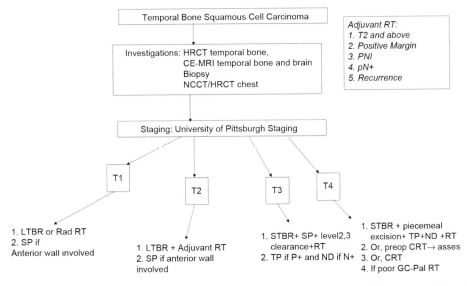

**Figure 11.15** Decision-making flowchart for temporal bone squamous cell carcinoma based on all the evidence collated. LTBR: lateral temporal bone resection; STBR: subtotal temporal bone resection; RT: radiotherapy; CRT: concurrent chemoradiation; SP: superficial parotidectomy; TP: total parotidectomy; P+: parotid involvement due to either direct spread or intraparotid nodes; GC: general condition; PNI: perineural invasion. *Note:* Total temporal bone resection at present has very limited evidence in its favour. CRT/preop CRT should instead be considered in the presence of petrous apex involvement.

(a)  (b)  (c)

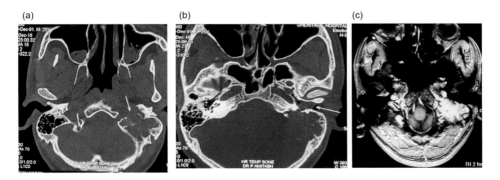

**Figure 11.16**  Expansile lytic lesion with soap bubble appearance involving the mastoid air cells and the ear canal (a and b). Lesion is extending to the posterior dura (c). Excision was done by subtotal temporal bone resection. Histopathology revealed giant cell tumour.

a parameningeal subsite, which have an unfavourable outcome compared with other head and neck RMS: 4-year OS 41% temporal bone, 91% orbit, 75% other sites (68).

### Other Soft Tissue or Bone Sarcoma and Tumours with Indeterminate Malignant Potential

A wide variety of soft tissue and bone sarcomas form the differential diagnosis for TBM, as enumerated in Table 11.1. These non-RMS sarcomas are relatively rare with less than 10% occurring in the skull base (69) (Figure 11.16). Imaging characteristics are summarized in Table 11.2. After histological confirmation, treatment of these tumours is by surgery followed by adjuvant radiation.

### Langerhans Cell Histiocytosis

The temporal bone is involved by LCH in 15–65% of the cases with 45% incidence of bilaterality (70, 71). Radiologically, the disease is centred over the mastoid with relative sparing of the middle ear and petrous apex. Typically there is osseous destruction of the mastoid air cells with no ossicular destruction (72). These radiological features together with paediatric age of onset and occasional multisystem disease raise the suspicion of LCH (Figure 11.17). Histopathological examination is supplemented with immunohistochemistry for CD1a, S100 and Langerin (CD 207) (73). LCH is not treated

surgically. Temporal bone is considered to be an unfavourable subsite, requiring intensive treatment with vinblastine, prednisolone and 6-mercaptopurine (74).

### Skull Base Osteomyelitis (SBO)

SBO is typically seen in an elderly immunocompromised patient. Patients present with long-standing history of earache and ear discharge refractory to standard medical management. Clinical examination reveals inflamed and oedematous external auditory canal, often obscuring the view of the tympanic membrane. Patients subsequently develop facial palsy followed by lower cranial nerve palsy. These features overlapping with TBM often give rise to a diagnostic dilemma (75). Biopsy from the granulation tissue followed by careful histopathological examination is required before ruling out malignancy (Figure 11.18). Radiological findings of some benign temporal bone tumours is depicted in Figure 11.19.

### METASTASES TO TEMPORAL BONE

Presence of otological symptoms with Facial nerve palsy in the background of a solid organ malignancy should raise the suspicion of metastasis to the temporal bone (76). Traditionally, metastases have been reported from lung, kidney, breast and thyroid. Radiologically metastatic spread to the temporal bone is found localized to the petrous

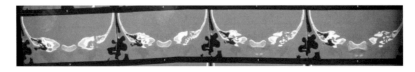

**Figure 11.17**  Expansile, lytic lesion of the temporal bone causing local osseous destruction. Extensive soft tissue infiltration is seen in the periauricular area. Histopathology revealed Langerhans cell histiocytosis.

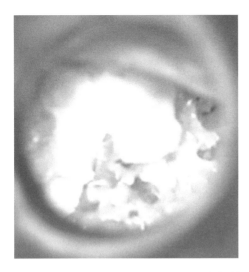

**Figure 11.18** Sequestrum in a case of skull base osteomyelitis.

apex, temporal squama, Facial nerve and internal auditory canal (76, 77). The abundance of metastatic lesions in the petrous apex reflect its vascularity and tendency for hematogenous spread from the above-mentioned tumours.

Apart from solid organ malignancy, metastasis can also occur from hematolymphoid malignancies. This is also known as granulocytic sarcoma, which implies extramedullary collection of immature myeloid cells (78). Patients may present with sudden onset facial palsy with features of mastoiditis on radiology. Unlike solid organ metastasis, granulocytic sarcoma has a predilection for the middle ear cleft and mastoid air cells. Granulocytic sarcoma is most frequently seen in cases on acute myeloid leukaemia (M2-subtype).

## FOLLOW-UP

Potential complications following a temporal bone resection include:

i. **Sequelae**

1. *Facial palsy or paresis:* The former is inevitable in the presence of direct infiltration of the nerve requiring sacrifice. Facial paresis can occur following a LTBR if Facial nerve rerouting has been performed.

2. Maximum conductive hearing loss following a LTBR.

3. Sensorineural hearing loss following STBR where labyrinthectomy and drilling of the vestibule is performed.

ii. **Complications**

1. Meningitis.

2. Cerebrospinal fluid otorrhea.

3. Flap necrosis (Figure 11.20).

4. Osteoradionecrosis.

5. Lower cranial nerve palsy.

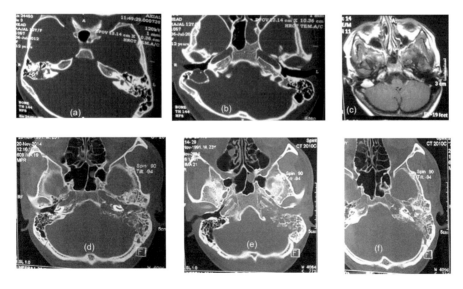

**Figure 11.19**  Differential diagnosis of benign temporal bone tumours. (a–c) Facial nerve schwannoma. There is multisegment involvement from second genu till the mastoid segment. Fusiform expansile lesion can be appreciated on both HRCT temporal bone and CE-MRI. (d–f) Endolymphatic sac tumour. Posteriorly based destructive tumour with no widening or destruction of the Jugular foramen points towards an endolymphatic sac tumour.

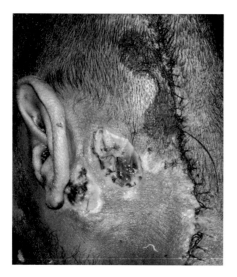

**Figure 11.20** Poorly designed incision can compromise vascularity of the skin flap leading to catastrophic skin flap necrosis and fistula formation.

iii. **Rehabilitation**

1. *Facial palsy:* Static procedures like lid loading with gold weight implant can be performed. Dynamic procedures include cable grafting with sural or greater auricular nerve when both proximal and distal segments are available, facial-ansa hypoglossi or facial-masseteric anastomosis when the proximal segment is unavailable (83) (Figure 11.21).

2. Osseintegrated implants for bone-anchored hearing mechanism can be used to rehabilitate hearing following LTBR. Ideally, there should be an interval of 6 months following adjuvant radiation if these implants are considered to minimize the risk of osteoradionecrosis (84).

## DISCUSSION

The temporal bone is an infrequent site for head and neck malignancy (2, 3). Owing to this, most experience available in literature is limited to single institution retrospective series with a heterogeneous mix of different histology. Lack of a harmonized staging system presents a unique challenge towards comparing outcomes across different studies. Squamous cell carcinoma is the most frequent histology encountered (6) and was the main focus of this chapter. Initial manifestations of this condition are like inflammatory diseases of the ear canal and mastoid air cells. This results in delay in diagnosis leading to frequent presentation at a locally advanced stage. TBM tends to recur at the local site rather than at the level of neck nodes or with distant metastasis (28). Therefore, surgical approach chosen should be robust to minimize margin positivity followed up with adjuvant treatment whenever appropriate. The minimum oncologically sound operation for TBM is a LTBR. In the absence of radiological involvement of the parotid gland in early-stage tumours, parotidectomy may be omitted if there is no anterior canal wall involvement.

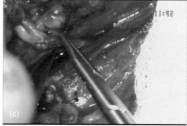

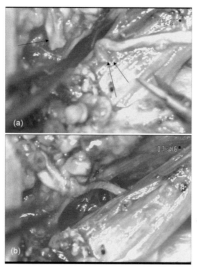

**Figure 11.21** Facial-ansa hypoglossi anastomosis. (a) Distal end of Facial nerve (single arrow) and distal end of ansa hypoglossi. (b) Coaptation of the nerves. (c) Epineurial suturing being performed with 8-0 nylon.

Similarly, cervical nodal dissection should be undertaken in T3-T4 tumours and in those with intra-parotid nodes. Since T2 by definition in the University of Pittsburgh staging involves bone erosion, adjuvant radiotherapy is indicated for all tumours T2 and beyond (38, 59).

STBR is indicated when the middle ear cleft is involved. There is insufficient evidence to recommend an en-bloc resection in these cases (48, 49). Similarly, TTBR is considered to be too morbid with high risk of potential perioperative mortality without significant impact on survival (65).

Radiotherapy is an organ preservation alternative for T1 tumours (61). Chemoradiation should be considered for inoperable cases (petrous apex involvement and ICA encasement) (60). Evidence in favour of preoperative chemoradiotherapy to reduce margin positivity in borderline operable cases is currently insufficient and is available in only one study (62).

Emphasis should be directed at identifying these tumours at an early stage as survival drops from 95–100% in stage I and II tumours to 47.5 to 29.5% in stage III and IV with a 5-year OS of 58–66.8% (Table 11.6). Facial nerve involvement, dural invasion, positive margins and lymph nodal involvement are important prognostic indicators (Table 11.5).

## CONCLUSION

TBM is challenging from both diagnostic and therapeutic aspects. Due to limited experience available in literature, these cases should preferably be managed at a specialized multidisciplinary setting with expertise available for lateral skull base surgery.

## KEY POINTS

1. LTBR is the minimum surgical procedure to be undertaken for tumours restricted to the external auditory canal.

2. Elective superficial parotidectomy is indicated for T3 and T4 and for the early-stage tumours with anterior canal wall involvement.

3. STBR is indicated if disease extends to middle ear cleft and mastoid air cells.

4. Piecemeal resection around critical neurovascular structures, drilling for margin at the level of bone and judicious use of frozen section is currently favoured over en-bloc resection for tumours that require more than a LTBR.

5. Adjuvant treatment is indicated for T2 and higher tumours.

6. Chemoradiation instead of TTBR should be considered for tumours with petrous apex involvement and ICA encasement

## REFERENCES

1. Bacciu A, Clemente IA, Piccirillo E, Ferrari S, Sanna M. Guidelines for treating temporal bone carcinoma based on long-term outcomes. Otol Neurotol. 2013; 34(5):898–907.

2. Testa JR, Fukuda Y, Kowalski LP. Prognostic factors in carcinoma of the external auditory canal. Arch Otolaryngol Head Neck Surg. 1997;123(7):720–4.

3. Crabtree JA, Britton BH, Pierce MK. Carcinoma of the external auditory canal. Laryngoscope. 1976; 86(3):405–15.

4. Gidley PW, Thompson CR, Roberts DB, DeMonte F, Hanna EY. The oncology of otology. Laryngoscope. 2012;122(2):393–400.

5. Myers EN, Suen JY, Myers JN, Hanna EY. Cancer of the Head and Neck, 5th ed. Philadelphia: Wolter Kluwers, 2017.

6. Gurgel RK, Karnell LH, Hansen MR. Middle ear cancer: a population-based study. Laryngoscope. 2009;119(10):1913–7.

7. Ramirez CC, Federman DG, Kirsner RS. Skin cancer as an occupational disease: the effect of ultraviolet and other forms of radiation. Int J Dermatol. 2005;44(2):95–100.

8. Isipradit P, Wadwongtham W, Aeumjaturapat S, Aramwatanapong P. Carcinoma of the external auditory canal. J Med Assoc. 2005;88(1):114–7.

9. Kuhel WI, Hume CR, Selesnick SH. Cancer of the external auditory canal and temporal bone. Otolaryngol Clin North Am. 1996;29(5):827–52.

10. Lobo D, Llorente JL, Suárez C. Squamous cell carcinoma of the external auditory canal. Skull Base. 2008;18(3):167–72.

11. Ruben RJ, Thaler SU, Holzer N. Radiation induced carcinoma of the temporal bone. Laryngoscope. 1977;87(10 Pt 1):1613–21.

12. Cahan WG, Woodard HQ, Higinbotham NL, Stewart FW, Coley BL. Sarcoma arising in irradiated bone: report of eleven cases. 1948. Cancer. 1998;82(1):8–34.

13. McRackan TR, Fang T-Y, Pelosi S, Rivas A, Dietrich MS, Wanna GB, et al. Factors associated with recurrence of squamous cell carcinoma involving the temporal bone. Ann Otol Rhinol Laryngol. 2014;123(4):235–9.

14. Bergmann K, Hoppe F, He Y, Helms J, Müller-Hermelink HK, Stremlau A, et al. Human-papillomavirus DNA in cholesteatomas. Int J Cancer. 1994;59(4):463–6.

15. Zhou H, Chen Z, Zhang W, Xing G. Middle ear squamous papilloma: a report of four cases analyzed by HPV and EBV in situ hybridization. Oncol Lett. 2014;7(1):41–6.

16. Tsai ST, Li C, Jin YT, Chao WY, Su IJ. High prevalence of human papillomavirus types 16 and 18 in middle-ear carcinomas. Int J Cancer. 1997;71(2):208–12.

17. Tsunoda A, Sumi T, Terasaki O, Kishimoto S. Right dominance in the incidence of external auditory canal squamous cell carcinoma in the Japanese population: does handedness affect carcinogenesis? Laryngoscope Investig Otolaryngol. 2017;2(1):19–22.

18. Levine H. Cutaneous carcinoma of the head and neck: management of massive and previously uncontrolled lesions. Laryngoscope. 1983;93(1):87–105.

19. Madsen AR, Gundgaard MG, Hoff CM, Maare C, Holmboe P, Knap M, et al. Cancer of the external auditory canal and middle ear in Denmark from 1992 to 2001. Head Neck. 2008;30(10):1332–8.

20. Leonetti JP, Smith PG, Kletzker GR, Izquierdo R. Invasion patterns of advanced temporal bone malignancies. Am J Otol. 1996;17(3):438–42.

21. Hosokawa S, Mizuta K, Takahashi G, Okamura J, Takizawa Y, Hosokawa K, et al. Surgical approach for treatment of carcinoma of the anterior wall of the external auditory canal. Otol Neurotol. 2012;33(3):450–4.

22. Wippold FJ. Head and neck imaging: the role of CT and MRI. J Magn Reson Imaging. 2007;25(3):453–65.

23. Gluth MB. Rhabdomyosarcoma and other pediatric temporal bone malignancies. Otolaryngol Clin North Am. 2015;48(2):375–90.

24. Zhang F, Sha Y. Computed tomography and magnetic resonance imaging findings for primary middle-ear carcinoma. J Laryngol Otol. 2013;127(6):578–83.

25. Ibrahim TF, Jahromi BR, Miettinen J, et al. Long-term causes of death and excess mortality after carotid artery ligation. World Neurosurg. 2016;90:116–22.

26. Roberson JB, Brackmann DE, Fayad JN. Complications of venous insufficiency after neurotologic-skull base surgery. Am J Otol. 2000;21(5):701–5.

27. Keller E, Ries F, Grünwald F, et al. [Multimodal carotid occlusion test for determining risk of infarct before therapeutic internal carotid artery occlusion.] Laryngorhinootologie. 1995;74(5):307–11.

28. Morris LGT, Mehra S, Shah JP, Bilsky MH, Selesnick SH, Kraus DH. Predictors of survival and recurrence after temporal bone resection for cancer. Head Neck. 2012;34(9):1231–9.

29. Grijalba Uche M, BonautMendía JF. [Metastases to the temporal bone. A report of two cases.] Acta Otorrinolaringol Esp. 1995;46(6):441–3.

30. Sabaté S, Mazo V, Canet J. Predicting postoperative pulmonary complications: implications for outcomes and costs. Curr Opin Anaesthesiol. 2014;27(2):201–9.

31. Amin MB, Edge S, Greene F, et al. (Eds.). AJCC Cancer Staging Manual, 8th ed. Springer International Publishing, American Joint Commission on Cancer, 2017.

32. Allanson BM, Low T-H, Clark JR, Gupta R. Squamous cell carcinoma of the external auditory canal and temporal bone: an update. Head Neck Pathol. 2018; 12(3):407–18.

33. Stell PM, McCormick MS. Carcinoma of the external auditory meatus and middle ear: prognostic factors and a suggested staging system. J Laryngol Otol. 1985;99(9):847–50.

34. Arriaga M, Curtin H, Takahashi H, Hirsch BE, Kamerer DB. Staging proposal for external auditory meatus carcinoma based on preoperative clinical examination and computed tomography findings. Ann Otol Rhinol Laryngol. 1990;99(9 Pt 1):714–21.

35. Moody SA, Hirsch BE, Myers EN. Squamous cell carcinoma of the external auditory canal: an evaluation of a staging system. Am J Otol. 2000; 21(4):582–8.

36. Higgins TS, Antonio SAM. The role of facial palsy in staging squamous cell carcinoma of the temporal bone and external auditory canal: a comparative survival analysis. Otol Neurotol. 2010;31(9):1473–9.

37. Lovin BD, Gidley PW. Squamous cell carcinoma of the temporal bone: a current review. Laryngoscope Investig Otolaryngol. 2019;4(6):684–92.

38. Gidley PW, Roberts DB, Sturgis EM. Squamous cell carcinoma of the temporal bone. Laryngoscope. 2010; 120(6):1144–51.

39. Sinha S, Dedmon MM, Naunheim MR, Fuller JC, Gray ST, Lin DT. Update on surgical outcomes of lateral temporal bone resection for ear and temporal bone malignancies. J Neurol Surg Part B Skull Base. 2017;78(1):37–42.

40. Gandhi AK, Roy S, Biswas A, et al. Treatment of squamous cell carcinoma of external auditory canal: a tertiary cancer centre experience. Auris Nasus Larynx. 2016;43(1):45–9.

41. Yin M, Ishikawa K, Honda K, et al. Analysis of 95 cases of squamous cell carcinoma of the external and middle ear. Auris Nasus Larynx. 2006;33(3):251–7.

42. Zanoletti E, Marioni G, Stritoni P, et al. Temporal bone squamous cell carcinoma: analyzing prognosis with univariate and multivariate models. Laryngoscope. 2014;124(5):1192–8.

43. Dean NR, White HN, Carter DS, Desmond RA, Carroll WR, McGrew BM, et al. Outcomes following temporal bone resection. Laryngoscope. 2010; 120(8):1516–22.

44. Chi F-L, Gu F-M, Dai C-F, Chen B, Li H-W. Survival outcomes in surgical treatment of 72 cases of squamous cell carcinoma of the temporal bone. Otol Neurotol. 2011;32(4):665–9.

45. Woolgar JA, Triantafyllou A, Lewis JS, et al. Prognostic biological features in neck dissection specimens. Eur Arch Otorhinolaryngol. 2013; 270(5):1581–92.

46. Mantravadi AV, Marzo SJ, Leonetti JP, Fargo KN, Carter MS. Lateral temporal bone and parotid malignancy with Facial nerve involvement. Otolaryngol Head Neck Surg. 2011;144(3):395–401.

47. Zhang T, Li W, Dai C, Chi F, Wang S, Wang Z. Evidence-based surgical management of T1 or T2 temporal bone malignancies. Laryngoscope. 2013;123(1):244–8.

48. Prasad SC, D'Orazio F, Medina M, Bacciu A, Sanna M. State of the art in temporal bone malignancies. Curr Opin Otolaryngol. 2014;22(2):154–65.

49. Sataloff RT, Myers DL, Lowry LD, Spiegel JR. Total temporal bone resection for squamous cell carcinoma. Otolaryngol Head Neck Surg. 1987; 96(1):4–14.

50. Cole JM. Glomus Jugulare tumor. Laryngoscope. 1977;87(8):1244–58.

51. Nadol JB, Schuknecht HF. Obliteration of the mastoid in the treatment of tumors of the temporal bone. Ann Otol Rhinol Laryngol. 1984;93(1 Pt 1):6–12.

52. Thomas DJ, King AR, Peat BG. Excision margins for nonmelanotic skin cancer. Plast Reconstr Surg. 2003;112(1):57–63.

53. Wolf DJ, Zitelli JA. Surgical margins for basal cell carcinoma. Arch Dermatol. 1987;123(3):340–4.

54. Schmults CD, Alam M, Chen P-L, Daniels GA, DiMaio D, Farma JM, et al. NCCN Guidelines Index Table of Contents. 2020, p. 88.

55. Narayan D, Ariyan S. Surgical considerations in the management of malignant melanoma of the ear. Plast Reconstr Surg. 2001;107(1):20–4.

56. Austin JR, Stewart KL, Fawzi N. Squamous cell carcinoma of the external auditory canal: therapeutic prognosis based on a proposed staging system. Arch Otolaryngol Head Neck Surg. 1994;120(11): 1228–32.

57. Ghavami Y, Haidar YM, Maducdoc M, et al. Tympanic membrane and ossicular-sparing modified lateral temporal bone resection. Otolaryngol Head Neck Surg. 2017;157(3):530 2.

58. Spector JG. Microsurgery of the skull base, by Ugo Fisch and Douglas Mattox with contributions by U. Aepple and A. Valavanis and drawings by Ivan Glitsch. Hard cover, 669 pages, 1,310 illustrations and color prints, and 15 tables. Published by Georg Thieme Verlag, price 440 DM., 1988. Laryngoscope. 1989;99(4):463.

59. Nam G-S, Moon IS, Kim JH, Kim SH, Choi JY, Son EJ. Prognostic factors affecting surgical outcomes in squamous cell carcinoma of external auditory canal. Clin Exp Otorhinolaryngol. 2018;11(4):259–66.

60. Morita S, Homma A, Nakamaru Y, et al. The outcomes of surgery and chemoradiotherapy for temporal bone cancer. Otol Neurotol. 2016;37(8):1174–82.

61. Ogawa K, Nakamura K, Hatano K, et al. Treatment and prognosis of squamous cell carcinoma of the external auditory canal and middle ear: a multi-institutional retrospective review of 87 patients. Int J Radiat Oncol Biol Phys. 2007;68(5):1326–34.

62. Nakagawa T, Kumamoto Y, Natori Y, et al. Squamous cell carcinoma of the external auditory canal and middle ear: an operation combined with preoperative chemoradiotherapy and a free surgical margin. Otol Neurotol. 2006;27(2):242–8; discussion 249.

63. Robbins KT, Pelliteri PK, Vicario D, et al. Targeted infusions of supradose cisplatin with systemic neutralization for carcinomas invading the temporal bone. Skull Base Surg. 1996;6(2):69–76.

64. Rasch CRN, Hauptmann M, Schornagel J, et al. Intra-arterial versus intravenous chemoradiation for advanced head and neck cancer: results of a randomized phase 3 trial. Cancer. 2010;116(9):2159–65.

65. Prasad S, Janecka IP. Efficacy of surgical treatments for squamous cell carcinoma of the temporal bone: a literature review. Otolaryngol Head Neck Surg. 1994;110(3):270–80.

66. Takenaka Y, Cho H, Nakahara S, Yamamoto Y, Yasui T, Inohara H. Chemoradiation therapy for squamous cell carcinoma of the external auditory canal: a meta-analysis. Head Neck. 2015;37(7):1073–80.

67. Maurer HM. The intergroup rhabdomyosarcoma study: update, November 1978. Natl Cancer Inst. 1981;(56):61–8.

68. Sbeity S, Abella A, Arcand P, Quintal MC, Saliba I. Temporal bone rhabdomyosarcoma in children. Int J Pediatr Otorhinolaryngol. 2007;71(5):807–14.

69. Lyos AT, Goepfert H, Luna MA, Jatte N, Malpica A. Soft tissue sarcoma of the head and neck in children and adolescents. Cancer. 1996;77(1):193–200.

70. Modest MC, Garcia JJ, Arndt CS, Carlson ML. Langerhans cell histiocytosis of the temporal bone: a review of 29 cases at a single center. Laryngoscope. 2016;126(8):1899–904.

71. D'Ambrosio N, Soohoo S, Warshall C, Johnson A, Karimi S. Craniofacial and intracranial manifestations of Langerhans cell histiocytosis: report of findings in 100 patients. AJR. 2008; 191(2):589–97.

72. Touska P, Juliano AF-Y. Temporal bone tumors: an imaging update. Neuroimaging Clin N Am. 2019; 29(1):145–72.

73. Harmon CM, Brown N. Langerhans cell histiocytosis: a clinicopathologic review and molecular pathogenetic update. Arch Pathol Lab Med. 2015; 139(10):1211–4.

74. Majumder A, Wick CC, Collins R, Booth TN, Isaacson B, Kutz JW. Pediatric Langerhans cell histiocytosis of the lateral skull base. Int J Pediatr Otorhinolaryngol. 2017;99:135–40.

75. Ganhewa AD, Kuthubutheen J. A diagnostic dilemma of central skull base osteomyelitis mimicking neoplasia in a diabetic patient. BMJ Case Rep. 2013;2013.

76. Song K, Park K-W, Heo J-H, Song I-C, Park Y-H, Choi JW. Clinical characteristics of temporal bone metastases. Clin Exp Otorhinolaryngol. 2019;12(1):27–32.

77. Gloria-Cruz TI, Schachern PA, Paparella MM, Adams GL, Fulton SE. Metastases to temporal bones from primary nonsystemic malignant neoplasms. Arch Otolaryngol Head Neck Surg. 2000;126(2):209–14.

78. Budhiraja S, Sagar P, Rajeshwari M, Kumar R. Rare initial presentation of acute myeloid leukemia as facial palsy. Indian J Med Paediatr Oncol 2018;39:555-7.

79. Sakthivel P, Singh CA, Thakar A, Thirumeni G, Raveendran S, Sharma SC. Masseteric-Facial nerve anastomosis: surgical techniques and outcomes – a pilot Indian study. Indian J Otolaryngol Head Neck Surg. 2020;72(1):92–7.

80. Nader M-E, Beadle BM, Roberts DB, Gidley PW. Outcomes and complications of osseointegrated hearing aids in irradiated temporal bones. Laryngoscope. 2016;126(5):1187–92.

# 12 Benign Neoplasms in Otology

*Smriti Panda, Chirom Amit Singh and Uma Patnaik*

## CONTENTS

## INTRODUCTION

In the practice of otology, the clinician comes across a variety of benign neoplasms. A working knowledge of the clinical features, etio-pathogenesis and management options available are essential for the ear, nose and throat (ENT) surgeon in order to successfully identify and manage these tumours. Treatment of these neoplasms usually requires a multidisciplinary approach and they are best managed at tertiary care centres and hence the clinician should also know when not to intervene. Various benign neoplasms are reported in the Temporal bone, we will describe a few important ones in this section (Table 12.1).

## PARAGANGLIOMAS

Paragangliomas are neuroendocrine tumours arising from the sympathetic and parasympathetic nervous system, commonly known as the Diffuse Neuroendocrine System (DNES). Embryologically, this system arises from the neural crest. Biochemical process giving rise to secretory behaviour can also be appreciated owing to the amine precursor and Uptake Decarboxylase System (APUD). Histologically, paragangliomas have unique features demonstrating architectural and immunohistochemical similarities to their cell of origin. A nesting or *Zellballen* pattern can be identified with two

## Table 12.1: Benign Tumours of the Temporal Bone

| | |
|---|---|
| Tumours of external auditory canal | Osteoma<br>Fibrous dysplasia<br>Nerve sheath tumour<br>Paraganglioma<br>Hemangioma |
| Tumours of middle ear | Adenoma<br>Meningioma<br>Chordoma<br>Paraganglioma<br>Hemangiopericytoma<br>Schwannoma |
| Tumour of inner ear | Paraganglioma<br>Lipoma<br>Schwannoma<br>Hemangioma<br>Hemangiopericytoma<br>Endolymphatic sac tumour |

main groups of cells: type I (chief cells) and type II (sustentacular) cells. Immunohistochemistry demonstrates positivity with synaptophysin, chromogranin and neuron-specific enolase and somatostatin in the chief cells and S-100 positivity in the sustentacular cells. Glenner and Grimley classified the paraganglion system into four subtypes (Table 12.2) (1).Temporal bone paraganglioma (TBG) arise either from the tympanic or mastoid canaliculi (tympano-mastoid) or from the Jugular bulb (tympano-Jugular).

### Aetiology

- *Hypoxia:* Type I cell hyperplasia has been noted in the carotid body of individuals living at a higher altitude and conditions that simulate hypoxia like chronic obstructive pulmonary disease and cyanotic heart disease (2, 3).

- *Genetic:* Traditional teaching of 10% incidence of familial paraganglioma (Rule of 10) has now been surpassed with a greater understanding of the molecular and genetic basis of paragangliomas. At present, familial paragangliomas constitute 40% of the overall

incidence of these tumours (4). Various clusters of genetic mutations underlying the development of paraganglioma have been identified as follows:

i. Cluster I – mutations in VHL, SDHx, HF2A, PHD1/2, FH and MDH2

ii. Cluster II – mutation in kinase receptor signalling and protein translation pathway – RET, NF-1

iii. Cluster III – Wnt-altered pathway

The genetic association of the succinate dehydrogenase gene has been most widely studied. Table 12.3 describes the salient features and Figure 12.1 shows the recommended screening strategy.

### Clinical Presentation

These tumours have a long history owing to their slow growth rate. The most common age of onset is the 5th decade (5). Tinnitus is the most common presenting feature in jugulotympanic paragangliomas. Tumours localized to the middle ear manifest as a visible polyp, hearing loss and otorrhea. Extension to the inner ear and petrous apex can result in sensorineural hearing loss and vertigo. Facial palsy signifies extensive intratemporal extension. Jugular foramen extension presents with lower cranial nerve weakness.

Various interesting eponymous clinical signs have been described for jugulotympanic paragangliomas:

1. *Brown's sign:* Blanching of the middle ear mass on pneumatic otoscopy

2. *Aquino sign:* Blanching of the middle ear mass on gently occluding carotid artery in the neck

3. *Rising sun sign:* Red mass in the middle ear occupying the hypotympanum

### Diagnostic Workup

A comprehensive preoperative evaluation should encompass high-resolution cross-sectional imaging, radiotracer studies to rule

## Table 12.2: Glenner and Grimley Classification of Paraganglioma

| S. No. | Type of Paraganglioma | Nature | Remarks |
|---|---|---|---|
| i | Branchiomeric | Parasympathetic | Associated with the vasculature of the head and neck till the arch of aorta |
| ii | Intravagal | Parasympathetic | |
| iii | Aortosympathetic | Sympathetic | |
| iv | Visceral autonomic | Sympathetic | |

**Table 12.3: Summary of the Features of Succinate Dehydrogenase (SDH) Gene Mutations**

| SDH Mutation | Locus | Transmission | Incidence in a Cohort of Paraganglioma (PGL) | Clinical Features | Multifocal | Bilateral Pheochromocytoma | Metastatic |
|---|---|---|---|---|---|---|---|
| SDHD | 11q23 | AD | 10.5% | PGL<br>Carney dyad<br>Renal cell carcinoma (RCC)<br>Pituitary adenoma | +++ | +/– | +/– |
| SDH AF2 | 11q12.2 | AD | <1 | PGL<br>Pheochromocytoma | ++ | None | +/– |
| SDHC | 1q23.3 | AD | 4 | PGL<br>Pheochromocytoma<br>Carney dyad | ++ | None | +/– |
| SDHB | 1p36.1 | AD | 20.6 | PGL<br>Carney Dyad<br>RCC<br>Pituitary adenoma | ++ | +/– | +++ |
| SDH A | 5p.15 | AR | 3 | PGL<br>Pheochromocytoma<br>Carney dyad<br>Pituitary adenoma | +/– | +/– | + |

*Abbreviations:* AD: Autosomal Dominant; AR: Autosomal Recessive.

out multicentricity, serum studies to identify secretory tumours and preoperative angiography and embolization when indicated.

*Cross-sectional Imaging:* On high-resolution computed tomography (HRCT), glomus tympanicum presents as a soft tissue density along the promontory with an intact Jugular bulb. Intact carotid-Jugular plate helps to differentiate glomus tympanicum from glomus jugulare. Erosion in case of the latter is known as the "Phelps Sign". In case of glomus tympanicum limited to the middle ear, HRCT may be unremarkable except of soft tissue along the promontory. Glomus jugulare tumours can be identified on HRCT by a destructive mass lesion centred over the Jugular foramen. The pattern of bone destruction is described as "moth-eaten" appearance. MRI reveals multiple flow voids, classically described as "salt and pepper" appearance. This contrasts with homogeneous enhancement of schwannomas (Figures 12.2 and 12.3).

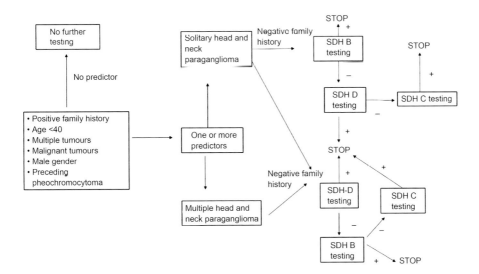

**Figure 12.1** Screening strategy for genetic mutation in head and neck paraganglioma.

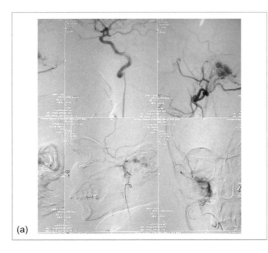
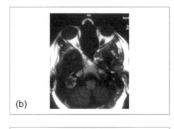
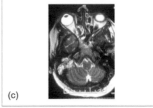

**Figure 12.2** Radiology in glomus jugulare. (a) Preoperative digital subtraction angiography showing tumour blush on cannulation of occipital and posterior auricular artery. (b) T1-weighted images showing tumour which is hypointense centrally with peripheral rim of hyperintensity. Tumour is closely abutting posterior fossa dura. (c) Salt and pepper appearance due to flow voids seen in T1-post contrast images.

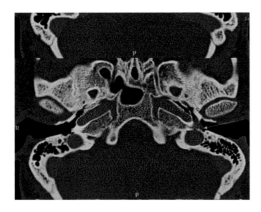

**Figure 12.3** HRCT Temporal bone showing glomus tympanicum. Soft tissue is seen in the region of the promontory. Thinned out intact bone is seen over the Jugular bulb.

*Radiotracer Studies:* Various radiotracer studies have been investigated in paragangliomas and found to be useful to identify multicentric tumours as well as a synchronous pheochromocytoma (Table 12.4) (6–9).

*Functional Evaluation:* The metabolic pathway of catecholamines is depicted in Figure 12.4. The battery of tests to assess the functional behaviour of paragangliomas include urinary and plasma catecholamines, urinary fractionated metanephrines, plasma-free metanephrines and urinary fractionated metanephrines. The salient features and indications for each of these investigations is enumerated in Table 12.5.

*Preoperative Angiography and Embolization:* Cerebral cross-circulation studies are a prerequisite before undertaking a lateral skull base approach for jugulotympanic paraganglioma. The principles of cerebral cross-circulation assessment have been described in the section dealing with malignant neoplasms in otology.

Temporal bone paragangliomas have a multi-compartmental vascular supply (10). The anterior tympanic artery supplies the region of the eustachian tube and carotid canal; the inferior tympanic artery is the main arterial supply for the region of the Jugular foramen and promontory. The superior compartment receives its supply from the middle meningeal and the accessory meningeal artery. Occipital and posterior auricular artery supplies the posterior compartment. The knowledge of the vascular compartment involved can facilitate superselective embolization. Indications for preoperative embolization include size greater than 3 cm, type C and D tumours according to Fisch staging. In such extensive tumours, preoperative embolization helps to devascularize the tumour and optimizing surgical conditions by reducing blood loss and operative time (11). Though overall considered to have an acceptable safety profile, reflux of embolized material has been described into high-pressure internal carotid system through intratumoural arteriovenous communications (12). Consequences of such an inadvertent event include stroke and cranial neuropathy.

**Table 12.4: Diagnostic Accuracy of Various Radiotracers Used for Diagnostic Purpose in Paraganglioma**

| Radiotracer | Mechanism | Sensitivity | Specificity | Comments |
|---|---|---|---|---|
| I123 or I131 MIBG | Type I amine uptake with localization to presynaptic adrenergic nerves on chromaffin tissue | 77–95% | 95–100% | Lower sensitivity in tumours above diaphragm, small tumours, necrosis, dopamine-secreting tumours and metastatic disease |
| In-111-pentetreotide | Detects tumours expressing SSTR, VIPomas, gastrinomas and paragangliomas | Reported sensitivity of 80–100% for carcinoids 87–89% for pheochromocytomas 60–90% for gastrinomas No specific data for head and neck paraganglioma | | Reduced detection of smaller lesions compared to DOTATATE PET |
| Ga-68 DOTANOC | Concentrates in tumour with high density of SSTR subtypes 2 and 5. This is coupled with a positron emitter and therefore can be picked up by a PET scanner | 90.4% | 85% | A 4-point scoring system is used to quantify uptake by comparing the ratio of tumour to liver uptake (Krenning score) |

*Abbreviations:* SSTR: Somatostatin receptor.

**Table 12.5: Summary of Biochemical Tests Required in the Preoperative Workup of a Paraganglioma**

| Biochemical Test | Upper Reference Limit | Sensitivity | Specificity |
|---|---|---|---|
| Plasma fractionated metanephrine (spot) | 0.47/1.1 nmol/l | 100% | 96% |
| 24-Hour unfractionated metanephrine | 1531 nmol/24 hours | 97.1% | 90.8% |
| Urinary VMA – 24 hours | <35 mic mol/24 hours | 93% | 75.6% |
| Chromogranin assay | 150 micg/l | 93% | 96% |

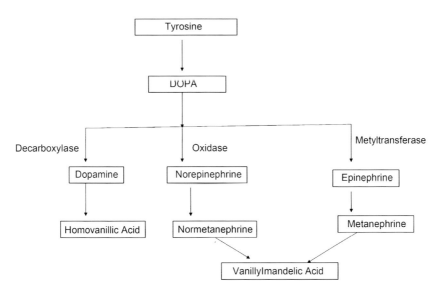

**Figure 12.4** Biochemical pathway involved in the metabolism of catecholamines.

## Table 12.6: **Glasscock and Jackson's Classification of Paraganglioma**

| S. No. | Tumour | Stage |
|---|---|---|
| 1 | Glomus tympanicum | Type 1 small mass limited to the promontory |
| | | Type 2 tumour completely filling the middle ear |
| | | Type 3 tumour filling the middle ear and mastoid |
| | | Type 4 tumour completely filling the middle ear, extending into the mastoid or through the external auditory canal. May also extend anteriorly to involve the carotid artery |
| 2 | Glomus jugulare | Type 1 small tumour involving the Jugular bulb, middle ear and mastoid |
| | | Type 2 tumour extending under the internal auditory canal. May have intracranial extension |
| | | Type 3 tumour extending to the petrous apex. May have intracranial extension |
| | | Type 4 tumour extending beyond the petrous apex into the clivus or infratemporal fossa. May have intracranial extension |

### Staging

There are three different classification systems for jugulotympanic paraganglioma which are being followed. These staging systems are useful in conveying the disease extent and for comparing treatment outcomes across different studies (Tables 12.6–12.8).

### Review of Literature

*Surgery*

The extent of surgery required for these tumours can be gross total resection (GTR) or subtotal resection (SR). Proponents of GTR believe that tumour recurrence is related to the extent of tumour resection. In a series of 53 Fisch class C

## Table 12.7: **Modified Fisch Classification for Paraganglioma**

| S. No. | Tumour | Class | |
|---|---|---|---|
| 1 | Tympanomastoid paraganglioma | *Class A:* Tumours confined to the middle ear | A1: Tumour margins clearly visible on otoscopic examination |
| | | | A2: Tumour margin not visible on otoscopy. Tumour may extend anteriorly to eustachian tube and/or posterior mesotympanum |
| | | *Class B:* Tumour confined to the tympanomastoid cavity without destruction of bone of the infralabyrinthine compartment of the Temporal bone | B1: Tumour involving middle ear with extension to the hypotympanum |
| | | | B2: Tumour involving middle ear with extension to the hypotympanum and mastoid |
| | | | B3 Tumour confined to the tympanomastoid compartment with erosion of carotid canal |
| 2 | TympanoJugular paragangliomas | *Class C:* Tumours extending beyond the tympanomastoid cavity, destroying bone of the infralabyrinthine and apical compartment of the Temporal bone and involving the carotid canal | C1: Tumours with limited involvement of the vertical portion of the carotid canal |
| | | | C2: Tumours invading vertical portion of the carotid canal |
| | | | C3: Tumour with invasion of the horizontal portion of the carotid canal |
| | | | C4: Tumour reaching the anterior foramen lacerum |
| | | *Class D:* Tumours with intracranial extension | Di1: Tumours with up to 2 cm intradural extension |
| | | | Di2: Tumours with more than 2 cm intradural extension |
| | | | Di3: Tumours with inoperable intradural extension |
| | | | De1: Tumours with up to 2 cm dural displacement |
| | | | De2: Tumours with more than 2 cm dural displacement |
| | | *Class V:* Tumours involving vertebral artery | Ve: Tumours involving extradural vertebral artery |
| | | | Vi: Tumours involving intradural vertebral artery |

### Table 12.8: de la Cruz Classification: Best Possible Surgical Approach Based on Tumour Extension

| S. No. | Tumour Extension | Surgical Approach |
|---|---|---|
| 1 | Tympanic | Transcanal |
| 2 | Tympano-mastoid | Mastoid-extended facial recess approach |
| 3 | Jugular bulb | Mastoid neck (possible Facial nerve rerouting) |
| 4 | Carotid artery | Infratemporal fossa |
| 5 | Transdural | Infratemporal fossa or intracranial |

*Source:* Surgery for Glomus Tumors, HYPERLINK "https://entokey.com/surgery-for-glomus-tumors-and-other-lesions-of-the-jugular-foramen/B9781416046653000494.htm" Chapter 49 Brackman DE, Arriaga MA in Otologic Surgery, eds Brackmann DE, Shelton C, Arriaga MA WB Saunders, Philadelphia. p579–593

and D tumours, GTR was possible in 83% with a recurrence rate of 10% (13). Updated results from the same group on 122 class C and D tumours revealed GTR rates of 86% with a 54% rate of new-onset lower cranial nerve palsy. The most commonly involved cranial nerve was the IX nerve (14). The otology group from Vanderbilt published results of total resection in 90% of 202 patients with a 35-year long follow-up. Though tumour recurrence rate was only 6%, new-onset cranial neuropathy occurred in 60% patients involving cranial nerves IX followed by XI, X and XII (15). The incidence of postoperative cranial neuropathy was found to be 8.7–13% in case of C4 and lower tumours and 63.6–81.8% in case of C4 and higher tumours (16).

In view of the postoperative morbidity consequent to a GTR, SR is advocated by many centres, especially for young patients with large tumours and functional preoperative cranial nerve status. Reserving this strategy for this group of patients, Jackson and colleagues did not experience tumour recurrence during a 45-month follow-up in a cohort of 12 patients (17). SR is also considered beneficial for patients aged >60 years and with multiple comorbidities (18, 19).

### Stereotactic Radiotherapy (SRS)

Radiosurgery for the treatment of skull base tumours was developed by Lars Leksel in 1951. This involves delivering a hypo-fractionated dose of radiotherapy using three-dimensional conformal plan with steep dose fall off. The techniques to deliver stereotactic radiation to the skull base include Gamma Knife (Cobalt-60), Linear Accelerator and Cyberknife. The prerequisites for the use of stereotactic radiosurgery in skull base paragangliomas are well-defined tumour margins, relatively small tumour volumes and lack of brain parenchymal invasion. To achieve local control without compromising the organs at risk, either a single fraction of 12–14 Gy or 50 Gy total dose in a fractionated manner can be considered. In a meta-analysis on 15 studies

conducted on radiosurgery in glomus tumour, the pooled local control rate for 511 patients was 95.4% over a median follow-up ranging between 27.4 and 148 months. The mean tumour volume considered eligible for stereotactic radiosurgery ranged between 3.6 and 133 ml (20). Ivan et al. performed a systematic review comparing various treatment modalities for skull base glomus tumours ($n = 869$) and found the best local control rates for patients having received SRS alone (95%), 86% for GTR, 69% for STR and 71% for STR+SRS. The rates of post-procedure cranial nerve IX–XI palsy was the least in the SRS only group (21).

### External Beam Radiotherapy

The recommended radiation dose to achieve local control in a skull base glomus is 40–50 Gy in 25 fractions. At present, the indications for external beam radiotherapy include the following:

i. As a primary treatment, modality in tumours deemed unresectable due to carotid encasement or poor venous cross-circulation.

ii. After subtotal resection.

iii. Salvage after surgical failure or relapse.

iv. In the adjuvant setting in case of malignant paraganglioma.

Literature is heterogeneous in terms of indication, radiation dose and technique and response assessment. Overall local control rates range between 95 and 100% with stabilization of tumour growth and cranial nerve palsy (22).

### Wait and Watch

A wait and scan policy is not routinely recommended. Alvarez-Morujo and colleagues considered this strategy in nine patients with multicentric paragangliomas. Significant interval change in size was noted for two patients during a 36-month follow-up period (23). This strategy may be reserved for patients with bilateral para-ganglioma at risk for bilateral lower cranial nerve weakness, elderly patients with multiple comorbidities and in small recurrent tumours.

### *Treatment Outcomes*

Jansen et al. performed a systematic review of treatment outcomes in jugulotympanic para-ganglioma. Of the18 studies reviewed, surgery was performed in 299 patients and radiotherapy in 83. Local control was 100% for class A and B tumours and risk of new-onset cranial nerve palsy was <1%. Post-treatment improvement in hearing and tinnitus was noted on an average in 11% class A patients and 3% of class B patients. For class C1-4, surgical cohort had a local control rate of 80–95%, not significantly different from the radiotherapy arm (84%). New-onset cranial nerve deficit was noted in 67–100% C1-4 patients post-surgery as opposed to none of the patients who were treated with radiotherapy (24).

### *Peptide Receptor Radionuclide Therapy (PRRT)*

The principal radionuclide used from a thera-peutic angle in case of unresectable or metastatic pheochromocytomas and paragangliomas is I-131 MIBG. It specifically concentrates in tis-sues expressing noradrenaline and monoamine vesicular transport system. A meta-analysis on 243 metastatic paragangliomas revealed response rates of complete response 3%, partial response 27% and stable disease 52%, respec-tively (25).

However, MIBG uptake was found to be poor in patients with SDH-x mutation and head and neck paraganglioma (26). Therapeutic soma-tostatin analogues like Y-90 DOTANOC and Lu-177 DOTANOC have been shown to have radiographic, biochemical and clinical response rates of 10.7%, 14.3% and 21.4%, respectively, in head and neck paragangliomas in a phase II (27).

### Surgical Management

Infratemporal fossa A approach for exposure of the Jugular foramen is depicted in Figure 12.5. The C-shaped incision used for this approach is similar in design to the incision described in the section on malignant neoplasms. A rectangular mucoperiosteal flap is elevated. For performing the cul-de-sac closure, the cartilaginous canal is transected circumferentially at the level of the spine of Henle. The mucoperiosteal flap is used to buttress the closure. Before doing so, the skin of the bony canal is excised. Sub-plastysmal flap is elevated in the neck. After retraction of the sternomastoid, posterior belly of digastric is identified. Vascular control is obtained at the level of internal Jugular vein and internal, exter-nal and common carotid arteries. Lower cranial nerves are identified and preserved.

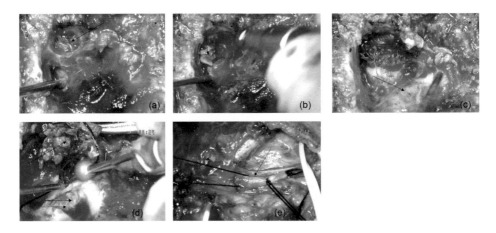

**Figure 12.5** Fisch type A approach for jugulotympanic paraganglioma. (a) Cortical mastoidectomy has been performed. Tumour is seen filling the external auditory canal (arrow) with an intact canal wall. Suction tip overlies the dome of the lateral semicircular canal. (b) Posterior canal wall is being lowered. Epitympanum has been exposed, revealing an intact ossicular chain. Subsequently, the incudostapedial joint is carefully dislocated. (c) A thin plate of bone is left over the sigmoid sinus (arrow). (d) Sigmoid sinus has been unroofed (double arrow). Tumour is seen in the area of the Jugular foramen (single arrow). (e) Upper end of internal Jugular vein is ligated in the neck followed by extraluminal packing of the sigmoid sinus. (Courtesy: Prof Suresh C Sharma, AIIMS, New Delhi.)

The Facial nerve is identified in its extratemporal course, superficial parotidectomy is performed and terminal branches of Facial nerve are delineated. A canal wall down mastoidectomy is performed. Facial nerve is identified and 270° decompression of the Facial nerve is performed from the geniculate ganglion to the stylomastoid foramen. Facial nerve is rerouted anteriorly into the parotid bed. Bone over the sigmoid sinus is drilled till a thin shell of bone is left to facilitate extraluminal packing. Infracochlear cell tracts are exenterated next.

Internal Jugular vein is ligated in the neck. For extradural tumours, lateral wall of sigmoid sinus is unroofed and excised with the tumour. During this procedure, bleeding is expected from the inferior petrosal sinus, which can be controlled with compression using hemostatic agents. In case of intracranial tumours requiring dural resection, a water-tight repair needs to be performed to avoid a CSF leak. A small dural defect can be plugged with fat. Larger defects need multilayer repair with the first layer of fascia, followed by obliteration of the cavity with fat and buttressed with pedicled temporalis or sternomastoid muscle.

In type C3 tumours, Fisch type B approach is used. This entails drilling of the anterior canal wall and exposure of the temporomandibular joint. Drilling is begun from the base of the zygoma followed by sacrifice of the middle meningeal artery and the mandibular nerve.

*Caveats in Surgical Management of Jugulotympanic Paraganglioma*

1. *Management of sigmoid sinus:* Extraluminal packing of the sigmoid sinus is favoured over intraluminal packing to avoid traumatizing the vein of Labbe.

2. *Management of the Facial nerve:* Anterior rerouting of the Facial nerve results in temporary paresis with 66.7–93% achieving House-Brackmann Grade I–II in the long term (28, 29). To circumvent this problem, "Intact Bridge" technique has been described for C-1 tumours. In this technique, fallopian canal is left intact in the vertical part followed by drilling of the infracochlear and infralabyrinthine cells.

### Differential Diagnosis

1. *Non-paraganglioma Jugular foramen tumours:* schwannoma, meningioma, primary neuroectodermal tumour and metastasis.

2. *Pseudomass of the Jugular foramen:*

   i. Jugular bulb flow variants due to slow, turbulent or jetting may cause diagnostic dilemma on T1-weighted and post-contrast images.

   ii. High-riding and dehiscent Jugular bulb can give the impression of a Jugular foramen paraganglioma.

   iii. *Internal Jugular vein thrombophlebitis:* Radiologically, mimics jugulotympanic paraganglioma by appearing as widened Jugular foramen. MRI findings typically include a halo of oedema around the vein with perivenous soft tissue enhancement.

### ENDOLYMPHATIC SAC TUMOURS

Endolymphatic sac tumour (ELST) was first described as a low-grade papillary adenocarcinoma, mimicking the histology of renal cell carcinoma, situated in the posteromedial aspect of the petrous bone (30). Heffner et al. are credited with the identification of the association of this tumour with the endolymphatic sac, giving the eponymous name of Heffner Tumour. These are rare tumours with less than 200 cases reported in literature (31).

### Aetiology

1. *Sporadic:* No genetic association, age at presentation is usually in the 5th–6th decade.

2. *Von Hippel-Lindau syndrome (VHL):* ELST in VHL has an incidence of 24% (32). These tumours have a predilection for bilaterality, presentation at a younger age and being more common in females. The genetic locus is located on the short arm of chromosome-3 transmitted in an autosomal dominant manner.

### Clinical Features

1. *Cochleo-vestibular dysfunction:* ELST can present as follows:

   a. *Sudden sensorineural hearing loss (SNHL):* Intralabyrinthine haemorrhage followed by inflammation and degeneration.

   b. *Gradual SNHL:* Direct invasion of otic capsule and development of endolymphatic hydrops.

   c. *Vertigo and aural fullness:* Obstruction of endolymphatic reabsorption and endolymphatic hydrops.

2. *Cranial neuropathy:* The most commonly involved cranial nerve is the Facial nerve involved in 5–33%, lower cranial nerves may get involved with tumour extension (33, 34).

## Table 12.9: Bambakidis and Magerian Grading of ELST

| Grade | Tumour Extent | Surgical Approach |
|-------|---------------|-------------------|
| I | Confined to Temporal bone, middle ear and or external auditory canal | Hearing preservation with retrolabyrinthine transdural approach |
| II | Extension into posterior fossa | Extended retrolabyrinthine and transdural approach. Translabyrinthine approach if no serviceable hearing |
| III | Extension into posterior fossa or middle fossa | Subtemporal craniotomy or petrosectomy |
| IV | Extension to clivus or sphenoid ring | Staged and anterior and posterior fossa technique |

3. *Signs of intracranial extension:* Disease extension into the posterior fossa can result in raised intracranial pressure and brainstem compression.

4. *Metastasis:* It is rare; there are however, reports of "Drop metastasis" to the spine (35).

### Radiology

HRCT reveals destructive bone lesion centred on the posteromedial aspect of the Temporal bone. Intratumoural haemorrhage characteristically gives rise to calcification and heterogeneous hyperdensity. The same is visualized as hyperintensity on contrast-enhanced T1-weighted sequences. On non-contrast T1 and T2 sequences, the appearance is heterogeneous with areas of hyperintensity mixed with hypointense areas.

### Staging and Surgical Approach

Bambakidis and Magerian in their retrospective evaluation of 103 ELST proposed their classification system with therapeutic implications, as shown in Table 12.9 (36). The tumour is identified in relation to the posterior semicircular canal. Excision is performed with 0.5 cm dural margin.

### Review of Literature

Bambakidis et al. have reported the outcomes of a large number of ELST in their literature review of 103 ELST (36). Tumours associated with VHL were found to be of lower grade than sporadic tumours. Complete resection was the most important determinant of long-term disease-free status. Oncological outcomes from notable series have been summarized in Table 12.10 (37–39).

## Table 12.10: Summary of the Oncological Outcomes of Notable Series

| Study | n | Follow-Up | Local Control |
|-------|---|-----------|---------------|
| Heffner 1989 | 16 | 61 months | 69% |
| Kim 2012 | 33 | 50 months | 91% |
| Carlson 2013 | 11 | 63 months | 91% |

Stereotactic radiotherapy with gamma knife may be considered for tumours that are unresectable and following subtotal resections.

### Differential Diagnosis

- *Paraganglioma:* Bulk of the lesion is centred over the Jugular foramen than the posteromedial aspect of the Temporal bone and destruction of the carotid-Jugular spine. Uptake on DOTANOC scan also differentiates it from ELST.

- *Choroid plexus papilloma:* Preoperative differentiation is difficult; it is diagnosed by IHC showing positive staining for transthyretin.

- *Eosinophilic granuloma.*

- *Metastasis:* Lytic skull base metastasis can originate from the thyroid, kidney and prostate.

- Meningioma.

- Primary bone tumour.

### VESTIBULAR SCHWANNOMA (VS)

VS is a cerebellopontine angle (CPA) tumour arising from the vestibular division of the VIII cranial nerve. It accounts for 75% of all CPA tumours and 5–10% of all intracranial neoplasms (40). Increased radiological surveillance has resulted in a steady rise in the incidence of VS (3.1 per million in 1976 to 19.4 per million in 2008) along with an increase in identification of smaller tumours (mean tumour size from 30 mm in 1979 to 10 mm in 2008) (41).

### Classification

- Small VS – less than 1.5 cm

- Medium VS – 1.5–0.5 cm

- Large VS – more than 2.5 cm

### Genetic Basis

Five percent of VS occur in the background of neurofibromatosis type 2 (NF2). Table 12.11

## Table 12.11: Salient Features of Sporadic and NF-2 Associated VS

| Features | Sporadic VS | NF-2 VS |
|---|---|---|
| Incidence of mutation in NF2 gene | 60% | 90% |
| Type of mutation | Point mutation and small deletion | Truncating mutations |
| Laterality | Unilateral | Bilateral |
| Associated tumours | None | Meningioma, astrocytoma, ependymoma |
| Age of onset | Middle age | Childhood |

enumerates the differences between the sporadic and NF2-associated VS (42).

### Imaging

Gadolinium-enhanced T1 images are recommended for screening as well as surveillance for VS. These tumours are hypointense on T1-weighted and hyperintense on T2-weighted images. Twenty percent interval change in volume signifies tumour growth. Cystic VS can be identified on T2-weighted sequences.

### Management and Outcomes

The following factors need to be considered before deciding on the appropriate treatment plan:

1. Sporadic or NF-2 associated
2. Size of the tumour
3. Preoperative functional status of cranial nerves
4. Patient and institutional preference

Surgical treatment options include subtotal resection or total resection. Approaches described include transotic and translabyrinthine (hearing ablative), retrosigmoid and middle fossa approach (hearing preserving). Small tumours restricted to the internal acoustic meatus are best approached through the middle fossa approach. With extension to the CP angle, this approach entails superior petrosal sinus ligation and Temporal lobe retraction. The translabyrinthine approach offers complete visualization of the Facial nerve and is well-suited for large tumours with no preoperative serviceable hearing. Retrosigmoid approach can be used for all tumour sizes, though extensive tumour removal requires cerebellar retraction. It is considered hearing preserving procedure for medially situated tumours. Indications for combined approach include the following:

1. Tumour greater than 4 cm
2. Extensive tumours involving the CP angle
3. Tumours traversing the intracranial compartments

Focus is now shifting towards subtotal resection to preserve function with radiotherapy reserved in cases demonstrating tumour growth on interval radiology.

For NF-2 associated VS, treatment is challenging as tumours are often found to be adherent to surrounding structures and the brainstem. Extent of surgery should be carefully determined as bilateral hearing loss and Facial nerve damage can be debilitating. For tumours larger than 3 cm, facial palsy occurred in 50% and hearing preservation was reported in 3 out of 11 (43, 44).

Zhang et al. published their results on the outcomes following surgical management of 1006 VS patients from 1990 to 2006 (45). The most favoured approach was the translabyrinthine followed by transotic. Retrosigmoid approach was commonly utilized for stage 2 tumours and middle fossa approach for stage 1 tumours. Success in terms of complete tumour removal was achieved in 99.4%. In 97.7% Facial nerve was anatomically intact with a House-Brackman score of I–II at 1 year in 85.1% of the patients. Hearing was preserved in 61.6% of the patients. Mortality rates were 0.3%. Though CSF leak was seen in 9%, meningitis occurred in only 1.2% of the patients.

The management options for VS < 3cm include surgery, SRS and observation with interval radiology. The International Stereotactic Radiosurgery Society (ISRS) recommends 11–14 Gy to the tumour margin for single-fraction SRS for tumours less than 3 cm and 4–5 Gy in five fractions, 3–4 Gy in ten fractions and 6 Gy in three fractions for fractionated SRS for tumours greater than 3–4 cm. There are currently no studies available to compare the outcomes between single fraction and fractionated SRS. Meta-analysis by Rykaczewski on 46 articles from 1998 to 2011 showed hearing preservation in 66.45% with a median dose of 12.4 Gy applied to the tumour periphery (46). Results from a single institution study on 829 patients treated with SRS, new-onset facial palsy was less than 1% and Trigeminal sensory loss was reported at 3.1% at the end of 5 years (47).

Conservative management consisting of watchful waiting with interval radiology may also be offered to patients with VS measuring less than 3cm in size. This is based on the premise that growth rate of VS is 0.66–1.9 mm per year (48–50).

Cystic VS arise due to cystic change in Antoni B component. This entity is known for its aggressive clinical course due to the expansion of the cystic component. Consensus is to avoid conservative management in these patients. Cystic VS are classified into intratumoural and peritumoural types. Cysts tend to be adherent to surrounding neurovascular structures making it difficult to preserve cranial nerve function postoperatively (51, 52). SRS in these cases offers a chance at better functional outcome with comparable tumour control rates. In a meta-analysis involving 246 patients, SRS in cases of cystic VS resulted in tumour control of 92% at a median follow-up of 49.7 to 150 months (53).

### Differential Diagnosis

Non-schwannoma CP angle lesions: Table 12.12 demonstrates the salient radiological features of these lesions (54).

A rare entity that needs to be considered in the differential diagnosis of VS is intracochlear schwannoma; these have been classified as intravestibular, intracochlear, intravestibulocochlear, transmodiolar, transmacular, transotic and tympanolabyrinthine by Kennedy et al. (55). These tumours commonly present with unilateral hearing loss, with less than 10% presenting with vestibular symptoms. Radiologically, features overlap with labyrinthitis. Intracochlear schwannomas are usually observed with serial MRI with surgery reserved for cases evolving to cause vestibular symptoms or encroaching onto internal auditory canal, CP angle and middle ear (56).

## TUMOURS OF THE FACIAL NERVE

Tumours arising from the Facial nerve include Facial Nerve Schwannoma (FNS), Facial nerve haemangioma, Facial nerve glomus and granular cell tumours. All of them present with long-standing history of progressive Facial nerve weakness interspersed with a waxing and waning course in few patients. Extension into the vestibule or internal auditory canal may lead to hearing loss and vestibular symptoms in due course of the disease.

### Facial Nerve Schwannoma

The site of origin FNS most commonly include the geniculate ganglion (60–66%) followed by tympanic (53%) and the labyrinthine segment (50.6–60%) (57). When tumour involves Facial nerve proximal and distal to the geniculate ganglion, MRI reveals a "hour-glass" appearance. Skip lesions are reported in 20% of the cases with the characteristic "beads on string" appearance on MRI (58). Treatment goal in case of FNS is the maintenance of Facial nerve function for as long as possible. Management options have undergone a paradigm shift overtime as seen from the data published by the House Ear Institute (59). Prior to 1995, 85% of all the cases underwent resection, 15% were managed by decompression. In contrast to those patients diagnosed after 1995, 29% were observed, 32.7% underwent decompression and resection was performed in only 27%. SRS can also be offered in case of FNS. Though tumour control rates to the tune of 83.3–100% have been reported, most studies claim no change in Facial nerve function and few reporting worsening of function post SRS (57).

### Facial Nerve Hemangioma (FNH)

FNH most commonly arises from the geniculate ganglion and often known as geniculate hemangioma. Apart from progressive Facial nerve palsy, symptoms may include facial twitching and sensorineural hearing loss. The latter is seen in 25% of the cases due to development of a cochlear fistula (60). FNH can be observed with interval radiology with surgery reserved for progressive Facial nerve palsy.

### Glomus Facialis

These are rare glomus tumours originating in the Facial nerve with sparing of the middle ear and the Jugular foramen on radiology (61, 62). Radiological and histological appearance is like primary jugulotympanic paraganglioma. Management strategy is to preserve Facial nerve function for the longest duration by following wait and watch in asymptomatic patients

## Table 12.12: Non-schwannoma CP Angle Lesions

| Tumour | Radiological Feature |
|---|---|
| VS and hemangioblastoma | T1 and T2 isointense, contrast enhancement with flow voids |
| Meningioma, hemangiopericytoma | Uniformly enhancing, hyperostosis and calcification |
| Epidermoid | CSF like intensity in T1 and T2, restriction on diffusion-weighted images |
| Lipoma | T1 hyperintense, non-enhancing, signal suppression on fat-suppressed images |
| ELST | T1 hyperintense, heterogeneous enhancement with contrast |
| Arachnoid cyst | CSF-like intensity on CT and MRI, may erode bone |

and resection with cable grafting following the onset of facial palsy.

## NON-PARAGANGLIOMA JUGULAR FORAMEN LESIONS

1. **Jugular Foramen Schwannoma**: Approximately 100 cases are reported in literature. These tumours tend to occur in the background of neurofibromatosis type 2.

2. **Jugular Foramen Meningioma:** These are third most common entity arising from the Jugular foramen. Location in the Jugular foramen presents unique challenges: transgression into three compartments (intradural, intrapetrous and extracranial), involvement of Facial nerve and involvement of lower cranial nerve (63).

3. **ELST**

4. **Chordoma:** Chordomas are tumours located in the midline arising from notochordal remnants. Jugular foramen chordomas have an incidence of 0.2% (64).

5. **Chondrosarcoma**: Skull base chondrosarcoma frequently arise from the petro-clival junction. These locally aggressive tumours are rarely situated in the Jugular foramen.

6. **Metastasis**: Incidence of skull base metastasis is 4% with adenocarcinomas from prostate, breast and kidney being the most common location of the primary tumour (65).

Radiology is the key to differentiate between these lesions (Table 12.13).

## KEY LEARNING POINTS

- The most common Jugular foramen tumour is the jugulotympanic paraganglioma.

- Infratemporal fossa approach described by Fisch is the preferred surgical approach to these tumours.

- Preoperative DSA to assess cerebral cross-circulation and embolization should be considered.

- The option of wait and watch should be provided to patients at risk of bilateral lower cranial nerve palsy.

- Stereotactic radiosurgery and external beam conformal radiotherapy are evolving treatment modalities with tumour growth stabilization properties and lower risk of new onset cranial nerve palsy.

- Vestibular schwannoma is the main CPA lesion confronted by a neurotologist. Factors to be taken into account when deciding treatment strategy include size, bilaterality, preoperative function status of the VII and VIII nerve complex.

- Surgery is invariably considered for tumours greater than 3–4 cm and those presenting with brainstem compression. Approaches include translabyrinthine, transotic, middle fossa approach and retrosigmoid approach.

- Options for tumours less than 3 cm include wait and watch with interval radiology, stereotactic radiosurgery and surgery.

- Primary Facial nerve tumours are governed by the treatment principle – to preserve Facial

## Table 12.13: Non-paraganglioma Jugular Foramen Lesions

| Tumour | Radiological Feature |
| --- | --- |
| Meningioma | Extra-axial, broad-based dural attachment, sclerosis of the surrounding bone on CT, uniform contrast enhancement on MRI. Jugular foramen schwannomas have an infiltrative growth pattern |
| Schwannoma | Cause widening of Jugular foramen. Margins are smooth with no bone destruction. MRI pattern is isointense on T1 and hyperintense on T2. No dural tail or flow voids seen. Usually follow the course of the lower cranial nerves. Uniform enhancement is also noted on T1-weighted images |
| Chordomas and chondrosarcoma | These tumours have identical radiological appearance except for relation with the midline. Chordomas are located along the midline while chondrosarcomas are parasagittal in location. These tumours cause irregular bone destruction with calcification. Tumours are isointense or hypointense on T1-weighted and hyperintense on T2-weighted images. Enhancement in post-gadolinium images is heterogeneous giving rise to "soap-bubble" appearance |
| Skull base metastasis | These tumours especially if originating from renal cell carcinoma show avid contrast enhancement but are distinguished from glomus tumours by their permeative pattern of destruction – in contrast to the tumour growth occurring along paths of least resistance in glomus tumours |

nerve function for as long as possible and to intervene surgically only in the presence of progressive worsening of Facial nerve function.

## REFERENCES

1. Shields TW, LoCicero J, Reed CE, Feins RH. *General Thoracic Surgery*. Lippincott Williams & Wilkins, 2011, 2664 p.

2. Arias-Stella J, Valcarcel J. Chief cell hyperplasia in the human carotid body at high altitudes: physiologic and pathologic significance. *Hum Pathol*. 1976;7(4):361–73.

3. Heath D, Edwards C, Harris P. Post-mortem size and structure of the human carotid body. *Thorax*. 1970; 25(2):129–40.

4. Gimenez-Roqueplo A-P, Dahia PL, Robledo M. An update on the genetics of paraganglioma, pheochromocytoma, and associated hereditary syndromes. *Horm Metab Res*. 2012;44(5):328–33.

5. Spector GJ, Sobol S, Thawley SE, Maisel RH, Ogura JH. Panel discussion: glomus jugulare tumors of the temporal bone. Patterns of invasion in the temporal bone. *Laryngoscope*. 1979;89(10 Pt 1):1628–39.

6. Milardovic R, Corssmit EPM, Stokkel M. Value of 123I-MIBG scintigraphy in paraganglioma. *Neuroendocrinology*. 2010;91(1):94–100.

7. Koopmans KP, Jager PL, Kema IP, Kerstens MN, Albers F, Dullaart RPF. 111In-octreotide is superior to 123I-metaiodobenzylguanidine for scintigraphic detection of head and neck paragangliomas. *J Nucl Med*. 2008;49(8):1232–7.

8. Papotti M, Bongiovanni M, Volante M, et al. Expression of somatostatin receptor types 1-5 in 81 cases of gastrointestinal and pancreatic endocrine tumors: a correlative immunohistochemical and reverse-transcriptase polymerase chain reaction analysis. *Virchows Arch Int J Pathol*. 2002;440(5):461–75.

9. Krenning EP, Valkema R, Kooij PP, et al. Scintigraphy and radionuclide therapy with [indium-111-labelled-diethyl triamine penta-acetic acid-d-Phe1]-octreotide. *Ital J Gastroenterol Hepatol*. 1999;31(Suppl 2):S219–23.

10. Murphy TP, Brackmann DE. Effects of preoperative embolization on glomus jugulare tumors. *Laryngoscope*. 1989;99(12):1244–7.

11. Valavanis A. Preoperative embolization of the head and neck: indications, patient selection, goals, and precautions. *AJNR Am J Neuroradiol*. 1986;7(5):943–52.

12. Rangel-Castilla L, Shah AH, Klucznik RP, Diaz OM. Preoperative onyx embolization of hypervascular head, neck, and spinal tumors: experience with 100 consecutive cases from a single tertiary center. *J Neurointerventional Surg*. 2014;6(1):51–6.

13. Sanna M, Jain Y, De Donato G, Rohit, Lauda L, Taibah A. Management of Jugular paragangliomas: the Gruppo Otologico experience. *Otol Neurotol*. 2004;25(5):797–804.

14. Bacciu A, Medina M, Ait Mimoune H, et al. Lower cranial nerves function after surgical treatment of Fisch class C and D tympanoJugular paragangliomas. *Eur Arch Otorhinolaryngol*. 2015;272(2):311–9.

15. Wanna GB, Sweeney AD, Haynes DS, Carlson ML. Contemporary management of Jugular paragangliomas. *Otolaryngol Clin North Am*. 2015;48(2):331–41.

16. Fayad JN, Keles B, Brackmann DE. Jugular foramen tumors: clinical characteristics and treatment outcomes. *Otol Neurotol*. 2010;31(2):299–305.

17. Jackson CG, Haynes DS, Walker PA, Glasscock ME, Storper IS, Josey AF. Hearing conservation in surgery for glomus jugulare tumors. *Am J Otol*. 1996;17(3):425–37.

18. Cosetti M, Linstrom C, Alexiades G, Tessema B, Parisier S. Glomus tumors in patients of advanced age: a conservative approach. *Laryngoscope*. 2008; 118(2):270–4.

19. Willen SN, Einstein DB, Maciunas RJ, Megerian CA. Treatment of glomus jugulare tumors in patients with advanced age: planned limited surgical resection followed by staged gamma knife radiosurgery: a preliminary report. *Otol Neurotol*. 2005;26(6):1229–34.

20. Sahyouni R, Mahboubi H, Moshtaghi O, et al. Radiosurgery of glomus tumors of temporal bone: a meta-analysis. *Otol Neurotol*. 2018;39(4):488–93.

21. Ivan ME, Sughrue ME, Clark AJ, et al. A meta-analysis of tumor control rates and treatment-related morbidity for patients with glomus jugulare tumors. *J Neurosurg*. 2011;114(5):1299–305.

22. Tran Ba Huy P. Radiotherapy for glomus jugulare paraganglioma. *Eur Ann Otorhinolaryngol*. 2014; 131(4):223–6.

23. Álvarez-Morujo RJG-O, Ruiz MÁA, Serafini DP, Delgado IL, Friedlander E, Yurrita BS. Management of multicentric paragangliomas: review of 24 patients with 60 tumors. *Head Neck*. 2016;38(2):267–76.

24. Jansen TTG, Timmers HJLM, Marres HAM, Kaanders JHAM, Kunst HPM. Results of a systematic literature review of treatment modalities for jugulotympanic paraganglioma, stratified per Fisch class. *Clin Otolaryngol*. 2018;43(2):652–61.

25. van Hulsteijn LT, Niemeijer ND, Dekkers OM, Corssmit EPM. (131)I-MIBG therapy for malignant paraganglioma and phaeochromocytoma: systematic review and meta-analysis. *Clin Endocrinol (Oxf)*. 2014;80(4):487–501.

26. Angelousi A, Kassi E, Zografos G, Kaltsas G. Metastatic pheochromocytoma and paraganglioma. *Eur J Clin Invest*. 2015;45(9):986–97.

27. Imhof A, Brunner P, Marincek N, et al. Response, survival, and long-term toxicity after therapy with the radiolabeled somatostatin analogue [90Y-DOTA]-TOC in metastasized neuroendocrine cancers. *J Clin Oncol*. 2011;29(17):2416–23.

28. Sanna M, Shin S-H, De Donato G, et al. Management of complex tympanoJugular paragangliomas including endovascular intervention. *Laryngoscope*. 2011; 121(7):1372–82.

29. Fisch U. Infratemporal fossa approach for glomus tumors of the temporal bone. *Ann Otol Rhinol Laryngol*. 1982;91(5 Pt 1):474–9.

30. Gaffey MJ, Mills SE, Fechner RE, Intemann SR, Wick MR. Aggressive papillary middle-ear tumor: a clinicopathologic entity distinct from middle-ear adenoma. *Am J Surg Pathol*. 1988;12(10):790–7.

31. Wick CC, Manzoor NF, Semaan MT, Megerian CA. Endolymphatic sac tumors. *Otolaryngol Clin North Am*. 2015;48(2):317–30.

32. Diaz RC, Amjad EH, Sargent EW, Larouere MJ, Shaia WT. Tumors and pseudotumors of the endolymphatic sac. *Skull Base*. 2007;17(6):379–93.

33. Friedman RA, Hoa M, Brackmann DE. Surgical management of endolymphatic sac tumors. *J Neurol Surg Part B*. 2013;74(1):12–9.

34. Hansen MR, Luxford WM. Surgical outcomes in patients with endolymphatic sac tumors. *Laryngoscope*. 2004;114(8):1470–4.

35. Tay KY, Yu E, Kassel E. Spinal metastasis from endolymphatic sac tumor. *AJNR Am J Neuroradiol*. 2007;28(4):613–4.

36. Bambakidis NC, Megerian CA, Ratcheson RA. Differential grading of endolymphatic sac tumor extension by virtue of von Hippel-Lindau disease status. *Otol Neurotol*. 2004;25(5):773–81.

37. Heffner DK. Low-grade adenocarcinoma of probable endolymphatic sac origin A clinicopathologic study of 20 cases. *Cancer*. 1989;64(11):2292–302.

38. Carlson ML, Thom JJ, Driscoll CL, et al. Management of primary and recurrent endolymphatic sac tumors. *Otol Neurotol*. 2013;34(5):939–43.

39. Kim HJ, Hagan M, Butman JA, et al. Surgical resection of endolymphatic sac tumors in von Hippel-Lindau disease: findings, results, and indications. *Laryngoscope*. 2013;123(2):477–83.

40. Niknafs YS, Wang AC, Than KD, Etame AB, Thompson BG, Sullivan SE. Hemorrhagic vestibular schwannoma: review of the literature. *World Neurosurg*. 2014;82(5):751–6.

41. Stangerup S-E, Tos M, Thomsen J, Caye-Thomasen P. True incidence of vestibular schwannoma? *Neurosurgery*. 2010;67(5):1335–40; discussion 1340.

42. Yao L, Alahmari M, Temel Y, Hovinga K. Therapy of sporadic and NF2-related vestibular schwannoma. *Cancers*. 2020;12(4):835.

43. MacNally SP, Rutherford SA, King AT, et al. Outcome from surgery for vestibular schwannomas in children. *Br J Neurosurg*. 2009;23(3):226–31.

44. Kim BS, Seol HJ, Lee J-I, et al. Clinical outcome of neurofibromatosis type 2-related vestibular schwannoma: treatment strategies and challenges. *Neurosurg Rev*. 2016;39(4):643–53.

45. Zhang Z, Nguyen Y, De Seta D, et al. Surgical treatment of sporadic vestibular schwannoma in a series of 1006 patients. *Acta Otorhinolaryngol Ital*. 2016;36(5):408–14.

46. Rykaczewski B, Zabek M. A meta-analysis of treatment of vestibular schwannoma using gamma knife radiosurgery. *Contemp Oncol Poznan Pol*. 2014;18(1):60–6.

47. Lunsford LD, Niranjan A, Flickinger JC, Maitz A, Kondziolka D. Radiosurgery of vestibular schwannomas: summary of experience in 829 cases. *J Neurosurg*. 2005;102(Suppl):195–9.

48. Hughes M, Skilbeck C, Saeed S, Bradford R. Expectant management of vestibular schwannoma: a retrospective multivariate analysis of tumor growth and outcome. *Skull Base*. 2011;21(5):295–302.

49. Yamakami I, Uchino Y, Kobayashi E, Yamaura A. Conservative management, gamma-knife radiosurgery, and microsurgery for acoustic neurinomas: a systematic review of outcome and risk of three therapeutic options. *Neurol Res*. 2003;25(7):682–90.

50. Daultrey CRJ, Rainsbury JW, Irving RM. Size as a risk factor for growth in conservatively managed vestibular schwannomas: the Birmingham experience. *Otolaryngol Clin North Am*. 2016;49(5):1291–5.

51. Charabi S, Tos M, Børgesen SE, Thomsen J. Cystic acoustic neuromas: results of translabyrinthine surgery. *Arch Otolaryngol Neck Surg*. 1994;120(12): 1333–8.

52. Thakur JD, Khan IS, Shorter CD, et al. Do cystic vestibular schwannomas have worse surgical outcomes? Systematic analysis of the literature. *Neurosurg Focus*. 2012;33(3):E12.

53. Ding K, Ng E, Romiyo P, et al. Meta-analysis of tumor control rates in patients undergoing stereotactic radiosurgery for cystic vestibular schwannomas. *Clin Neurol Neurosurg*. 2020;188:105571.

54. Friedmann DR, Grobelny B, Golfinos JG, Roland JT. Nonschwannoma tumors of the cerebellopontine angle. *Otolaryngol Clin North Am*. 2015;48(3): 461–75.

55. Kennedy RJ, Shelton C, Salzman KL, Davidson HC, Harnsberger HR. Intralabyrinthine schwannomas: diagnosis, management, and a new classification system. *Otol Neurotol*. 2004;25(2):160–7.

56. Magliulo G, Colicchio G, Romana AF, Stasolla A. Intracochlear schwannoma. *Skull Base*. 2010;20(2): 115–8.

57. McRackan TR, Wilkinson EP, Rivas A. Primary tumors of the Facial nerve. *Otolaryngol Clin North Am*. 2015;48(3):491–500.

58. Mowry S, Hansen M, Gantz B. Surgical management of internal auditory canal and cerebellopontine angle Facial nerve schwannoma. *Otol Neurotol.* 2012;33(6):1071–6.

59. Wilkinson EP, Hoa M, Slattery WH, et al. Evolution in the management of Facial nerve schwannoma. *Laryngoscope.* 2011;121(10):2065–74.

60. Mangham CA, Carberry JN, Brackmann DE. Management of intratemporal vascular tumors. *Laryngoscope.* 1981;91(6):867–76.

61. Dutcher PO, Brackmann DE. Glomus tumor of the facial canal: a case report. *Arch Otolaryngol Head Neck Surg.* 1986;112(9):986–7.

62. Petrus LV, Lo WM. Primary paraganglioma of the Facial nerve canal. *AJNR Am J Neuroradiol.* 1996;17(1):171–4.

63. Sanna M, Bacciu A, Falcioni M, Taibah A, Piazza P. Surgical management of Jugular foramen meningiomas: a series of 13 cases and review of the literature. *Laryngoscope.* 2007;117(10):1710–9.

64. Chen QQ, Liu Y, Chang CD, Xu YP. Chordoma located in the Jugular foramen: case report. *Medicine (Baltimore).* 2019;98(21):e15713.

65. Hayward D, Morgan C, Emami B, Biller J, Prabhu VC. Jugular foramen syndrome as initial presentation of metastatic lung cancer. *J Neurol Surg Rep.* 2012; 73(1):14–8.

# 13 Endoscopes in Otology

*Sasikanth CM and Manikandan A*

## CONTENTS

## INTRODUCTION

From the use of loupes in the early 20th century, the rudimentary Operating Microscope of Swedish otologist Carl Olof Nylen, to the more advanced binocular otological microscope introduced by Carl Zeiss in 1953, better visualization of the ear anatomy and understanding of various diseases has resulted in introduction and refinement of surgical techniques in otology. The widespread use of the operating microscope spawned many "microscopic otologists" who practiced and taught large incision, wide exposure surgery, which still remains standard practice.

As early as 1967, Mer et al. used rigid endoscopes to visualize and describe middle ear anatomy. Significant work in endoscopic ear surgery started only after 1990. Two decades later, it is still seen as a significant departure from conventional ear surgery. This chapter aims to provide an overview of the various indications, techniques, advantages and disadvantages of endoscope use in routine otological practice.

*Advantages of Endoscopic Ear Surgery:*

- Better visibility and illumination even in narrow, confined spaces of the middle ear.

- Ease of access – direct transcanal access to disease.

- Avoidance of large incisions and dissection through normal tissue and excessive bone removal to reach small disease. Hence, negligible wound morbidity.

- Ability to visualize "difficult areas" which are hidden to microscopic view, thereby reducing the incidence of disease recidivism.

*Disadvantages:*

- Difficult dissection because of "single-hand technique". This, however, is a relative problem in beginners. The learning curve is shorter for surgeons well-versed in endoscopic sinus surgery, the basic skill of handling the endoscope and single-handed dissection being the same, albeit in a more confined space and with finer instruments.

- Thermal damage to tissues from heat dissipated by the tip of the endoscope has been documented, especially when a xenon light source was used. Such damage can however be avoided by using bare minimum light settings needed for good visualization, not keeping the scope in the operating field for too long continuously and frequent irrigation with saline.

- Absence of binocularity and consequent loss of depth perception.

## REVIEW OF LITERATURE

It has been more than two decades since the first use of endoscopes in middle ear surgeries and endoscopic ear surgery is slowly gaining acceptance among the otologists in the last few years (1, 2). Various middle ear surgeries like myringotomy, tympanoplasty, ossiculoplasty, cholesteatoma surgery and stapes surgery are increasingly being done by Transcanal Endoscopic Ear Surgery (TEES).

The microscope and its limitations have long dictated the perception of middle ear diseases and their management. Microscope requires an adequate amount of light in a straight line to reach the plane of surgery for better visualization. This needs wider exposure which is achieved by soft tissue retraction and/or bone drilling. However, endoscopes provide a better visualization as the light beam is transmitted from the tip of the instrument. With the increasing use of endoscopes, many of the limitations of microscopes have been overcome. This has resulted in better understanding of the disease process and a paradigm shift in the surgical management of middle ear diseases.

TEES transforms the external auditory canal as the direct portal of access to various areas of tympanic cavity like mesotympanum, attic, hypotympanum, facial recess, sinus tympani and eustachian tube. Most surgical failures in cases of chronic otitis media squamous operated through conventional post-aural approach occur because of difficulty in removing the disease in the hard-to-reach hidden areas of the tympanic cavity and not because of the mastoid cavity (3). In contrast, TEES provides a panoramic and magnified view of all these areas of tympanic cavity which facilitates the surgeon in addressing these areas effectively.

Transcanal endoscopic tympanoplasty is the most frequently done surgeries among all endoscopic ear surgeries. The success rate in endoscopic tympanoplasty in terms of graft uptake ranges between 90% and 98% (4, 5). Various studies have shown that the success rate in terms of graft uptake and hearing improvement are similar in endoscopic and microscopic approaches. The endoscopic surgery, however, has various added advantages like reduced surgical time, less operative bleeding, pain, morbidity and hospital stay (6).

Endoscopes are also increasingly being used in cholesteatoma surgeries either as the sole approach or as a part of combined endoscopic-microscopic approach (3). The role of endoscope in localization of residual cholesteatoma in the hidden areas of tympanic cavity also makes it ideal for second look surgeries. Use of endoscope reduces the need for open cavity and canal wall down mastoidectomy as many cases of COM squamous can be managed with TEES involving minimal tissue dissection. Thomassin et al. reported a reduction in incidence of residual cholesteatoma when endoscope was used in canal wall up or canal wall down procedures for cholesteatoma (7, 8). Tarabichi stated that limited attic cholesteatomas can be removed by TEES without the need for trans-mastoid approach. Complete removal of attic disease along with preservation of the ossicles is more likely to be achieved with the endoscope. However, if the cholesteatoma sac extends beyond the body of incus into the aditus and mastoid, this approach

will not suffice, and exploration of mastoid is required for disease removal (9). Endoscopic cholesteatoma surgery is associated with lesser incidence of postoperative morbidity and better outcomes (10).

Paediatric cholesteatoma of tympanic cavity can be managed by minimally invasive TEES. Marchioni et al. reported that chances of ossicular preservation are high and recurrence rate is low in paediatric cholesteatoma patients operated by TEES when compared with microscopic canal wall up approach (11). Various studies have reported that significant improvement in the air-bone gap and lesser rate of residual disease were demonstrated in paediatric cholesteatoma patients who underwent TEES (12–14).

## DISCUSSION

The endoscope has found various applications in present-day otology practice. The common and significant uses are discussed in this section.

### OPD Procedures

The key to good endoscopic ear surgery is the achievement of excellent eye-hand coordination in the narrow confines of the ear. The author advocates an adequate period of endoscope use for routine outpatient procedures:

- Aural toileting
- Ear wax removal
- Removal of foreign bodies from the external auditory canal

The endoscope, coupled with a camera unit and display monitor, helps in better visualization and documentation of preoperative findings and postoperative results.

### Myringotomy and Grommet Insertion

Otitis media with effusion is a common condition encountered in paediatric patients. Myringotomy with insertion of grommet is indicated in chronic cases, often along with adenoidectomy. The endoscopic technique of myringotomy and insertion of the ventilation tube does not require elaborate and often cumbersome process of setting up the operating microscope and changing the position of the patient. This significantly reduces the total operating time. Studies have shown that the results are similar to the microscopic technique (15).

### Endoscopic Myringoplasty

Endoscopic repair of the tympanic membrane is the simplest TEES procedure with the least complications. The absence of a large external incision with the resultant wound morbidity makes it more acceptable to the patient.

Two basic techniques of graft placement are as follows:

- Myringoplasty through creation of a tympanomeatal flap.

- Myringoplasty through the existing perforation without raising a tympanomeatal flap (direct technique).

The choice of graft also varies

- Temporalis fascia harvested through a small temporal incision

- Tragal perichondrium

- Composite graft – tragal cartilage with perichondrium

The author follows the direct technique with the use of a composite graft in all cases. A zero degree 3-mm endoscope is used for the whole procedure. If required, a 30° endoscope is introduced through the perforation to visualize the ossicular chain and middle ear ventilation pathways. The raising of a flap is reserved only for cases where ossiculoplasty is required. Steps of endoscopic myringoplasty are depicted in Figures 13.1–13.3. The avoidance of a flap has the following advantages:

- Less operating time

- No bleeding

- Faster healing

- No granulation tissue due to exposure of bone

However, the main disadvantage of not lifting a flap is that the graft is not tucked in and there are more chances of graft displacement and hence failure of surgery.

### Ossiculoplasty

Inspection and reconstruction of the ossicular chain, when necessary, is an integral part of tympanoplasty procedure. Repair of the ossicular chain may be done using

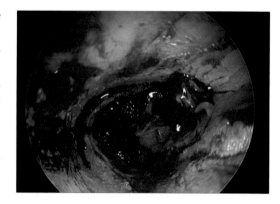

**Figure 13.2** Baring of handle of malleus and creation of gel foam bed.

- Autologous grafts

- Homografts

- Alloplastic materials

The endoscopic technique can be used to correct all types of ossicular defects using any type of material for repair. Various studies have compared endoscopic ossiculoplasty to the conventional microscopic technique and using various types of graft materials. Superior visualization and better early audiological outcome were the only advantages found in the endoscopic technique. Long-term outcomes and incidence of complications were found to be comparable to the microscopic technique (16).

### Stapes Surgery

The surgical management of otosclerosis has evolved over the past century, from the stapes mobilization and extraction procedures, fenestration of the horizontal semicircular canal, to the present stapedectomy and stapedotomy procedures with prosthesis insertion. The introduction of the operating microscope in ear surgery

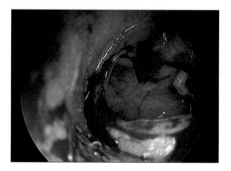

**Figure 13.1** Large central perforation with ossicular chain.

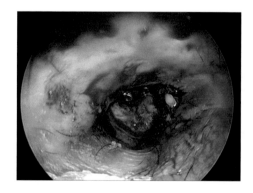

**Figure 13.3** Graft placement.

aided in refinement of the procedure and all further improvements evolved around this technique. The main limitation of the microscope is its restricted visibility in a straight line. Even a minor bony overhang of the posterior wall of the external auditory canal or the chorda tympani nerve in its normal position can impair visibility of the operative field. This invariably requires bone curetting and manipulation of the chorda tympani nerve. The superstructure of the stapes, the anterior crus in particular, is also not visible thereby making its removal a blind procedure. Congenital malformations of the stapes and Facial nerve canal dehiscence are few more conditions when working with a microscope is difficult. Results with endoscopic stapedotomy have been found to be comparable with those using an operating microscope (17, 18). All the above shortcomings are circumvented by the endoscope. The manoeuvrability and better magnification help in studying the anatomy better. The main disadvantage of the endoscopic technique is the difficulty in placing the prosthesis with a single hand. Some surgeons use improvised "endoscope holders", thereby making both hands available for such intricate manoeuvres. The postoperative care and surgical outcomes are comparable with the standard microscopic techniques. Steps of endoscopic stapes surgery are depicted in Figures 13.4–13.6.

### Endoscopic Surgery for Cholesteatoma

Endoscopes are now used by many surgeons in the surgical management of cholesteatoma.

The endoscope can be employed in the following ways:

- Exclusively endoscopic cholesteatoma surgery

- Along with the microscope mainly to look for residual disease

- Limited access "Second Look" procedures

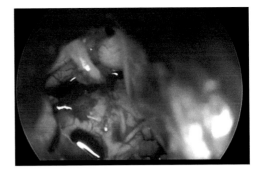

**Figure 13.5** View of oval window after stapes removal.

*Exclusively Endoscopic Cholesteatoma Surgery:* Tarabichi was one of the earliest proponents of transcanal endoscopic cholesteatoma surgery along with reconstruction with tragal cartilage. His study of 168 cases with a 2-year follow-up period showed very low recurrence rates (19).

The main technique involves a direct transcanal access to disease, "Following and Removing" the cholesteatoma from and around various structures in the middle ear with minimal bone removal if necessary to access disease. This is followed by reconstruction of bony defect and ossiculoplasty using tragal cartilage and tympanoplasty with composite tragal cartilage-perichondrium graft.

The main advantages of this technique are as follows:

- The ease of access without dissection of healthy soft tissue and bone.

- Ensuring complete disease removal due to better field of vision and visibility of "Hidden Areas" like the sinus tympani, facial recess, eustachian tube orifice and anterior epitympanum.

- In many cases ossicular preservation is also possible without compromising disease removal.

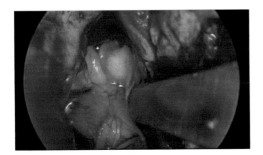

**Figure 13.4** Ascertaining diagnosis of otosclerosis (fixed stapes).

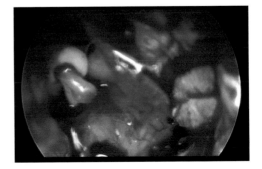

**Figure 13.6** Piston in place.

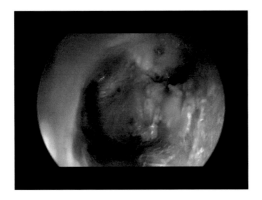

**Figure 13.7** Attic cholesteatoma with attic wall erosion.

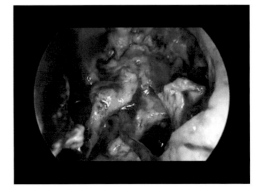

**Figure 13.9** Cholesteatoma dissected off the ossicles.

Steps of endoscopic cholesteatoma surgery are depicted in Figures 13.7–13.10. Extensive mastoid disease is not amenable to this technique and an intact canal wall/canal wall down mastoidectomy may be required in such cases. In spite of these distinct advantages, this modality still remains controversial in the surgical management of cholesteatoma.

*Endoscope-Assisted Mastoid Surgery:* The microscopic canal wall down or intact canal wall techniques remain the standard surgical modalities for management of cholesteatoma. In spite of all the advantages of the endoscopic technique, certain situations warrant the use of the microscope for ease of dissection and complete disease removal:

- Extensive mastoid cholesteatoma
- Congenital external ear anomalies/ atresia of the external auditory canal with cholesteatoma
- Complications like dehiscence of lateral semicircular canal or tegmen of mastoid

The endoscopic dissection commences via the transcanal route with dissection of the cholesteatoma from the mesotympanum/epitympanum towards the aditus. This is followed by the microscope-assisted mastoidectomy and dissection of the mastoid portion of the cholesteatoma sac. After removal of the cholesteatoma, the endoscope is again introduced to visualize any residual disease.

*Limited Access Second-look Procedures:* A second-look procedure is a common practice, especially after intact canal wall surgery for cholesteatoma, to detect recurrent disease. This usually involves the same amount of surgical exposure as the initial procedure. Alternatively, the mastoid cavity can be visualized with an endoscope introduced through a small post-aural incision. Recurrent disease, if any, may be removed with appropriate instruments and by increasing the exposure.

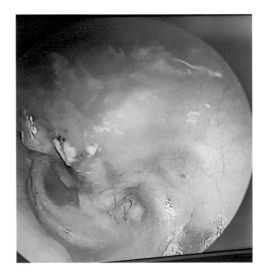

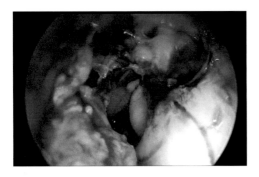

**Figure 13.8** Cholesteatoma sac after TM flap elevation.

**Figure 13.10** Postoperative status at 40 days.

## MIDDLE EAR NEOPLASMS

Paragangliomas are the commonest primary neoplasms seen in the middle ear. The second commonest are the adenomatous tumours, which may be benign (adenomas) or malignant (adenocarcinomas). All these tumours have very similar clinical presentations and radiological findings.

The treatment of these tumours is complete surgical removal. The surgical approach depends on the extent of the disease and involvement of certain areas. Tumours confined to the central part of the middle ear cleft are amenable to a purely transcanal approach. With the endoscopic technique, all the "difficult areas", namely the anterior epitympanum, hypotympanum, sinus tympani and facial recess regions can be visualized and accessed. Extension of the tumour to the mastoid necessitates a "combined transcanal post-aural approach". The basic surgical exposure and technique is the same as in cholesteatoma surgery. The main difference is in the highly vascular nature of these tumours, especially glomus tumours. Liberal infiltration of the external auditory canal with adrenaline solution, placing adrenaline-soaked cotton pledgets in the surgical field, shrinking the tumour with bipolar diathermy and frequent irrigation with warm saline solution are adequate for a clean and clear endoscopic operative field.

The main advantages of endoscope use are as follows:

- Improved visualization and better dissection of the tumour from its attachments

- Preservation of the ossicles

- Avoiding damage to vital structures like the Facial nerve

The main drawback of the endoscopic technique is the single-handed dissection. The help of a second surgeon may be required for suctioning blood and cautery smoke. Irrespective of the surgical technique, the patients are followed up periodically for recurrence.

## ENDOSCOPES IN MANAGEMENT OF CEREBELLOPONTINE (CP) ANGLE LESIONS

Endoscopes are used in the management of CP angle lesions as an alternative to the operating microscope or in combined techniques where the visualization with the microscope is limited in certain areas. The current approaches are associated with significant patient morbidity due to large incisions, bone removal, craniotomy and brain retraction. Exclusively endoscopic techniques in the management of inner ear and petrous apex lesions are still in their evolutionary stages with very limited indications and fewer proponents (20).

The main endoscopic approaches are as follows:

- Trans-canal endoscopic infra-cochlear route for lesions located and extending inferior to the cochlea with normal preoperative hearing thresholds.

- Trans-canal endoscopic trans-vestibular and trans-cochlear route for lesions associated with pre-op hearing loss.

The exclusively trans-canal approaches are planned when the lesion is small. Though this approach is less invasive than the conventional approaches, the main deterrent is the risk of haemorrhage after tumour removal and the limited access to the medial end of the IAC to control it.

*Combined Approaches* – combined microscopic-endoscopic approaches are the commonest approaches for most lesions of the inner ear, petrous apex and IAC.

There are two common routes:

- Trans-mastoid

- Retro-sigmoid

The latter is usually a purely neurosurgical approach. The endoscope is usually used only for visualization.

## CONCLUSION

Endoscopic ear surgery is now seen as a paradigm shift from the conventional ear surgery techniques. But most of the advanced applications of the endoscope in otology are still in their nascent stages, making it just an adjunct and not a replacement to the operating microscope.

Nevertheless, the significantly low morbidity and rate of complications of the endoscopic procedures make it more acceptable to the patients. With better TEES-specific instruments, refinement of current techniques and more structured training process, it is likely to gain more popularity and acceptance in the near future.

## KEY POINTS

1. The introduction of endoscopes in otology has changed the established knowledge of middle ear anatomy, physiology and pathology of diseases, leading to introduction of newer surgical techniques and refinement of older ones.

2. Though many of the endoscopic ear surgery procedures can be carried out with existing

ear surgery instruments and rigid Hopkins 4- or 3-mm endoscope used in sino-nasal surgery, a wide variety of endoscopes in different lengths, diameters and angles of view along with TEES-specific instruments are also available.

3. The endoscope has found use in routine outpatient procedures like oto-endoscopy, aural toileting and removal of foreign bodies.

4. The surgical utility of the endoscope has encompassed a wide range of procedures, starting from myringotomy to the excision of skull base tumours at the other end of the spectrum.

5. Though the endoscope has many distinct advantages over the operating microscope, it has still not replaced it as the instrument of choice in many otological procedures.

6. Ongoing research, innovations in techniques and instrumentation are likely to make the endoscope find wider application in otology.

## REFERENCES

1. Mohindra S, Panda NK. Ear surgery without microscope: is it possible. Indian J Otolaryngol Head Neck Surg. 2010;62:138–41.

2. Raj A, Meher R. Endoscopic transcanal myringoplasty: a study. Indian J Otolaryngol Head Neck Surg 2001; 53:47–9.

3. Kapadiya M, Tarabichi M. An overview of endoscopic ear surgery in 2018. Laryngoscope Investig Otolaryngol. 2019;4:365–73.

4. Tarabichi M. Endoscopic transcanal middle ear surgery. Indian J Otolaryngol Head Neck Surg. 2010;62(1):6–24.

5. Pap I, Toth I, Gede N, et al. Endoscopic type I tympanoplasty is as effective as microscopic type I tympanoplasty but less invasive: a meta-analysis. Clin Otolaryngol. 2019;44(6):942–53.

6. Plinkert P, Lowenheim H. Trends and perspectives in minimally invasive surgery in otorhinolaryngology: head and neck surgery. Laryngoscope. 1997;107(11 Pt 1): 1483e–9.

7. Thomassin JM, Korchia D, Doris JM. Endoscopic-guided otosurgery in the prevention of residual cholesteatomas. Laryngoscope. 1993;103:939–43.

8. Thomassin JM, Braccini F. Role of imaging and endoscopy in the follow up and management of cholesteatomas operated by closed technique. Rev Laryngol Otol Rhinol (Bord). 1999;120(2):75–81.

9. Tarabichi M. Endoscopic management of limited attic cholesteatoma. Laryngoscope. 2004;114(7):1157–62.

10. Das A, Ghosh D, Sengupta A, et al. Endoscopic versus microscopic management of attic cholesteatoma: a randomized controlled trial. Laryngoscope. 2020;130(10):2461–6.

11. Marchioni D, Soloperto D, Rubini A, et al. Endoscopic exclusive transcanal approach to the tympanic cavity cholesteatoma in pediatric patients: our experience. Int J Pediatr Otorhinolaryngol. 2015;79(3):316–22.

12. Hunter JB, Zuniga MG, Sweeney AD, et al. Pediatric endoscopic cholesteatoma surgery. Otolaryngol Head Neck Surg. 2016;154(6):1121–7.

13. James AL. Endoscopic middle ear surgery in children. Otolaryngol Clin North Am. 2013;46(2): 233–44.

14. Jang CH, Jung EK, Sung CM, et al. Minimally invasive transcanal myringotomy for pediatric early stage congenital cholesteatoma. Int J Pediatr Otorhinolaryngol. 2016;90:1–4.

15. Martellucci S, Pagliuca G, de Vincentiis M, et al. Myringotomy and ventilation tube insertion with endoscopic or microscopic technique in adults: a pilot study. Otolaryngol Head Neck Surg. 2015; 152(5):927–30.

16. Manzoor NF, Nassiri AM, Rivas A. Endoscopic ossiculoplasty. Curr Otorhinolaryngol Rep. 2019;7:244–247.

17. Surmelioglu O, Ozdemir S, Tarkan O, Tuncer U, Dagkiran M, Cetik F. Endoscopic versus microscopic stapes surgery. Auris Nasus Larynx. 2017;44(3):253–7.

18. Isaacson B, Hunter JB, Rivas A. Endoscopic stapes surgery. Otolaryngol Clin North Am. 2018;51(2):415–28.

19. Tarabichi, M. Transcanal endoscopic management of cholesteatoma, Otol Neurotol. 2010;31(4):580–8.

20. Mattox DE. Endoscopy-assisted surgery of the petrous apex. Otolaryngol Head Neck Surg. 2004;130(2):229–41.

# 14 Anaesthesia Techniques in Otology

*Deepak Dwivedi and Gunjan Dwivedi*

## CONTENTS

## INTRODUCTION

Ear surgeries involve all age groups and include procedures on the external ear, middle ear, inner ear and the mastoid. The procedures may be of short duration or may be complex, involving the skull base requiring greater expertise and time. The anaesthesia required for such procedures may vary from short to prolonged duration, depending on the type of the surgery.

*External Ear Surgeries:* These surgeries include removal of the foreign bodies, preauricular abnormalities and external auditory meatus reconstruction.

*Middle Ear Surgeries:* Otitis media is the second most common illness during childhood (1). The incidence increases in certain congenital conditions like craniofacial abnormalities, cleft palate and Down's syndrome. Prolonged duration of nasotracheal intubation in paediatric critically ill patients is also associated with a higher incidence of middle ear effusions (2). The aetiology includes the repeated upper respiratory tract infections, dysfunction of the eustachian tube (ET) either due to its short length or partial obstruction due to the adenoids, all leading to the negative pressure in the middle ear and persistence of the effusion. If it remains untreated, its sequalae include risk of development of cholesteatoma, perforation, deafness and damage to the ossicular chain (3). The treatment options for these children depend on the stage at which they present. Children present early benefit with myringotomy with or without insertion of a grommet. This helps in aerating and equalizing the pressure in

the middle ear (1, 3). Those who present later in childhood may require definitive surgery in the form of tympanoplasty to eradicate the disease from the middle ear and to reconstruct the hearing mechanism if required.

Middle ear surgeries in adults include tympanoplasty with or without mastoidectomy (canal wall up or down, depending on the extent of the disease), stapedotomy and stapedectomy for improving the hearing (3).

*Cochlear Implantation/Inner Ear Surgery:* Patients with severe sensorineural hearing loss (SNHL) benefit from the cochlear implants. The aetiology of severe SNHL includes absent sensory neuroepithelium of the cochlea either due to genetic or infective pathology or secondary to cochlear ossification and ageing. The procedure is best performed before the age of 30 months to give the best chance of development of the speech in these children (3). The procedure involves the placement of electrodes through a cochleostomy after accessing the middle ear through the facial recess following cortical mastoidectomy (2).

## ANAESTHESIA CONSIDERATIONS

Major concerns for the otologic surgery include the need for providing a bloodless field, incorporation of the Facial nerve monitoring, patient positioning and choice of anaesthesia. Impact of nitrous oxide use in the middle ear surgery, airway management and concerns regarding the prevention of postoperative nausea and vomiting (PONV) are the other factors (1, 3, 4).

## Preoperative Concerns

Preoperative evaluation and assessment in patients with hearing loss is challenging as history taking and communication becomes difficult; therefore, a relatively quiet place is preferred (3). A detailed systemic examination is mandatory to rule out any neurological and cardiovascular comorbidities and precaution must be exercised in patients with advanced age where atherosclerosis-related changes in the carotids and the neck have implications during the positioning. Presence of anaemia, hypovolemia and any other contraindication to the hypotensive anaesthesia needs to be endorsed and communicated to the surgeons (3, 4).

Children presenting for the ear surgeries may have associated adenoid hypertrophy and can have history of recurrent upper respiratory tract infection rendering their airway being hyperreactive (2). History of obstructive sleep apnoea and snoring should be elicited; one needs to be careful in such patients as they are more sensitive to sedatives and CNS depressant drugs used in general anaesthesia (GA). Extubation should be done once the patient is fully awake to prevent postoperative adverse airway events and hypoxemia in these patients. Associated congenital anomalies, e.g. craniofacial abnormality, Down's syndrome and cleft palate, render the airway management difficult and require alternative difficult airway management algorithms and protocols to be in place and practised beforehand for the better outcome (2). Likewise, congenital deafness is known to be associated with prolonged QT interval in isolation or as a part of syndrome, namely Jervell Lange-Nielsen syndrome mandating a preoperative ECG in such cases. Children with sensorineural deafness are very anxious, and therefore it is always better to have parent accompanying the child till the operating room (OR) until the induction sequence is completed (3).

## Techniques of Anaesthesia

*Local Anaesthesia:* The choice of anaesthesia depends on many factors – duration of surgery, patient's cooperation and preference, surgeons' expertise and choice. Procedures like tympanoplasty, myringotomy, stapedectomy and external ear minor procedures can be safely done under local anaesthesia. The drug commonly used is 2% lignocaine with adrenaline (1: 200,000). Auriculotemporal nerve, vagus (auricular branch), Facial nerve, greater auricular nerve and the lesser occipital nerve are the sensory nerves supplying the ear (Figure 14.1) (5). "Plester's injection technique" is commonly employed for the local anaesthesia block, which includes eight steps. Step 1 in which the local anaesthetic injection is given in the postauricular fold (Figure 14.2), steps 2–4 involve further advancing the needle from the entry point at step 1 in three directions – superior, inferior and posterior – to the external canal of the ear (Figure 14.3) and steps 5–8 involve dividing the ear canal into four quadrants followed by the injection into each quadrant in a step-wise manner (Figure 14.4) (6).

Local anaesthesia has several advantages of being less expensive and safer allowing the assessment of hearing and detecting vertigo

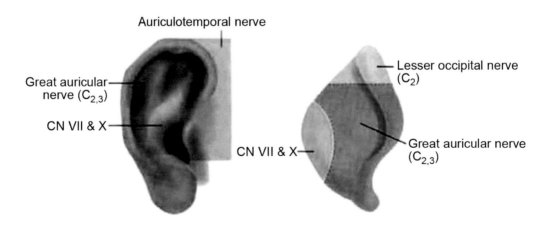

**Figure 14.1** Nerve supply of the pinna.

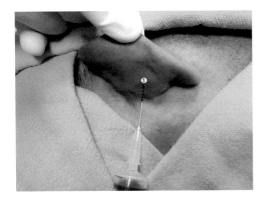

**Figure 14.2** Plester injection technique – step 1 shows postauricular injection.

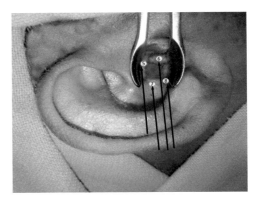

**Figure 14.4** Plester injection technique, steps 5–8 show stepwise injection in four quadrants of the ear canal.

during surgery. Other advantages include early recovery from the procedure with lesser incidence of PONV (4, 7). In a survey by Yung et al. of patients undergoing middle ear surgery under local anaesthesia, patients experienced noise disturbance in nearly 30%, anxiety was reported by 24% and claustrophobia was complained by 9.3% of the patients (6). However, 89% of the respondents were in favour of local anaesthesia. In a similar prospective study by Caner et al., 73% of the respondents who underwent middle ear surgery under local anaesthesia were satisfied with the technique, though around 33% people complained about the noise as the distressing feature followed by the anxiety (7). To overcome the discomfort and anxiety as a limiting factor of local anaesthesia technique, it has

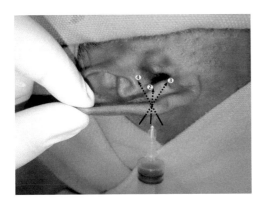

**Figure 14.3** Plester injection technique – steps 2–4 show needle advanced further from the step 1 directed superior, posterior and inferior to external ear canal.

been successfully combined with the sedation leading to the concept of "monitored anaesthesia care" (MAC) (4). Thota et al. used propofol with fentanyl combination and found it ideal due to its positive impact on recovery profile and PONV when compared with fentanyl and midazolam infusion (8).

*General Anaesthesia:* The majority of the procedures in otology are still performed under GA. The simple reason is the preference of the patient and surgeon, and requirement of immobilization during the use of the microscope (4). Prolonged procedures with uncomfortable position of the head with the face covered under the drapes and the complete avoidance of the pain and discomfort due to multiple needle pricks during the administration of the LA go in favour of GA. Preoperative anxiety can be taken care of with intravenous midazolam (0.02–0.03 mg/kg). Standard monitoring (pulse oximetry, ECG, capnography, non-invasive blood pressure and temperature) should be done; additional monitoring depends on the availability and includes depth of anaesthesia and the neuromuscular monitoring. Issues involved in GA include choice of the technique (total intravenous anaesthesia or balanced anaesthesia technique), effect of anaesthesia on middle ear pressure (MEP) and cochlear implantation.

**Balanced Anaesthesia Technique:** It includes the use of propofol (2 mg/kg) for the induction and the inhalational agents (sevoflurane, desflurane or isoflurane) for the maintenance with oxygen and nitrous oxide or with air. Short or intermediate acting muscle relaxants are used for aiding the intubation and opioids like fentanyl or remifentanil are used for analgesia (4).

**Total Intravenous Anaesthesia Technique (TIVA):** It is a technique which completely avoids the use of the inhalational agent for the induction as well as for the maintenance of anaesthesia. TIVA requires specialized pump known as target-controlled infusion pumps to administer drug based on its pharmacokinetic model incorporating various algorithms to achieve the desired effect (9). The drugs, most commonly used are propofol, an induction agent combined with the ultrashort acting opioid remifentanil (9). The advantages of TIVA are smooth emergence, lesser incidence of Post Operative Nausea and Vomiting (PONV) and ability to allow monitoring and testing of the somatosensory and motor-evoked potential (9). Mukherjee et al. in their double-blind study on 100 patients for middle ear surgery compared TIVA technique with balanced anaesthesia technique and concluded that incidence of PONV was 34% in the balanced anaesthesia group as compared to 17% in the TIVA group (10).

### Effect of Anaesthesia on Middle Ear Pressure (MEP)

Anaesthesia agents cause change in the MEP which can result in serous otitis media and hemotympanum, affect the uptake of the graft and have an adverse effect on the ossicular chain (11). Various factors affecting MEP include patient position, changes in ET and hypo/hyperventilation. Aetiology includes gas exchange between the mucosa of the middle ear and submucous connective tissue (11). Carbon dioxide can increase the MEP by the simple diffusion across the membrane into the middle ear cavity; therefore, there is always a need to maintain normo-capnia during anaesthesia. Normal range of MEP is between −200 to +200 decapascals (daPa) (11). Sade et al. concluded that gas diffusion through the middle ear mucosa is proportional to the diffusion coefficient of the gases (12). Ikarashi et al. showed that apart from the varied diffusion coefficient of the gases, it is the vascularity of the mucosa which affects the tympanomastoid cavity volume (13). Deniz et al. in their study observed that among sevoflurane and desflurane, the former cause less change in MEP (11). Ozturk et al. compared MEP in children where one group received TIVA and the other group received inhalational anaesthesia, the results showed increase of 80 daPa MEP in the inhalational group (14). Ozcan et al. conducted a clinical study where TIVA and low-flow

anaesthesia were considered superior to high-flow anaesthesia with desflurane concerning its effect on MEP (15).

### Anaesthesia Concerns for Cochlear Implantation Surgery

A comparison of GA with inhalational agents and TIVA during the testing of the integrity of the cochlear implant demonstrated favourable results with TIVA (4). Cochlear implant functioning is checked by electrical stimulation, which includes electrically Elicited Stapedius Reflex Threshold (ESRT) that represents the maximum loud sound tolerated without discomfort and electrically elicited compound action potential (ECAP). Inhalational agents show a linear relationship with ESRT threshold and hence TIVA was considered an ideal technique for determining these reflex thresholds (16–19).

### Airway Management

Airway managed with endotracheal intubation during GA is associated with sore throat, cough and potentially dental injuries due to laryngoscopy (4). Depth of anaesthesia required in cases of GA with endotracheal intubation is more, which in turn leads to delayed emergence with increased incidence of post-extubation adverse airway events. Studies have shown successful use of the supraglottic devices, e.g. laryngeal mask airway (LMA) and proseal LMA for the prolonged surgeries of ENT with lesser complications (20). It is also advisable to be prepared for the difficult airway management in a syndromic child coming for cochlear implantation and other otologic surgeries (21).

### Positioning

Position commonly used for the middle ear surgery is head elevation of 15–20°, which helps in lowering the venous pressure and providing an oligemic surgical field (3, 4). Care has to be taken in elderly patients with carotid stenosis due to atherosclerosis or in patients of rheumatoid arthritis and Down's syndrome where extensive rotation can increase the risk of the C1 and C2 subluxation. A lateral tilt of the table will be beneficial in such subsets of patients (22, 23).

### Nitrous Oxide

Blood gas coefficient of 0.46 makes nitrous oxide highly diffusible when compared to nitrogen in the air-filled cavities, including the middle ear cavity (24, 25). The passive egress of the gas occurs through the patent ET, but in cases of the ET dysfunction there is an increased pressure leading to the distension of middle ear cavity, which will affect the overlay graft for tympanoplasty (3, 4). Caution has to be followed at the time of placement of the graft and nitrous oxide should preferably be avoided. At the end of the surgery when nitrous oxide is stopped, it diffuses out from the middle ear cavity and makes the pressure sub-atmospheric, thereby adversely affecting the integrity of the ossicular chain and may lead to graft displacement.

### Surgical Field

Microscopic surgery requires an oligemic surgical field as any evident bleeding will completely obscure the field of vision. The physical measures adopted initially are sufficient in majority of the patients in providing dry surgical field. Measures include 15° head up position, which facilitates the venous drainage (1, 3, 4). Balanced anaesthesia technique or TIVA technique when used to maintain adequate depth of anaesthesia blunt the adrenergic response and prevents the obscuring of the surgical site with the blood (4).

If the physical measures are not enough, then comes the role of the pharmacological agents which because of their innate properties limit the blood loss and aid in keeping the surgical field dry. The mean arterial pressure value between 50 and 55 mmHg and systolic pressure between 80 and 90 mmHg is ideal in providing controlled hypotension (3, 4). In patients with known hypertension, the recommendation is to decrease not greater than 30% from the baseline values. Careful selection of the patients is mandatory to prevent end organ damage in patients with cardiovascular disease as the microcirculation of the tissue gets affected and is not well-tolerated by this subset of patients.

The various pharmacological agents include vasodilators, beta-blockers, alpha-2 agonists and magnesium sulfate. Vasodilators like sodium nitroprusside and nitroglycerine are no longer preferred as these agents, especially sodium nitroprusside, have a narrow therapeutic index and need close invasive monitoring. The adverse effects include lactic acidosis, cyanide poisoning, rebound hypertension and tachyphylaxis (26). Nitroglycerine when compared to sodium nitroprusside is not very effective and the effect sets in slowly (26). Cantarella et al. compared the hemodynamic effects of remifentanil and nitroglycerine for producing controlled hypotension in patients undergoing middle ear surgery targeting the MAP between 50 and 70 mmHg. The results showed that both are effective in maintaining the dry surgical field, but nitroglycerine was associated with more tachycardia (27).

β-Blockers like labetalol and esmolol have been used for creating a dry surgical field. Labetalol is a selective α1 antagonist and non-selective β1 and β2 antagonists, while esmolol is a selective β1-blocker. Labetalol when compared to esmolol is capable of antagonizing the action of topical epinephrine used for creating the dry field by its α1 antagonist action. Both are capable of reducing heart rate and MAP. Lavere et al. conducted a randomized control trial and compared blood loss and validated surgical field visibility score between esmolol and labetalol and concluded that either of the two can be used, depending on the cost and choice. β-Blockers are contraindicated in patients of diabetes mellitus, bronchial asthma, chronic obstructive pulmonary disease, sinus bradycardia, stroke and end-stage kidney disease (28).

Alpha-2 Adrenoreceptor Agonists (Clonidine and Dexmedetomidine) look very promising for providing Hypotensive anaesthesia due to their properties and action on reducing the central Catecholamine secretions, anaesthesia and analgesia sparing effects with minimal respiratory depression and a predictable Hemodynamics (29). Caution is against its effect leading to moderate hypotension and bradycardia, which can be prevented by administering the drug through the continuous infusion and avoiding the boluses as well as not to be used in patients on β-blockers with heart rate on the lower side or in patients of Sinus Bradycardia. Gupta et al. in their prospective study used infusion of Dexmedetomidine with stable hemodynamics at the rate of 0.5 µg/kg/hour after the induction of anaesthesia and discontinued 20 minutes before the completion of the surgery. The assessment done by the surgeons about the surgical field intraoperatively graded it as grade 1, i.e. minimal bleeding requiring intermittent suction only (30). Double-blinded trial by Modir et al. compared Remifentanil, Dexmedetomidine and Magnesium Sulfate for providing the dry surgical field and recovery in the postoperative period. Dexmedetomidine loading dose used was 1 µg/kg in 100 ml normal saline, which was administered over 10 minutes followed by the continuous infusion of the 0.4 µg/kg/hour. The results showed Dexmedetomidine to be superior to the other two drugs in providing relatively an ideal operating condition with the controlled hemodynamics, although with delayed recovery (31).

Remifentanil, a µ-receptor agonist opioid, has an ultrashort duration of action which makes it suitable for TIVA. It maintains the autoregulation of the microcirculation of the middle ear, limits the blood flow to the middle ear, decreases the blood pressure and improves the visualization of the operative field (32). Remifentanil has a disadvantage of producing hyperalgesia in the immediate postoperative period once the infusion is discontinued. Ryu et al. when compared remifentanil and magnesium sulfate for middle ear surgery concluded that both provide good surgical conditions, but magnesium sulfate has an advantage in the postoperative period by providing good analgesia and minimal PONV and shivering (33).

Magnesium sulfate is a calcium antagonist and prevents egress of calcium ions from sarcoplasmic reticulum, which is responsible for the vasodilation. It enhances prostacyclin synthesis and inhibits the activity of angiotensin-converting enzyme. Antagonizing action on $N$-methyl-D-aspartate receptor is responsible for its analgesic action (4). Aboushanab et al. concluded that both magnesium sulfate and dexmedetomidine are capable of producing deliberate hypotension during middle ear surgery but magnesium sulfate has an advantage of early recovery (34). In the study, magnesium sulfate was loaded in the dose of 50 mg/kg in 100 ml and was administered over 10 minutes following the induction of anaesthesia. This was followed by the continuous infusion of magnesium sulfate at the rate of 15 mg/kg/hour till the end of the surgery (34). Magnesium is known to have a minimal effect over the cardiac output and has a favourable effect on the hemodynamics as it lowers the HR and MAP without resulting in reflex tachycardia and hypertension (35). It potentiates the action of the neuromuscular blockers as it blocks acetylcholine release necessary to reverse this block.

### Facial Nerve Monitoring

Facial nerve due to its course in the temporal bone is vulnerable to damage during middle ear surgery, more so in the diseased middle ear. It is prudent to monitor the Facial nerve intraoperatively to protect it from injury during the middle ear surgery. If GA is used with endotracheal intubation, it is recommended to use the initial dose of the short intermediate acting muscle relaxants, e.g. atracurium and mivacurium (36). Muscle relaxation should be reversed or allowed to wear off before the electromyography (EMG) of the Facial nerve is instituted to prevent the interference with its evoked potential measurement (36). Cai et al. correlated peripheral neuromuscular monitoring along with the Facial nerve EMG where EMG-evoked signals could be generated at even 50% neuromuscular blockade (NMB), thus concluding that partial NMB is feasible with neurophysiological monitoring of the Facial nerve (37). TIVA with propofol and remifentanil obviates the use of muscle relaxant when the LMA is inserted, but will require the depth of anaesthesia monitoring in such cases. Choe et al. concluded that for the microsurgery of the ear, Facial nerve monitoring was unimpeded with the minimal use of the neuromuscular blocking agents targeting the TOF (twitching) count of more than 1 with TIVA technique (38). Mangia et al. used local anaesthesia with sedation for otologic surgeries where they successfully did the Facial nerve monitoring and suggested this technique in patients with the higher risks of anaesthesia (39).

### Postoperative Nausea and Vomiting

Middle ear surgery has a reported incidence of PONV between 62% and 80% without the prophylactic antiemesis (4). The predisposing factors include younger age, prolonged duration of surgery, use of nitrous oxide in GA, vestibular system stimulation directly by the drill or during suction and irrigation as well as prolonged preoperative fasting intervals (3). TIVA technique with the use of propofol is associated with lesser incidence of PONV when compared to inhalational agents (40, 41). 5HT$_3$ receptor antagonist like ondansetron, romesetron etc. are used at the end of the surgery as a prophylaxis against the PONV (42, 43). Usmani et al. and Panda et al. have shown that the combination of ondansetron (0.1 mg/kg) and dexamethasone (0.15 mg/kg) is superior to drugs used in isolation (44, 45). Vestibular symptoms leading to PONV is common following the middle ear surgery as well as post cochlear implantation (46). It is amenable to and treated with betahistine, which is structurally an analogue belonging to histamine with H3 antagonist and H1 agonist activity (46).

### Postoperative Analgesia

Multimodal analgesia is adopted for the effective pain relief in the postoperative period. It includes use of paracetamol with opioids and NSAIDS/COX-2 inhibitors. The local infiltration with the local anaesthetics with epinephrine administered at the beginning of the surgery is helpful in augmenting the postoperative analgesia. Topical application of the pledgets soaked with local anaesthetic can be used for aiding the pain relief. Pairaudeau et al. have used absorbable haemostatic sponges soaked with 0.5% levobupivacaine (3).

Voronov et al. compared regional block by targeting the auricular branch of the vagus nerve with intranasal instillation of fentanyl in paediatric age group undergoing myringotomy. Auricular branch of vagus nerve provides sensory supply to the external auditory meatus as well as to the inferior aspect of the tympanic membrane. The nerve was targeted by averting the tragus and advancing the needle till it made contact with the cartilage after the penetration, where 0.25% bupivacaine with 1:200,000 adrenaline was injected with the volume not exceeding 0.2 ml (47). Role of pre-emptive analgesia was studied by Suresh et al. when they compared the greater auricular nerve (GAN) block given preoperatively for tympanomastoid surgeries with the postoperative administration of the same block and concluded that GAN block does not offer any benefit as far as the postoperative analgesia is concerned (48). Suresh et al. demonstrated the effectiveness of the GAN block, which was administered post-surgery to have opioid sparing effect, the quality of the analgesia was similar to the 0.1 mg/kg of morphine (49). Analogues of gabenoids like gabapentin and pregabalin are known to have analgesic, anticonvulsant and anxiolytic properties. Dhakal et al. administered 150 mg of pregabalin preemptively to the patients undergoing myringoplasty and found it to be an effective modality to reduce and limit the postoperative pain and lessen the consumption of the analgesics (50).

## CONCLUSION

Local anaesthesia with or without conscious sedation is a viable alternative to GA for simple otologic surgeries of the external ear and the middle ear cavity. TIVA has been preferred over inhalational anaesthesia as it provides good surgical conditions, unabated Facial nerve monitoring, smoother recovery and lesser incidence of PONV. Caution must be exercised while using nitrous oxide due to its effect on the MEP dynamics. Dexmedetomidine has been successful providing the dry surgical field for the surgeons with controlled hemodynamics. Supraglottic devices like proseal LMA could obviate endotracheal intubation and have proven their role in airway management for prolonged ear surgeries without increasing the risk of adverse airway events. Combination of dexamethasone and 5HT3 receptor antagonist has reduced the incidence of PONV substantially in patients undergoing ear surgeries.

## REFERENCES

1. Ravi R, Howell T. Anaesthesia for paediatric ear, nose and throat surgery: continuing education in anaesthesia. Crit Care Pain. 2007;7:33–37.

2. Landsman IS, Werkhaven JA, Motoyama EK. Anesthesia for pediatric otorhinolaryngologic surgery. In: Davis PJ, Cladis FP, Motoyama EK, editors. Smith's Anesthesia for Infants and Children, 8th ed. Philadelphia: Elsevier Mosby, 2011, p. 786–8.

3. Pairaudeau C, Mendonca C. Anaesthesia for major middle ear surgery. BJA Educ. 2019;19:136–43.

4. Liang S, Irwin MG. Review of anesthesia for middle ear surgery. Anesthesiol Clin. 2010;28:519–28.

5. Taha Al-Dabooni SI, Hammood HR, Abd Al Fekhrane RA. Anesthesia techniques for otologic surgery. Int J Adv Res Biol Sci. 2018;5:126–38.

6. Yung MW. Local anaesthesia in middle ear surgery: survey of patients and surgeons. Clin Otolaryngol Allied Sci. 1996;21(5):404–8.

7. Caner G, Olgun L, Gultekin G, Aydar L. Local anesthesia for middle ear surgery. Otolaryngol Head Neck Surg. 2005;133(2):295–7.

8. Thota RS, Ambardekar M, Likhate P. Conscious sedation for middle ear surgeries: a comparison between fentanyl-propofol and fentanyl-midazolam infusion. Saudi J Anaesth. 2015;9:117–21.

9. Nimmo AF, Absalom AR, Bagshaw O, et al. Guidelines for safe practice of total intravenous anaesthesia (TIVA), Joint Guidelines from the Association of Anaesthetists and the Society for Intravenous Anaesthesia. Anaesthesia. 2019;74:211–24.

10. Mukherjee K, Seavell C, Rawlings E, et al. A comparison of total intravenous with balanced anaesthesia for middle ear surgery: effects on postoperative nausea and vomiting, pain, and conditions of surgery. Anaesthesia. 2003;58(2):176–80.

11. Deniz E, Hekimoglu Şahin S, Sut N. Effects of general anaesthesia on the middle ear pressure. Turk J Anaesthesiol Reanim. 2019;47(2):92–7.

12. Sade J, Luntz M, Levy D. Middle ear gas composition and middle ear aeration. Ann Otol Rhinol Laryngol. 1995;104:369–73.

13. Ikarashi F, Tsuchiya A. Middle ear gas exchange via the mucosa: estimation by hyperventilation. Acta Otolaryngol. 2008;128:9–12.

14. Ozturk O, Demiraran Y, Ilce Z, Kocaman B, Guclu E, Karaman E. Effects of sevoflurane and TIVA with propofol on middle ear pressure. Int J Pediatr Otorhinolaryngol. 2006;70:1231–4.

15. Ozcan AD, Yungul AE, Muderris T, et al. Effect of total intravenous anesthesia and low and high flow anesthesia implementation on middle ear disease. Bio Med Res. 2018;2018:8214651.

16. Bajwa SJ, Kulshrestha A. The cochlear implantation surgery: a review of anesthetic considerations and implications. Int J Health Allied Sci. 2013;2:225–9.

17. Crawford MW, White MC, Propst EJ, et al. Dose-dependent suppression of the electrically elicited stapedius reflex by general anesthetics in children undergoing cochlear implant surgery. Anesth Analg. 2009;108:1480–7.

18. Schultz A, Berger FA, Weber BP, et al. Intraoperative electrically elicited stapedius reflex threshold is related to the dosage of hypnotic drugs in general anesthesia. Ann Otol Rhinol Laryngol. 2003;112:1050–5.

19. Hejazi MS, Moghaddam YJ, Pour MN, Banaii M, Abri R, Taghizadieh N. Evaluation of volatile and intravenous anesthetics, effects on the threshold of neuroresponse telemetry and the threshold of acoustically evoked stapedial reflex in children undergoing cochlear implant surgery. J Anaesthesiol Clin Pharmacol. 2018;34(2):177–81.

20. Safaeian R, Hassani V, Movasaghi G, Alimian M, Faiz HR. Postoperative respiratory complications of laryngeal mask airway and tracheal tube in ear, nose and throat operations. Anesth Pain Med. 2015;5(4):e25111.

21. Huang AS, Hajduk J, Rim C, Coffield S, Jagannathan N. Focused review on management of the difficult paediatric airway. Indian J Anaesth. 2019;63:428–36.

22. Harley EH, Collins MD. Neurologic sequelae secondary to atlantoaxial instability in Down syndrome: implications in otolaryngologic surgery. Arch Otolaryngol Head Neck Surg. 1994;120:159–65.

23. MacArthur A, Kleiman S. Rheumatoid cervical joint disease: a challenge to the anaesthetist. Can J Anaesth. 1993;40:154–9.

24. Tandon U, Dwivedi D. Nitrous oxide. Int J Clin Anesthiol. 2018;6(1):1089.

25. Brown SM, Sneyd JR. Nitrous oxide in modern anaesthetic practice. BJA Educ. 2016;16:87–91.

26. Mishra A, Singh RB, Choubey S, Tripathi RK, Sarkar A. A comparison between nitroprusside and nitroglycerine for hypotensive anesthesia in ear, nose, and throat surgeries: a double-blind randomized study. Med J DY Patil Univ. 2015;8:182–8.

27. Cantarella G, La Camera G, Di Marco P, Grasso DC, Lanzafame B. Controlled hypotension during middle ear surgery: hemodynamic effects of remifentanil vs nitroglycerin. Ann Ital Chir. 2018;89:283–6.

28. Lavere F, Rana NA, Kinsky MP, Funston JS, Mohamed SS, Chaaban MR. Blood loss and visibility with esmolol vs. labetalol in endoscopic sinus surgery: a randomized clinical trial. Clin Med Insights Ear, Nose Throat. 2019;12:1–8.

29. Durmus M, But AK, Dogan Z. Effect of dexmedetomidine on bleeding during tympanoplasty or septorhinoplasty. Eur J Anaesthesiol. 2007;24:447–53.

30. Gupta K, Bansal M, Gupta PK, Pandey MN, Agarwal S. Dexmedetomidine infusion during middle ear surgery under general anaesthesia to provide oligaemic surgical field: a prospective study. Indian J Anaesth. 2015;59:26-30.

31. Modir H, Modir A, Rezaei O, Mohammadbeigi A. Comparing remifentanil, magnesium sulfate, and dexmedetomidine for intraoperative hypotension and bleeding and postoperative recovery in endoscopic sinus surgery and tympanomastoidectomy. Med Gas Res. 2018;8(2):42–7.

32. Degoute CS. Controlled hypotension: a guide to drug choice. Drugs. 2007;67(7):1053–76.

33. Ryu JH, Sohn IS, Do SH. Controlled hypotension for middle ear surgery: a comparison between remifentanil and magnesium sulphate. Br J Anaesth. 2009;103:490-5.

34. Aboushanab OH, El-Shaarawy AM, Omar AM, Abdelwahab HH. A comparative study between magnesium sulphate and dexmedetomidine for deliberate hypotension during middle ear surgery. Egypt J Anaesth. 2011;27:227–32.

35. Akkaya A, Tekelioglu UY, Demirhan A, et al. Comparison of the effects of magnesium sulphate and dexmedetomidine on surgical vision quality in endoscopic sinus surgery: randomized clinical study. Rev Bras Anestesiol. 2014;64:406–12.

36. Cengiz M, Ganidagli S, Alatas N, San I, Baysal, Z. Partial neuromuscular blockage levels with mivacurium during mastoidectomy allows intraoperative Facial nerve monitoring. ORL 2008;70(4):236–41.

37. Cai YR, Xu J, Chen LH, Chi FL. Electromyographic monitoring of Facial nerve under different levels of neuromuscular blockade during middle ear microsurgery. Chin Med J (Engl). 2009;122(3):311–4.

38. Choe WJ, Kim JH, Park SY, Kim J. Electromyographic response of Facial nerve stimulation under different levels of neuromuscular blockade during middle-ear surgery. J Int Med Res. 2013;41(03):762–70.

39. Mangia LRL, Santos VM, Mansur TM, Wiemes GRM, Hamerschmidt R. Facial nerve intraoperative monitoring in otologic surgeries under sedation and local anesthesia: a case series and literature review. Int. Arch. Otorhinolaryngol. 2020;24(1):e11–7.

40. Fujii Y, Tanaka H, Kobayashi N. Prevention of postoperative nausea and vomiting with antiemetics in patients undergoing middle ear surgery, comparison of a small dose of propofol with droperidol or metoclopramide. Arch Otolaryngol Head Neck Surg. 2001;127(1):25–8.

41. Lee DW, Lee HG, Jeong CY, Jeong SW, Lee SH. Postoperative nausea and vomiting after mastoidectomy with tympanoplasty: a comparison between TIVA with propofol-remifentanil and balanced anesthesia with sevoflurane-remifentanil. Korean J Anesthesiol. 2011;61(5):399–404.

42. Gan TJ, Diemunsch P, Habib AS, et al. Consensus guidelines for the management of postoperative nausea and vomiting. Anesth Analg. 2014;118:85–113.

43. Shaikh SI, Nagarekha D, Hegade G, Marutheesh M. Postoperative nausea and vomiting: a simple yet complex problem. Anesth Essays Res. 2016;10:388–96.

44. Usmani H, Siddiqui RA, Sharma SC, et al. Ondansetron and dexamethasone in middle ear procedures. Indian J Otolaryngol. 2003;55(2):97–100.

45. Panda NB, Bharadwaj N, Kapoor P, Chari P, Panda NK. Prevention of nausea and vomiting after middle ear surgery: combination of ondansetron and dexamethasone is the right choice. J Otolaryngol. 2004;33:88–92.

46. Mukhopadhyay S, Niyogi M, Ray R, Mukhopadhyay BS, Dutta M, Mukherjee M. Betahistine as an add-on: the magic bullet for postoperative nausea, vomiting and dizziness after middle ear surgery? J Anesthesiol Clin Pharmacol. 2013;29:205–10.

47. Voronov P, Tobin MJ, Billings K, Cote CJ, Iyer A, Suresh S. Postoperative pain relief in infants undergoing myringotomy and tube placement: comparison of a novel regional anesthetic block to intranasal fentanyl – a pilot analysis. Paediatr Anaesth. 2008;18(12):1196–201.

48. Suresh S, Barcelona SL, Young NM, Heffner CL, Cote CJ. Does a preemptive block of the great auricular nerve improve postoperative analgesia in children undergoing tympanomastoid surgery? Anesth Analg. 2004;98:330–3.

49. Suresh S, Barcelona SL, Young NM, et al. Postoperative pain relief in children undergoing tympanomastoid surgery: is a regional block better than opioids? Anesth Analg. 2002;94:859–62.

50. Dhakal A, Shrestha BL, Pokharel M, Rajbhandari P, Karmacharya S. Effect of preemptive pregabalin for postoperative pain relief in myringoplasty. Indian J Otol. 2018;24:257–60.

# 15 Imaging in Otology

*Virender Malik, Dhanalakshmi B and Abha Kumari*

## CONTENTS

## INTRODUCTION

Imaging has played an ever-increasing role at all echelons in patients with ear diseases, from accurate diagnosis, guiding management, surgical planning, prognostication to evaluation in postoperative setting.

High-resolution computed tomography (HRCT) of the temporal bone, with its excellent resolution, easy availability and cost-effectiveness is accepted as the imaging investigation of choice in the evaluation of most external and middle ear diseases. The anatomical details are visualized in great detail with the current CT scanners (Figure 15.1). Magnetic Resonance Imaging (MRI) outscores HRCT for fluid and soft tissue characterization and evaluation of diseases involving the membranous labyrinth, nerves, intracranial extension and associated subtle neuroparenchymal abnormalities.

In this chapter, we discuss the role of conventional and established cross-sectional imaging (HRCT and MRI) techniques in evaluation of common ear diseases, the promising newer CT and MRI techniques in evaluation of cholesteatoma and Ménière's disease and a few of the potentially useful imaging techniques, presently in the research stage.

## DISCUSSION

### External Ear Diseases

Although most of the lesions involving external ear (auricle and External Auditory Canal [EAC]) are accessible clinically, the role of cross-sectional imaging is to evaluate extent of the lesion and associated abnormalities in middle and inner ear, assess feasibility for surgery and to rule out complications. HRCT of temporal bone, because of its high resolution and excellent bone evaluation capability, is a useful imaging tool to diagnose and guide management for external ear diseases.

The role of imaging in EAC atresia is not only in accurate diagnosis but also in surgical planning by identifying imaging features, which are pointers to operative contraindications and technically difficult surgery so that the patients can be explained about the prognosis preoperatively (1–3). A representative case of complete absence of EAC, with an associated smaller volume middle ear cavity, is illustrated in Figure 15.2.

HRCT shows characteristic differences in the morphological appearances of the pattern of bony overgrowth in osteochondroma and osteoma, easily differentiating the two (4). The HRCT distinctly identifies most of the complications of Malignant Otitis Externa (MOE), such as temporalis abscess, TM joint involvement and temporal bone osteomyelitis, whereas MRI outscores former in assessment of intracranial extension. The CT features like diffuse EAC erosion and soft tissue enhancement and absence of restriction of diffusion on MRI suggest a diagnosis of MOE over cholesteatoma (5, 6).

The characteristic imaging features of common external ear diseases, including MOE, osteochondroma, osteoma, cholesteatoma, keratosis obturans and squamous cell carcinoma (SCC) are summarized in Table 15.1.

### Middle Ear Diseases

HRCT is the imaging modality of choice to assess ossicular status and middle ear cavity. However, to differentiate various types of

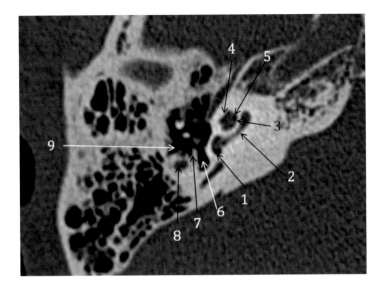

**Figure 15.1** Normal anatomy. High-resolution CT axial image shows round window niche (1); basal turn of the cochlea (2); interscalar septum (3); apical turn of the cochlea (4); middle turn of the cochlea (5); sinus tympani (6); pyramidal eminence (7); mastoid portion of the Facial nerve (8); facial recess (9).

middle ear effusions, soft tissue component delineation, detection of cholesteatoma (both primary and residual) and intracranial complications, MRI is preferred (7, 8).

*Chronic Otitis Media (COM):* In COM, HRCT clearly demonstrates soft tissue attenuation contents filling the middle ear, causing post-inflammatory ossicular chain fixation and erosion and can identify the exact extent of local spread as well as resultant complications. Although presence of bony erosions and restriction of diffusion on MRI favours cholesteatoma, they are encountered in cases of COM mucosal also (7). The disruption of the normal appearance of "ice cream cone" in epitympanum, "two parallel lines" in upper part of mesotympanum and "two dots" in lower part of mesotympanum on axial CT images are useful features indicating possibility of ossicular erosion. Representative cases of COM mucosal and cholesteatoma are illustrated in Figures 15.3 and 15.4, respectively.

In the setting of unequivocal cholesteatoma (based on clinical and otoscopic evaluation), HRCT as the primary and sole imaging technique suffices prior to first-stage surgery. However, if infection, inflammation and/or complications as fistula to lateral semicircular canal (LSCC) is suspected, evaluation with MRI is needed to differentiate the infection or inflammation from cholesteatoma and also

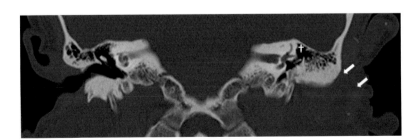

**Figure 15.2** EAC atresia. High-resolution coronal CT image demonstrates complete absence of left external auditory canal (EAC), blue arrows point to anticipated region of EAC. Also, the left middle ear cavity is smaller in volume (blue dagger). The inner ear and inner auditory canal are typically normal (as in present case), due to formation of these structures earlier in gestation.

## Table 15.1: **Key Features of External Ear Diseases**

| Disease | Key Imaging Characteristics | Remarks |
|---|---|---|
| EAC atresia | HRCT help assess detailed evaluation of the following : *Contraindication to surgery*: Atretic oval and or round window[1] *Technically difficult surgery*: Small-volume middle ear cavity, poorly pneumatized temporal bone, unfavourable course of Facial nerve[2] | *Poor surgical outcome*: If associated middle and inner ear dysplasia[3] |
| EAC osteochondroma | *CT*: Mostly bilateral, broad-based, bony overgrowth of the bony EAC[4] | Most common benign tumour of EAC Also called as Surfer's ear ( cold wind and water exposure) |
| EAC osteoma | *CT*: Mostly unilateral, solitary pedunculated bony overgrowth, most commonly at bony cartilaginous junction | Large osteoma may be associated with ear wax, debris or secondary cholesteatoma |
| Malignant otitis externa (MOE) | *CT*: Thickened and enhancing mucosa of EAC and auricle together with destructive appearance of the tympanic and mastoid bone strongly suggest MOE[5] *Temporalis abscess*: Diffuse muscle thickening with defined hypodense area *TM joint involvement*: Widened joint space with articular margins irregularity *Temporal bone osteomyelitis*: Increased bone density and linear periosteal reaction *MRI*: Better to assess intracranial extension | *Predisposing conditions*: Old, diabetic and immunocompromised state High morbidity and mortality DD: Cholesteatoma and squamous cell carcinoma of EAC |
| EAC cholesteatoma | *High-resolution bone window CT*: Well localized, soft tissue density eroding one of the walls of the EAC, no enhancement on PC images[6] *Follow-up CT*: Slow growing lesion *MRI*: Diffusion restriction present | DD MOE (rapidly growing, more diffuse EAC erosion, enhancement of the soft tissue, no restriction of diffusion)[5,6] |
| Keratosis obturans (KO) | *CT*: Well-demarcated soft tissue mass within bony EAC, diffusely enlarging (may cause smooth scalloping of surrounding bone but without causing bony erosion or periostitis.[5] Usually bilateral | Associated with sinusitis and bronchiectasis DD EAC cholesteatoma (bony erosion present, mostly unilateral) |

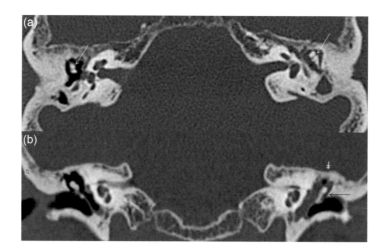

**Figure 15.3**   Chronic otitis media. Axial (a) and coronal (b) HRCT images show soft tissue attenuation contents causing opacification of the middle ear on left side with preserved middle ear ossicles (arrow in part a), tegmen tympani (two-headed arrow in part b) and scutum (arrows in part b). For comparison, note normal air-filled middle ear cavity (arrow in part a) on right side.

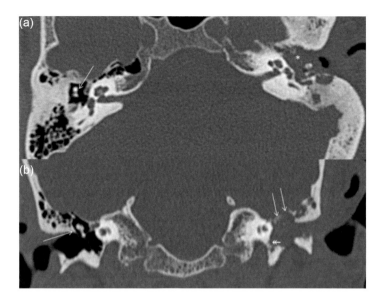

**Figure 15.4** Cholesteatoma. Axial (a) and coronal (b) HRCT images show opacification of the middle ear and mastoid on left side with soft tissue attenuation contents (asterix in part a). Note destruction of the tegmen tympani and scutum (arrows in part b) and lateral wall of Jugular fossa (two-headed arrow in part b) on left side. For comparison, note normal air-filled middle ear cavity and ossicles (arrow in part a) and scutum (arrow in part b) on right side.

assess the status of membranous labyrinth (9). In a postoperative patient with suspected residual or recurrent cholesteatoma, CT cannot reliably differentiate between effusion, granulation component, scar tissue and cholesteatoma.

The role of diffusion-weighted imaging (DWI) in cholesteatoma is currently well-established (10). Non-echoplanar imaging (non-EPI) sequences demonstrating diffusion restriction in cholesteatoma tissue make MRI a far better investigation in such settings. Despite shorter scan duration needed with echoplanar than with non-EPI techniques, the latter are preferred owing to less air-bone susceptibility distortion while assessing skull base and ear diseases (11). Current non-EPI techniques such as HASTE and PROPELLER sequences achieve high-resolution images and demonstrate high and low signal with cholesteatoma (keratin) and non-cholesteatoma tissue (inflammatory fluid and granulation tissue), respectively, on employing high b-values in DWI (12).

The high incidence of residual and recurrent disease following canal wall up (CWU) surgery for cholesteatoma mandates a second look surgery. Considering the financial implication and morbidity associated with a second look surgery, the disease detection on imaging would be a better option. Non-EPI, besides gaining acceptance as the most accurate imaging sequence in

primary cholesteatoma, is also considered a very useful imaging tool for detection of postoperative cholesteatoma (13). Recent studies highlight and emphasize the effectiveness of DWI as an alternative to second look surgery, even in children where the disease is usually more aggressive and has higher residual and recurrence potential (14). Although presently most institutions follow an annual surveillance for 3–5 years, the specific duration is based on individual patient's disease recurrence risk assessment (15).

The role of follow-up DWI in patients following canal wall down (CWD) surgery for cholesteatoma is usually limited to non-visualized disease on otomicroscopic examination, as in setting of disease extension (to petrous apex [PA] or mastoid tip) and opaque tympanic membrane reconstruction (16).

Potential false negatives in the setting of a residual/recurrent cholesteatoma (lesion <3 mm in size, auto-atticotomy and movement artefacts) mandates correlation with conventional T1 and T2 W images, clinical presentation and serial monitoring (15).

Although CT remains the established primary modality for diagnosis and surgical planning of primary cholesteatoma, the DWI finds its role in setting of non-visualized disease on otoscopic examination (opaque tympanic membrane and stenosed EAC), presence of high-risk retraction pockets and CT depicting completely filled middle ear cleft with a soft tissue attenuation lesion (17). Fused CT DWI images and 3D fusion maps may better guide the surgeon to plan the optimal approach for disease clearance and also to select a less invasive procedure such as transcanal endoscopic surgery in subset of cholesteatoma patients (18, 19).

*Otosclerosis:* In otosclerosis, the histopathologically proven replacement of normal dense enchondral bone with the islands of vascular, demineralized haversian bone in the initial phase and the presence of sclerotic bone in the later phase is depicted distinctly on HRCT as areas of bone resorption and sclerosis, respectively.

Of the various CT grading systems for otosclerosis, the one proposed by Symons and Fanning, describing progressive grades as limited fenestral involvement, patchy localized cochlear disease and diffuse confluent cochlear involvement of the otic capsule shows good inter- and intraobserver agreement and has gained wide acceptance (20–22). Representative case of otosclerosis is illustrated in Figure 15.5.

HRCT of the temporal bone, accepted as the imaging investigation of choice, plays an important role, not only in the initial diagnosis and surgical planning but also in prognostication of patients with otosclerosis (23, 24). Use of semiautomated histograms to assess CT bone density and multiplanar reconstructions paralleling the stapes crus help in detection of earliest bone resorption changes (25, 26).The demonstration of limited fenestral and advanced cochleariform disease with HRCT guides the surgeon to decide on stapes surgery versus cochlear implant as the most appropriate surgical modality in otosclerosis patients (23, 27). HRCT depicting lower Hounsfield density values in the otospongiotic foci, presence of higher disease grade and

osseous resorption involving superior semicircular canal is associated with poorer surgical outcomes (24).

The characteristics imaging features of common middle ear diseases are summarized in Table 15.2.

### Petrous Apex Lesions

The PA is a pyramid-shaped, anatomically complex region, bounded laterally by inner ear, medially petro-occipital fissure, petro-sphenoidal fissure anteriorly, posterior cranial fossa posteriorly, middle cranial fossa superiorly and the Jugular bulb and inferior petrosal sinus inferiorly. PA is divided by the internal auditory canal (IAC) into a larger anterior portion and a smaller posterior portion, with former typically containing bone marrow and the latter dense otic capsule.

The non-amenability of PA to direct examination makes role of cross-sectional imaging crucial in accurate diagnosis and guiding treatment. The normal imaging appearance of the anterior part of PA is variable due to differing contents, with marrow, air and sclerosis noted in 60%, 33% and 7%, respectively. Pneumatization of PA due to extension of air cells along various tracts communicating directly with the middle ear or mastoid account for spread of disease between these regions. Asymmetric pneumatization is noted in 5–10% of individuals and should be borne in mind while interpreting the images (28–30). Detailed evaluation of images is essential to identify pseudolesions in PA region, and therefore prevent unnecessary and potentially invasive surgeries.

The characteristic imaging features of common PA lesions like pseudolesions, cholesterol granuloma, petrous apicitis (31–33) and tumours (34–38) among others are summarized

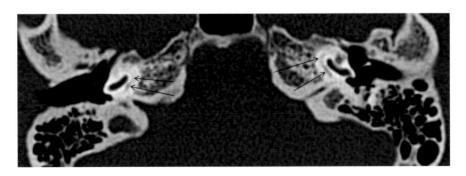

**Figure 15.5** Otosclerosis. Axial HRCT image shows well-defined lucency surrounding the cochlea bilaterally (more conspicuous on left) producing a "fourth turn" or "double ring" sign appearance.

## Table 15.2: **Key Features of Common Middle Ear Diseases**

| Disease Process | Key Imaging Characteristics | Remarks |
|---|---|---|
| Acute otitis media (uncomplicated) | *CT:* Opacities in middle ear and mastoid, with possible fluid levels, preserved mastoid trabeculae and overlying cortex | Imaging is usually not necessary in uncomplicated acute otitis media |
| Complicated mastoiditis (CM) | *CT:* Partial-to-complete opacification of mastoid air cells (incipient mastoiditis) → erosion of bony septae of mastoid air cells (coalescent mastoiditis) → erosion of lateral wall (subperiosteal abscess), sigmoid plate (epidural abscess) Mass with perilesional fat stranding or rim-enhancing collection deep to SCM (Bezold abscess) or within digastric triangle ( Citelli abscess) *MRI:* T1 C+ – mucosal contrast enhancement in majority. Better demonstration of intracranial extension | Presence of postauricular erythema, tenderness and oedema suggests possibility of CM → imaging crucial to exclude complications *Petrous apicitis:* Middle ear/mastoid infection → persistent air cell tracts → petrous apex infection |
| Chronic otitis media (COM) mucosal | *CT:* Demonstration of PIOF – peristapedial tent (fibrous tissue in the niche of oval window), tympanosclerosis (focal calcified densities in middle ear cavity, tendons and ossicular chain), lamellar structures of high density (most commonly in epitympanum) Demonstration of PIOE: long and lenticular process of incus, followed by stapes head | Erosions are far less common in COM without associated acquired cholesteatoma |
| Cholesteatoma | *CT:* Pars flaccida cholesteatoma – erosion of scutum, long process of incus, tegmen tympani and LSCC Pars tensa cholesteatoma – erosion of bony Facial nerve canal and stapedial suprastructure | Pars flaccida cholesteatoma more common than the tensa cholesteatoma In a postoperative patient with suspected residual or recurrent cholesteatoma, MRI-DWI is the investigation of choice |
| Otosclerosis | *CT:* Shows well-defined lucencies most commonly in region of fissula ante fenestram ( fenestral disease), followed by cochlear involvement (retrofenestral disease) *Grades of involvement:* Grade 1 – limited fenestral involvement, grade 2 – patchy localized cochlear disease, grade 3 – diffuse confluent involvement of otic capsule | Most commonly bilateral |

*Abbreviations:* PIOF: Post-Inflammatory Ossicular Chain Fixation; PIOE: Post-Inflammatory Ossicular Chain Erosion; LSCC. Lateral Semicircular Canal.

in Table 15.3. A representative case of cholesterol granuloma is illustrated in Figure 15.6.

### Inner Ear Diseases

*Labyrinthine Ossificans (LO):* HRCT temporal bone and heavily T2-weighted MRI sequence, such as constructive interference in steady state (CISS) of the inner ear, are considered complementary in diagnosis and evaluation of labyrinthine ossificans. Early detection of LO is important as the chances of success of cochlear implantation decrease with increasing degree of osseous obliteration of membranous labyrinth.

MRI, in the early pre-ossification stage of LO, demonstrates intermediate or low signal in the normally T2 hyperintense membranous labyrinth, contributing to the timely diagnoses and early surgical planning in these patients (39).

*Paediatric SNHL:* In the setting of paediatric SNHL, HRCT can be an acceptable primary imaging modality in patients with unilateral or asymmetric SNHL or mixed hearing loss, whereas in those with auditory neuropathy spectrum disorder (ANSD) evaluating with MRI to assess cochlear nerve, auditory pathways, and brain structures is advisable (40).

## Table 15.3: **Key Features of Common Petrous Apex Lesions**

| Disease Process | Key Imaging Characteristics | Remarks |
|---|---|---|
| **Pseudolesions** **Asymmetric pneumatization (AP)** | Asymmetric pneumatization (AP) → resultant asymmetric fatty marrow → fat signal intensity on all sequences | Avoid mistaking for CG ( both hyper I on T1WI), FS sequence (complete loss of signal with FS techniques in AP), normal trabeculated bone on CT in AP |
| **Petrous apex effusion** | T1 iso to hypo I, T2 very Hyper I (like CSF), no CE | Rarely thin rim enhancement |
| **Developmental lesions** **Cholesterol granuloma (CG)** | Hyper I on both T1WI and T2WI, peripheral low signal due to hemosiderin rim on T2WI, remains high signal with FS techniques | Most common cystic lesion of the petrous apex  Repeated Haemorrhages common  Hydrated mucocoele may have identical MRI signal on both T1WI and T2WI |
| **Cholesteatomas** | *CT:* Non-enhancing, expansile PA lesion  *MRI:* T1 hypo I, T2 hyper I, diffusion restriction | Congenital more common than acquired type |
| **Inflammatory lesions** **Petrous apicitis** | *CT:* Opacification of petrous air cells in early stage, bone destruction in later stages  *MRI:* T1 hypo I, T2 hyper I, CE in pneumatized anterior petrous apex[31] | Medial extension of acute otitis media into a pneumatized petrous apex  *Presentation:* Acute febrile illness and some or all of symptoms of Gradenigo triad (ear pain, VI cranial nerve palsy and facial pain)[32] |
| **Complicated petrous apicitis** | *Meningitis:* Enhancement of adjacent duramater and cranial nerves  *Abscess:* Ring enhancement and restricted diffusion on DWI | *Gallium SPECT:* Useful for evaluating response to therapy[33] |
| **Tumours** **Paraganglioma (PG)** | *CT:* Typical moth-eaten or permeative bone changes  *MRI:* Salt-and-pepper appearance  Intense CE on both CT and MRI [34] | PG (Jugular foramen or middle ear) → preformed air cell tracts → petrous apex |
| **Chondrosarcoma (CS)** | *CT:* Typically centred at synchondroses, destructive petrous apex mass with arcs and rings of calcification  *MRI:* T1 hypo I, T2 very hyper I, heterogeneous post CE[35,36] | Degeneration of remnants of enchondral cartilage along skull base synchondroses (petroclival and petrosphenoidal) → CS |
| **Chordomas** | *CT:* Locally destructive soft tissue masses centred in clivus, extending laterally to involve PA, tumoral calcification  *MRI:* T1 hypo I, T2 hyper I, may show characteristic honeycomb enhancement pattern[37] | Originate from embryologic remnants of notochord |
| **Endolymphatic sac tumour (ELST)** | *CT:* Soft tissue masses with prominent intratumoral calcification, permeative bone erosion along posterior surface of petrous bone  *MRI:* Areas of T1 hyper I common (met Hb, hemosiderin and cholesterol crystals )[38] | Locally aggressive tumours, arise from proximal rugose portion of endolymphatic sac  Repeated intratumoural haemorrhage  If bilateral, associated with VHL |
| **Metastases** | *CT:* Aggressive lytic lesion destroying the skull base  *MRI:* Depicts soft tissue extent of lesion, low to intermediate signal intensity on T1WI and variable signal intensity on T2WI.  Intratumoral flow voids (in highly vascular metastases from renal, thyroid carcinoma, melanoma) | Most common site for metastases in temporal bone is PA  Most common from breast, lung, prostate, and renal cell carcinomas  Slow blood flow through PA marrow → allows filtering and deposition of tumour cells |
| **Osseous dysplasias** Fibrous dysplasia | *CT:* Benign expansion of involved bones, relative preservation of cortical integrity, characteristic ground-glass internal matrix  *MR:* May show appearances mimicking malignant process | Disorganized arrangement of bone trabeculae mixed with fibrous tissue and cysts  Craniofacial investment more common in polyostotic type FD |

*Abbreviations:* SPECT: Single Photon Emission Computed Tomography; VHL: Von Hippel-Lindau Syndrome; Hypo I: Hypointense; Hyper I: Hyperintense

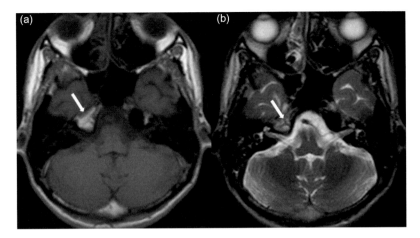

**Figure 15.6** Cholesterol granuloma. Axial MRI images show conspicuous high signal intensity lesion on T1 (arrow in part a) and mildly increased signal intensity on T2 (arrow in part b) and remain high signal on fat suppression and show no post contrast enhancement (not shown). The higher signal intensity is due to cholesterol component and methemoglobin.

MRI, by identifying abnormalities in the inner ear and/or the vestibulocochlear nerve in approximately 20% of patients with congenital SNHL, plays an integral role in evaluation and management of this entity (41). High-resolution 3D T2WI images enable detailed evaluation of the vestibulocochlear nerve, membranous labyrinth and any associated brain anomalies (42). Minute labyrinthine structures as the lamina spiralis and interscalar septum which are not well seen on CT are clearly visualized on 3T scanner, high-resolution, T2WI sequences (43). HRCT plays an important role in surgical planning, by allowing detailed evaluation of the temporal bone, and identification of anatomical variants which may influence surgery. Cone beam CT techniques provide superior resolution and entail lower radiation dose exposure, the latter being of paramount importance in paediatric setting.

For potential CI candidates, detailed evaluation using dual approach (both CT and MRI) is advisable for accurate diagnosis, effective surgical planning and prognostication. For determining electrode position and status in post CI setting, the skull radiographs (modified Stenver's or Towne's view) are fairly accurate (44, 45). Although conventional X-rays provide useful information about position of the electrode array in setting of post-cochlear implantation imaging, the computed tomography (high-resolution or cone beam) provides a more detailed and accurate evaluation of electrode position, confirmation of dislocation (scalar or cochlear), fold over (tip or basal) and malposition of the electrode array (44, 45). The

early identification of an inadvertent positioning of the electrode array facilitates decision for the revision surgery and consequently a better clinical outcome.

Representative cases of some of common inner ear malformations are illustrated in Figure 15.7 (complete labyrinthine aplasia), Figure 15.8 (common cavity), Figure 15.9 (incomplete partition type 1) and Figure 15.10 (isolated dilatation of vestibular aqueducts).

Radiological features of SNHL classification in children, based on morphology of cochlea, vestibule, SSC, IAC and Facial nerve canal, are summarized in Table 15.4.

### Ménière's Disease

Making a clinical diagnosis of Ménière's disease is challenging, despite the battery of audiological, vestibular and electrophysiological tests available to the otolaryngologist. This difficulty is accentuated in atypical presentation of the disease, and hence there is a need for a reliable diagnostic imaging modality (56).

The endolymphatic compartment in inner ear comprises a smaller component of the total inner ear fluid, as scala media in cochlea and saccule and utricle in the vestibule (57). Despite clear demonstration of labyrinth's fluid-containing structures for many years using MRI sequences like CISS, the inability of conventional MRI to distinguish endolymphatic from the perilymphatic compartments is a shortcoming (58). Nakashima et al. were the first group to distinctly demonstrate in 2007 endolymphatic hydrops in MD patients, with FLAIR sequence imaging on a 3T MRI, 24 hours following

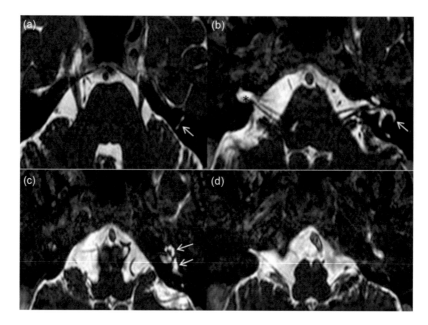

**Figure 15.7** Congenital labyrinthine aplasia. Serial axial heavily T2W MRI images (CISS) of inner ear show absence of cochlea, vestibule, semicircular canals, vestibular and cochlear aqueducts on the right side. A small cystic structure (asterisk in part b) is seen replacing these structures on right side. The left ear shows normal appearance of superior semicircular canal (arrow in part a), vestibule and lateral semicircular canal (arrows in part b) and cochlea (arrow in part c) for comparison. Part (d) showing inferior most aspect of left inner ear structures.

intratympanic administration of Gadolinium (59). The drawbacks such as long waiting period before imaging, lesser degree of perilymph enhancement, dependence on normal permeability of round window and inability to assess and compare both ears simultaneously with intratympanic route of administration led the researchers to focus on further studies with intravenous route of administration. A 4-hour delay between intravenous gadolinium administration and imaging demonstrated greater degree of perilymph enhancement (60–62). Until recently, the role of imaging was largely limited to exclusion of clinical MD mimickers. However, presently data is available supporting and emphasizing importance of application of 3 T MRI at 4 hours post-intravenous gadolinium using 3D FLAIR sequences for diagnosis and grading of the associated EH (63–65).

Various semiquantitative grading systems assessing the degree of EH, based on relative areas of the non-enhanced endolymphatic space

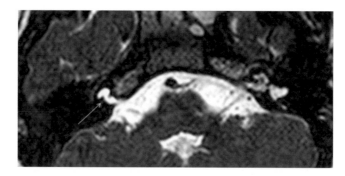

**Figure 15.8** Common cavity. Axial heavily T2W MRI images (CISS) of inner ear show a single bilobed fluid-filled structure (arrow) representing cochlea and vestibule. Compare it with normal appearance of cochlea and vestibule on the left side.

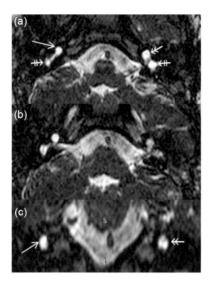

**Figure 15.9** Incomplete partition type I (right). (a) Axial and (c) coronal heavily T2W MRI images (CISS) of inner ear show complete loss of normal cochlear morphology on right side, appearing as a cystic structure (arrow). On the left side, although complete absence of modiolus is noted, the interscalar septae are well-visualized as hypointense structures (two-headed arrow). Both vestibules are dilated (arrow with double stroke), left being more conspicuous than right. (b) Bilateral vestibular aqueducts are not dilated.

versus the contrast-enhanced perilymph space, have been reported and have shown encouraging results (64, 65). Although the current diagnostic criteria of MD do not include MRI for diagnosis and grading of EH, the documentation of good clinico-radiological correlation using 4 hours delayed MR imaging method and the grading methods along with ongoing further imaging developments would result in

greater role of MR imaging in diagnosis and therapeutic decisions-making of MD patients. The incorporation of MRI in the diagnostic criteria of MD is likely to make it more robust.

### Imaging in Temporal Bone Injury

Early identification and extent delineation of the fractures and dislocations is essential to managing the temporal bone injury and preventing complications. HRCT with multiplanar bone window reformats is the imaging modality of choice in the setting of temporal bone injury. The traditional classification, based on the main direction of fracture plane, grouped temporal bone fractures as transverse, longitudinal and mixed (66). Currently, classification based on presence or absence of otic capsule involvement is considered more clinically relevant and better predictor of more serious complications, including Facial nerve paralysis, Cerebrospinal Fluid (CSF) leaks and SNHL (67). HRCT with 3D reconstruction elegantly demonstrates temporal bone fractures and dislocations of ossicular chain, otic capsule involvement, Facial nerve canal and carotid canal injury. CT or MR angiography is usually undertaken for fractures extending through the carotid canal to assess for associated vascular complications such as dissection, pseudoaneurysm and arteriovenous fistula formation (68). CT or MR venography is performed where fractures appear to involve the regions of venous sinuses.

Also, the "indirect signs" suggestive of temporal fracture, including intracranial air adjacent to temporal bone, air within TM joint, pneumolabyrinth, opacification of mastoid air cells and EAC are well-demonstrated on HRCT.

### NEWER IMAGING TECHNIQUES

Despite steady improvements in the resolutions of CT and MRI, the detection of a few of

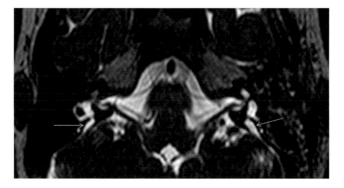

**Figure 15.10** Isolated dilatation of bilateral vestibular aqueducts. Axial heavily T2W MR images (CISS) show dilatation of bilateral vestibular aqueducts, left > right (arrows on both sides).

## Table 15.4: Key Features of Inner Ear Malformations Common Petrous Apex Lesions

| Disease | Cochlea | Vestibule | SCC | IAC | Facial N. Canal | Associated Features |
|---------|---------|-----------|-----|-----|-----------------|---------------------|
| Complete labyrinthine aplasia | Absent | | | Aplastic/ hypoplastic[46] | Aberrant[47] | Variable hypoplasia of middle ear cavity, petrous bone and PCF[47] |
| Rudimentary otocyst | Absent | Absent | Tiny parts +/– may be present | *Absent[48] | Absent | *Tiny (mms) ovoid or round cavity within the otic capsule[48] |
| Cochlear aplasia with normal labyrinth | Absent | Normal | Normal | Hypoplasia | Aberrant | Frequently symmetrical |
| Cochlear aplasia with dilated vestibule (CADV) | Absent | Variably dilated | Variably dilated | Hypoplasia | Aberrant | Frequently asymmetrical CADV vs. CC (CAVD: normally sited IAC, cochlear promontory absent)[43] |
| Common cavity (CC) | Common cavity of cochlea and vestibule, wider (>10 mm average) than tall (>7 mm average)[46] | | Often horizontal SCC | IAC opens into centre of CC | Aberrant | CC versus CADV (CC: IAC opens into centre of CC, cochlear promontory present)[43] |
| Type-1 IP | Normal size, cystic outline, no modiolus/ISS | Mostly enlarged vestibule but normal VD | Often horizontal SCC | Enlarged* | Normal | No internal structure in whole of cochlea,* "figure of 8"appearance#[46] |
| Type-2 IP (most common form of IP, Mondini's deformity) | Normal size, cystic apex, normal modiolus/ISS | Mildly dilated vestibule, dilated VD | Normal | Normal | Normal | No internal structure in upper cochlea + enlarged VA*[49] |
| Type-3 IP (rarest form of IP) | Normal size, no modiolus, ISS present but dysplastic | Normal | Normal | Bulbous, direct cochlear connection | Aberrant | Only ISS present (no modiolus) + bulbous IAC,* high CSF leak risk[50] |
| Cochlear hypoplasia type 1 (CH-1) | Small, bud-like, no ISS/modiolus[51] | Normal | Normal | Direct cochlear connection | Normal | Most severe form of CH |
| Cochlear hypoplasia type 2 (CH-2) | Small, normal outline, defective ISS/modiolus | Normal | Normal | Direct cochlear connection | Normal | Appear like small IP-2 |
| Cochlear hypoplasia type 3 (CH-3) | Small (<2 turns), "unwound cochlea",## [52] small modiolus, short ISS | Hypoplasia | Hypoplasia | Normal | Normal | Tapered basal cochlear turn |

| Disease | Cochlea | Vestibule | SCC | IAC | Facial N. Canal | Associated Features |
|---|---|---|---|---|---|---|
| Cochlear hypoplasia type 4 (CH-4) | Small, hypoplastic apical and middle turns | Normal | Normal | Normal | Aberrant[53] | Normal basal cochlear turn |
| Dysplastic SCC | Mostly normal, rarely abnormal | Normal | Dysplastic | Normal | Normal | SCC typically short and wide, LSCC most commonly affected |
| Enlarged VA | Isolated enlarged VA is rare, >80% have associated inner ear anomaly[54] | | | | | Most common radiological abnormality in patients with early onset SNHL, dilated osseous VA,© dilated endolymphatic duct and sac†[55] bilateral in 90% |

*Abbreviations:* SCC: Semicircular Canal; IP: Incomplete Partition; LSCC: Lateral Semicircular Canal; #: in type 1 IP, the cystic cochlea if associated with dilated vestibule confers a characteristic "figure of 8" appearance; *: key imaging features; ©: axial measurement midway between the common crus and external aperture is >1 mm or the measurement at the operculum is >2 mm; †: On thin section T2W MRI, endolymphatic duct and sac are considered dilated if diameter exceeds that of ascending portion of the adjacent posterior SCC; ##: unwound cochlea – anterior offset of apical and middle turns from basal turn.

pathologies such as less than 3-mm residual or recurrent cholesteatoma, loosened stapedotomy piston and other prosthesis from the ossicles is beyond the resolution of currently available cross-sectional technology (69). Also, other than the important concerns as the artefacts due to implants (metallic or magnetic) and ionizing radiation from CT imaging, inability to assess dynamic properties of otologic structures are few of the limitations of current imaging modalities.

A few relatively newer imaging techniques that have lately shown promise in various clinical settings include cone-beam CT (CBCT), MRI non-EPI DWI sequences, MRI 3D FLAIR hydrops sequences and MRI multi-echo fast field echo sequences (mFFE).

Compared to MDCT, CBCT has the advantage of lower radiation dose, better spatial resolution, holds promise in early detection of sub-millimetric otosclerotic foci, evaluation of ossicular discontinuity and fixation, inner ear malformations, semicircular canal dehiscences and identifying electrode position (post-cochlear implantation) (70). However, increased image artefacts, examination and computational time and inaccuracies in estimation of bone density are a few of limitations with CBTC.

MRI non-EPI DWI sequences and MRI 3D FLAIR hydrops sequences have proven their clinical utility in detecting cholesteatoma and Ménière's disease, respectively. mFFE by enabling visualization of cochlear nuclei can prognosticate usefulness of brainstem implant electrode placement in setting of bilateral congenital deafness due to bilateral aplasia of the cochlear nerves. However, indistinct visualization of cochlear nuclei until sufficient myelination of surrounding structures is achieved (age of 2 years) is a limitation with mFFE (71, 72).

A few interesting techniques, though presently in experimental stage, include X-ray microtomography (micro-CT), high-frequency ultrasound (HFUS) and optical coherence tomography (OCT). Micro-CT, a useful research tool, provides very high resolution (with semi-histological quality), optimal for visualization of tissues of the inner ear tissues, its main drawback being high radiation dose (73).

HFUS can evaluate dynamic movement of the middle ear structures and could be a powerful tool to assess an implant interaction with cochlear inner structures. Currently, a 64-element phased array which can visualize the cochlea (through round window) is under development (74).

OCT works by splitting light into a reference and sample arm, provides depth-resolved images of the optical reflectivity of tissue structures and has potential clinical application not only in assessment of tympanic membrane but also in evaluation of the middle ear structures (75, 76).

## CONCLUSION

Imaging plays an ever-increasing role in otology, with current imaging techniques providing excellent anatomical information but still have limitations in resolution of very small structures and lack functional assessment. Several new imaging modalities which are presently in research stage may enter the mainstream use over the next decade.

## REFERENCES

1. Gassner EM, Mallouhi A, Jaschke WR. Preoperative evaluation of external auditory canal atresia on high-resolution CT. AJR Am J Roentgenol. 2004; 182:1305–12.

2. Lambert PR, Dodson EE. Congenital malformations of the external auditory canal. Otolaryngol Clin North Am. 1996;29:741–60.

3. Yeakley JW, Jahrsdoerfer RA. CT evaluation of congenital aural atresia: what the radiologist and the surgeon need to know. J Comput Assist Tomogr. 1996;5:724–31.

4. Turetsky DB, Vines FS, Clayman DA. Surfer's ear: exostoses of the external auditory canal. AJNR Am J Neuroradiol. 1990;11(6):1217–8.

5. Persaud RA, Hajioff D, Thevasagayam MS, et al. Keratosis obturans and external ear canal cholesteatoma: how and why we should distinguish between these conditions. Clin Otolaryngol Allied Sci. 2004;29(6):577–81.

6. Heilbrun ME, Salzman KL, Glastonbury CM, et al. External auditory canal cholesteatoma: clinical and imaging spectrum. AJNR Am J Neuroradiol. 2003;24(4):751–6.

7. Lemmerling MM, De Foer B, VandeVyver V, Vercruysse J-P, Verstraete KL (2008) Imaging of the opacified middle ear. Eur J Radiol. 66:363–71.

8. Vercruysse JP, De Foer B, Somers T, Casselman J, Offeciers E. Magnetic resonance imaging of cholesteatoma: an update. B-ENT. 2009;5:233–40.

9. De Foer B, Vercruysse JP, Spaepen M. Diffusion-weighted magnetic resonance imaging of the temporal bone. Neuroradiology. 2010;52:785–807.

10. Lingam RK, Connor SEJ, Casselman JW, et al. MRI in otology: applications in cholesteatoma and Ménière's disease. Clin Radiol. 2018;73:35–44.

11. Muzaffar J, Metcalfe C, Colley S, et al. Diffusion-weighted magnetic resonance imaging for residual and recurrent cholesteatoma: a systematic review and meta-analysis. Clin Otolaryngol. 2016;42(3)536–43.

12. Mas-Estelles F, Mateos-Fernandez M, Carrascosa-Bisquert B, et al. Contemporary non-echo-planar diffusion-weighted imaging of middle ear cholesteatomas. Radio Graphics. 2012;32:1197–213.

13. Lingam RK, Bassett P. A meta-analysis on the diagnostic performance of non-echo-planar diffusion-weighted imaging in detecting middle-ear cholesteatoma: 10 years on. Otol Neurotol. 2017; 31:521–8.

14. Nash R, Wong PY, Kalan A, et al. Comparing diffusion weighted MRI in the detection of postoperative middle-ear cholesteatoma in children and adults. Int J Pediatr Otorhinolaryngol. 2015;79:2281–5.

15. Lingam RK, Nash R, Majithia A, et al. Non-echoplanar diffusion weighted imaging in the detection of postoperative middle-ear cholesteatoma: navigating beyond the pitfalls to find the pearl. Insights Imaging. 2016;75:669–78.

16. Nash R, Kalan A, Lingam RK, et al. The role of diffusion-weighted magnetic resonance imaging in assessing residual/recurrent cholesteatoma after canal wall down mastoidectomy. Clin Otolaryngol. 2016;41:307–9.

17. Migirov L, Wolf M, Greenberg G, et al. Non-EPI DW MRI in planning the surgical approach to primary and recurrent cholesteatoma. Otol Neurotol. 2014;35:121–5.

18. Yamashita K, Hiwatashi A, Togao O, et al. High-resolution three-dimensional diffusion-weighted MRI/CT image data fusion for cholesteatoma surgical planning: a feasibility study. Eur Arch Otorhinolaryngol. 2015;272:3821–4.

19. Watanabe T, Ito T, Furukawa T, et al. The efficacy of color mapped fusion images in the diagnosis and treatment of cholesteatoma using transcanal endoscopic ear surgery. Otol Neurotol. 2015;36:763–8.

20. Marshall AH, Fanning N, Symons S, et al. Cochlear implantation in cochlear otosclerosis. Laryngoscope. 2005;115:1728–33.

21. Lee TC, Aviv RI, Chen JM, et-al. CT grading of otosclerosis. AJNR. 2009;30(7):1435–9.

22. Rotteveel LJ, Proops DW, Ramsden RT, Saeed SR, van Olphen AF, Mylanus EA. Cochlear implantation in 53 patients with otosclerosis: demographics, computed tomographic scanning, surgery, and complications. Otol Neurotol. 2004;25:943–52.

23. Burmeister J, Rathgeb S, Herzog J. Cochlear implantation in patients with otosclerosis of the otic capsule. Am J Otolaryngol. 2017;38(5):556–59.

24. Whetstone J, Nguyen A, Nguyen-Huynh A, et al. Surgical and clinical confirmation of temporal bone CT findings in patients with otosclerosis with failed stapes surgery. AJNR. 2014;35:1195–1201.

25. Yamashita K, Yoshiura T, Hiwatashi A, et al. The radiological diagnosis of fenestralotosclerosis: the utility of histogram analysis using multidector row CT. Eur Arch Otorhinolaryngol. 2014;271:3277–82.

26. Mori N, Toyama Y, Kimura N, et al. Detection of small fenestralotosclerotic lesions by high-resolution computed tomography using multiplanar reconstruction. Auris Nasus Larynx. 2013;40:36–40.

27. Virk J, Singh A, Lingam R. The role of imaging in the diagnosis and management of otosclerosis. Otol Neurotol. 2013;34:55–60.

28. Connor SE, Leung R, Natas S. Imaging of the petrous apex: a pictorial review. Br J Radiol. 2008;81(965): 427–35.

29. Isaacson B, Kutz JW, Roland PS. Lesions of the petrous apex: diagnosis and management. Otolaryngol Clin North Am. 2007;40(3):479–519.

30. Chaljub G, Vrabec J, Hollingsworth C, Borowski AM, Guinto FC Jr. Magnetic resonance imaging of petrous tip lesions. Am J Otolaryngol. 1999;20(5):304–313.

31. Koral K, Dowling M. Petrous apicitis in a child: computed tomography and magnetic resonance imaging findings. Clin Imaging. 2006;30(2):137–9.

32. Davé AV, Diaz-Marchan PJ, Lee AG. Clinical and magnetic resonance imaging features of Gradenigo syndrome. Am J Ophthalmol. 1997;124(4):568–70.

33. Lee YH, Lee NJ, Kim JH, Song JJ. CT, MRI and gallium SPECT in the diagnosis and treatment of petrous apicitis presenting as multiple cranial neuropathies. Br J Radiol. 2005;78(934):948–51.

34. Ong CK, Fook-Hin Chong V. Imaging of Jugular foramen. Neuroimaging Clin N Am. 2009;19(3):469–82.

35. Nemec S, Donat M, Hoeftberger R, Matula C, Czerny C. Chondrosarcoma of the petrous apex: a diagnostic and therapeutic challenge. Eur J Radiol Extra. 2005;54:87–91.

36. Oghalai JS, Buxbaum JL, Jackler RK, McDermott MW. Skull base chondrosarcoma originating from the petroclival junction. Otol Neurotol. 2005;26(5):1052–60.

37. Brown RV, Sage MR, Brophy BP. CT and MR findings in patients with chordomas of the petrous apex. AJNR Am J Neuroradiol. 1990;11(1):121–4.

38. Janse van Rensburg P, van der Meer G. Magnetic resonance and computed tomography imaging of a grade IV papillary endolymphatic sac tumour. J Neurooncol. 2008;89(2):199–203.

39. Coelho DH, Roland JT. Implanting obstructed and malformed cochleae. Otolaryngol Clin North Am. 2012;45(1):91–110.

40. Roche JP, Huang BY, Castillo M, Bassim MK, Adunka OF, Buchman CA. Imaging characteristics of children with auditory neuropathy spectrum disorder. Otol Neurotol. 2010;31:780–88.

41. Sennaroglu L. Cochlear implantation in inner ear malformations: a review article. Cochlear Implants Int. 2010;11:4–41.

42. Kanona H, Stephenson K, D'Arco F, Rajput K, Cochrane L, Jephson C. Computed tomography versus magnetic resonance imaging in paediatric cochlear implant assessment: a pilot study and our experience at Great Ormond Street Hospital. J Laryngol Otol. 2018;132:529–33.

43. Sennaroğlu L, Bajin MD. Classification and current management of inner ear malformations. Balkan Med J. 2017;34:397–411.

44. Colby CC, Todd NW, Harnsberger HR, Hudgins PA. Standardization of CT depiction of cochlear implant insertion depth. AJNR Am J Neuroradiol. 2015;36(2):368–71.

45. Fernandes V, Wang Y, Yeung R, et al. Effectiveness of skull X-ray to determine cochlear implant insertion depth. J Otolaryngol Head Neck Surgery. 2018;47(1):50–6.

46. Joshi VM, Navlekar SK, Kishore GR, Reddy KJ, Kumar ECV. CT and MR imaging of the inner ear and brain in children with congenital sensorineural hearing loss. Radiographics. 2012;32:683–98.

47. Ozgen B, Oguz KK, Atas A, Sennaroglu L. Complete labyrinthine aplasia: clinical and radiologic findings with review of the literature. AJNR Am J Neuroradiol. 2009;30:774–80.

48. Sennaroglu L. Histopathology of inner ear malformations: do we have enough evidence to explain pathophysiology? Cochlear Implants Int. 2016;17:3–20.

49. Lo WW. What is a 'Mondini' and what difference does a name make? AJNR Am J Neuroradiol. 1999; 20:1442.

50. Huang BY, Zdanski C, Castillo M. Pediatric sensorineural hearing loss, Part 2: syndromic and acquired causes. AJNR Am J Neuroradiol. 2012;33:399–406.

51. Sennaroglu L, Saatci I. A new classification for cochleovestibular malformations. Laryngoscope. 2002;112:2230–41.

52. Hsu A, Desai N, Paldino MJ. The unwound cochlea: a specific imaging marker of branchio-oto-renal syndrome. AJNR Am J Neuroradiol. 2018;39:2345–9.

53. Sennaroğlu L, Bajin MD, Pamuk E, Tahir E. Cochlear hypoplasia type four with anteriorly displaced Facial nerve canal. Otol Neurotol. 2016;37:407–9.

54. Mafee MF, Charletta D, Kumar A, Belmont H. Large vestibular aqueduct and congenital sensorineural hearing loss. AJNR Am J Neuroradiol. 1992;13:805–19.

55. D'Arco F, Talenti G, Lakshmanan R, Stephenson K, Siddiqui A, Carney O. Do measurements of inner ear structures help in the diagnosis of inner ear malformations? A review of literature. Otol Neurotol. 2017;38:384–92.

56. Muzzi E, Rinaldo A, Ferlito A. Ménière disease: diagnostic instrumental support. Am J Otolaryngol. 2008;29:188–94.

57. Liu F, Huang W, Meng X, et al. Comparison of noninvasive evaluation of endolymphatic hydrops in Meniere's disease and endolymphatic space in healthy volunteers using magnetic resonance imaging. Acta Otolaryngol. 2012;132:234–40.

58. Casselman JW, Kuhweide R, Deimling M, et al. Constructive interference in steady state 3D FT MR imaging of the inner ear and cerebellopontine angle. AJNR Am J Neuroradiol. 1993;14:47–57.

59. Nakashima T, Naganawa S, Sugiura M, et al. Visualization of endolymphatic hydrops in patients with Meniere's disease. Laryngoscope. 2007;117:415–20.

60. Kim TY, Park DW, Lee YJ, et al. Comparison of inner ear contrast enhancement among patients with unilateral inner ear symptoms in MR images obtained 10 minutes and 4 hours after gadolinium injection. AJNR Am J Neuroradiol. 2015;36:2637–42.

61. Sano R, Teranishi M, Yamazaki M, et al. Contrast enhancement of the inner ear in magnetic resonance images taken at 10 minutes or 4 hours after intravenous gadolinium injection. Acta Otolaryngol. 2012;132:241–6.

62. Tagaya M, Teranishi M, Naganawa S, et al. 3 Tesla magnetic resonance imaging obtained 4 hours after intravenous gadolinium injection in patients with sudden deafness. Acta Otolaryngol. 2010;130:665–9.

63. Pakdaman MN, Ishiyama G, Ishiyama A, et al. Blood-labyrinth barrier permeability in Ménière disease and idiopathic sudden sensorineural hearing loss: findings on delayed postcontrast 3D-FLAIR MRI. AJNR Am J Neuroradiol. 2016;37:1903–8.

64. Baráth K, Schuknecht B, Naldi AM, Schrepfer T, Bockisch CJ, Hegemann SC. Detection and grading of endolymphatic hydrops in Ménière disease using MR imaging. AJNR Am J Neuroradiol. 2014;35(7):1387–92.

65. Bernaerts A, Vanspauwen R, Blaivie C, et al. The value of four stage vestibular hydrops grading and asymmetric perilymphatic enhancement in the diagnosis of Ménière's disease on MRI. Neuroradiology. 2019;61:421–29.

66. Ishman SL, Friedland DR. Temporal bone fractures: traditional classification and clinical relevance. Laryngoscope. 2004;114 (10):1734–41.

67. Little SC, Kesser BW. Radiographic classification of temporal bone fractures: clinical predictability using a new system. Arch Otolaryngol Head Neck Surg. 2006;132 (12):1300–4.

68. Resnick DK, Subach BR, Marion DW. The significance of carotid canal involvement in basilar cranial fracture. Neurosurgery. 1997;40(6):1177–81.

69. Juliano AF, Ginat DT, Moonis G. Imaging review of the temporal bone: Part I. Anatomy and inflammatory and neoplastic processes. Radiology. 2013;269:17–33.

70. Lagleyre S, Sorrentino T, Calmels MN, et al. Reliability of high-resolution CT scan in diagnosis of otosclerosis. Otol Neurotol. 2009;30(8):1152–9.

71. Sennaroglu L, Colletti V, Manrique M, et al. Auditory brainstem implantation in children and non-neurofibromatosis type 2 patients: a consensus statement. Otol Neurotol. 2011;32:187–91.

72. Sennaroğlu L, Sennaroğlu G, Yücel E, et al. Long-term results of ABI in children with severe inner ear malformations. Otol Neurotol. 2016;37:865–72.

73. Postnov A, Zarowski A, De Clerck N, et al. High resolution micro-CT scanning as an innovative tool for evaluation of the surgical positioning of cochlear implant electrodes. Acta Otolaryngol. 2006;126:467–74.

74. Bezanson A, Adamson R, Brown J. Fabrication and performance of a miniaturized 64-element high-frequency endoscopic phased array. IEEE Trans Ultrason Ferroelectr Freq Control. 2014;61:33–43.

75. MacDougall D, Rainsbury J, Brown J, Bance M, Adamson R. Optical coherence tomography system requirements for clinical diagnostic middle ear imaging. J Biomed Opt. 2015;20(5):056008.

76. Chang EW, Kobler JB, Yun SH. Subnanometer optical coherence tomographic vibrography. Opt Lett. 2012;37(17):3678–80.

# 16 Tools and Technology in Otology

*Sabarigirish K and Uma Patnaik*

## CONTENTS

## INTRODUCTION

Technology is ever evolving and the field of otology like every other field of modern medicine is continuously changing with these technological advances. There are various areas where technological advances have revolutionized the outlook towards contemporary clinical practice. We will discuss some of these recent advances in this chapter which are gradually changing the practice of otology as they continue to evolve themselves.

We will cover the topic under the following subheads:

- *Tools:* Hyper-efficient diagnostic, therapeutic and point-of-care tools which improve outcomes and patient safety like LASER.

- *Technology:* Revolutionary technology like three-dimensional modelling and tissue printing, which will alter the current practice.

- *Biomaterials:* Nanotechnology-based biomaterials coupled with tissue engineering that is replacing current ones in implants, prostheses and stents.

- *Molecular biology:* Proteomics-based big data which is significantly changing our appreciation of ear disorders and their pathogenicity mechanisms.

- *Information technology and Artificial Intelligence (AI):* Digital solutions such as virtual care and big data based customized care are becoming integral to digital care. Machine Learning (ML) and deep neural network based applications have already started becoming diagnostic adjuncts.

- *Simulation:* Simulated and augmented reality combined with haptics is being used for treatment planning and surgical training.

## TOOLS

### Laser

*Laser* stands for light amplification by stimulated emission of radiation. Surgical lasers are devices that cause light amplification and create coherent light beams ranging from the far infrared to the ultraviolet parts of the spectrum. The light of the laser has similar characteristics to visible light, in that it can be reflected by mirrors and focused through lenses (1).

The history of lasers began when Theodore Maiman invented the ruby laser in 1960 (2). Otolaryngologists realized the potential of laser very early and considered different methods for use of pulsed laser systems in treating disorders of middle ear and labyrinth (3, 4). The first application of lasers in otology was reported in 1967, when Sataloff attempted to use a neodymium laser for stapedotomy (4). Research keeps on growing towards finer use of lasers in otology.

### Laser Physics

There are three major differences between a laser and a lamp light. The laser is

1. Monochromatic – one wavelength or colour (if the energy is in the visible spectrum).

2. Coherent – the photons or waves travel in step or in-phase with one another.

3. Collimated – most important property. It enables light to be focused on smallest possible spot (diffraction limited).

### Laser–Tissue Interactions

1. *Photoablative:* When molecular bonds are divided.

2. *Photochemical:* When laser light interacts with photosensitizers to produce chemical and physical reactions. This forms the basis for photodynamic therapy.

3. *Photomechanical:* When the laser energy is pulsed to disrupt tissue or stones by the mechanism of shock waves.

4. *Photothermal:* Conversion of absorbed laser light into heat. The tissue effect can be cutting, coagulation or vaporization, depending on the laser wavelength and the laser delivery device. The photothermal mechanism is predominant in laser use in otolaryngology and examples include $CO_2$ and the argon laser for stapedotomy.

### Types of Lasers

*Argon laser:* Its wavelength is 514 and 488 nm. It is operated by continuous wave (CW) mode and can be delivered through optical fibres. It is mainly used in treating vascular cutaneous lesions because of its absorption by melanin and haemoglobin (7). It is used in otology to perform stapedotomy procedures because of its ability to be focused on a small spot size (8). Other otological application included lysis of middle ear adhesions and spot welding of grafts in tympanoplasty (9, 10).

*Potassium titanyl phosphate (KTP) laser:* Its wavelength is 532 nm. It can be delivered through a micromanipulator or optical fibres using a handheld probe. Examples of handheld KTP laser applications include stapedotomy and excision of acoustic neuromas (11, 12). Use of a micromanipulator facilitates middle ear laser surgery because it is more convenient.

*$CO_2$ laser:* It is the workhorse of ear, nose and throat (ENT) practice. It operates at 10.6 μm. The invisible $CO_2$ laser beam has a coaxial helium-neon laser beam to act as indicator. It is used in stapedotomy and myringotomy procedures. It is also used for ablation of residual/recurrent cholesteatoma in COM squamous surgery. In 1998, Fink et al. reported efficient propagation of infrared energy through a hollow-core fibre lined with an omnidirectional dielectric mirror, which led to the development of the OmniGuide $CO_2$ laser system. In this system, the mirror, which consists of alternating layers of high and low refractory index materials, is precisely calibrated to guide light generated by the $CO_2$ laser through the flexible fibre in a helium medium. Helium flowing through the fibre also acts as a coolant (13).

*(Holmium-yttrium aluminium garnet (Ho-YAG) laser:* This laser has wavelength of 2.1 μm. It is a pulsed laser in near-infrared region. This laser is used for Facial nerve decompression.

*Diode laser:* It operates in red to near-infrared region of spectrum, used for photodynamic therapy and tissue welding (14).

### Specific Applications in Otology

*Stapes Surgery:* In inner ear surgery, the bone has to be ablated efficiently without thermal load of the small perilymphatic fluid compartment and damage to underlying vestibular structures.

Laser systems may be classified as continuous wave lasers, such as the argon and carbon dioxide lasers, or pulsed lasers, such as the erbium-yttrium-aluminium-garnet lasers, YAG, Holmium-YAG or Erbium-Yttrium-Scandium-Gallium-Garnet.

The application of all of these laser systems in stapedotomy has been reported by different authors (15–17).

Lasers in stapes surgery are being used to divide the stapedius tendon, divide the anterior and posterior crura and perforate the footplate. The ideal laser for stapes surgery should not penetrate deeply into the perilymph. It should be conducted through optical fibres, allowing easy manipulation, and should have good water absorption, equating to high bone ablation efficiency.

In this regard, argon laser has been found to be better in primary as well as revision stapes surgery. It can be delivered using micromanipulator or fibre-optic micro-handpiece with a divergent beam at the tip called as endo-otoprobe. The risk of penetration into perilymph is minimal in the hands of experienced surgeon and at a low power setting. The recommended power is 1 W at 0.2 second pulses or less (18, 19).

The use of KTP laser for stapes surgery was first described in the mid-1980s. Like the argon laser, it does not get completely absorbed by bone and has the risk of penetration through footplate, damage to inner ear structures and iatrogenic sensorineural hearing loss. It is highly absorbed by haemoglobin and is effective at achieving a bloodless surgical field. A comparative study done by Vincent et al. showed results following stapedotomy performed using flexible KTP and $CO_2$ laser, complication rate was negligible in both groups (20). The $CO_2$ laser group had a favourable outcome with mean AB gap of 3.1 dB as compared to KTP group where mean AB gap was 4.3 dB. KTP laser has been shown to be useful in revision stapes surgery.

The suitability of $CO_2$ laser for stapes surgery was demonstrated by Lesinski and Palmer. $CO_2$ laser achieved better hearing results and fewer complications than conventional surgery (21). The advantage is that it has got minimal depth of penetration and hence less collateral tissue damage.

Clinically there is not enough evidence to support the use of any one laser above the other, although the choice of laser depends on surgeon preference and institutional protocol (22).

*Cochlear Implant Surgery:* Lasers have been used in performing cochleostomy during cochlear implant surgery. Jan Kiefer et al. compared the effects of cochleostomies performed with a diamond drill or alternatively with two types of lasers that are currently applied in otology: the erbium-YAG laser and the $CO_2$ laser with flash-scan technology. They found that the best results in terms of preservation of cochlear function were obtained with the diamond drill. Hearing loss observed with the $CO_2$ laser was slightly greater, although differences to the group of drilling were not statistically significant (23).

Mechanical ablation of the bone with a diamond drill caused minimal hearing loss, probably because of minimal thermal damage and acoustic stress to the inner ear structures; it may result in inadvertent direct mechanical damage (23).

*Cholesteatoma Surgery:* Lasers facilitate ablation of microscopic and macroscopic cholesteatoma matrix from ossicles, close to the Facial nerve and areas that are difficult to access using conventional instruments. Fibre-optic-based lasers are preferred to facilitate accurate delivery and minimize collateral damage. Use of lasers has

been shown to decrease residual disease, but it has been associated with higher incidence of facial palsy (24).

*Vestibular Schwannoma Surgery:* The OmniGuide $CO_2$ laser is a safe and effective tool when used as an adjunct in the resection of medium to large vestibular schwannomas. This device is most useful as a cutting tool and as an aid to piecemeal tumour removal rather than as a tissue vaporizer. The benefit of the OmniGuide laser may be greatest for very large or giant tumours or for very firm tumours resistant to cutting using microscissors (13).

## TECHNOLOGY
### Three Dimensional Printing

3D printing, also known as rapid prototyping, is a nascent technology that is being rapidly adapted in otology for resident training and patient treatment planning. With significant decline in the costs and rapid improvements in technology, use of 3D printing in otology is on the rise. However, many otological applications for 3D printing are currently in preliminary stages, mostly in proof-of-concept stages or are being evaluated in animal models.

Using DICOM data from computed tomography (CT), magnetic resonance imaging (MRI) and ultrasound (US), 3D models are generated utilizing computer-aided design (CAD) software and exported as files such as an. STL files, compatible with 3D printers (25). 3D printer fabricates the solid objects encoded in the. STL file, layer-by-layer, beginning at the base of the object and finishing at the top, using one of the many printing techniques available today. The resolution of the printed model depends equally on the intricacy of the printing technique as well as on the quality of CAD data utilized.

### Applications in Otology

1. *Perioperative planning:* Full-scale 3D replicas of complex otological structures are far superior to the 2D radiological images for preoperative planning by surgeons in complicated surgical procedures in complex anatomical situations (26). In addition to visualization, these models made with appropriate materials give the surgeon an opportunity to practice the intended surgery, get a tactile feedback and anticipate errors with the currently available technology. It even helps the surgeon to customize equipment to further optimize operative interventions.

2. *Patient education:* 3D models of anatomical structures are also useful for patient education as it is easier for patients to understand pathology and surgical interventions without the complexities of interpreting complex radiological images, which may intuitively aid in giving the informed consent. A comparison of preoperative and projected postoperative models may also be used to manage expectations of the patients, especially in the areas of surgical correction of external ear anomalies.

3. *Surgical training:* With the increasing non-availability of immediate post-mortem temporal bones, surgical training of residents by conventional cadaveric temporal bone dissection is gradually becoming obsolete. Three-dimensional printed temporal bones are expected to obviate this widening gap, despite the current difficulties replicating middle ear bones and retained powders within mastoid air cells. Therefore, there is a need to integrate 3D printed temporal bone dissections into resident education, enabling the resident to practice these skills, thus lessening the danger to patients. Many centres have validated the transference of dissection skills to live operating theatres following dissections on 3D printed temporal bones (27–29). During implementation, participants were asked to qualitatively evaluate these training exercises in terms of realism, anatomical accuracy, utility and efficacy. Despite using different materials in the 3D printing process, results were largely similar with positive feedback from trainees.

Three-dimensional models can be printed with specific pathologies and anomalies to best prepare for a specific operation. This can increase exposure to rare pathologies that residents may not otherwise encounter in their training. Training models such as the Electric Phantom (ElePhant) allow for training with real-time feedback. ElePhant utilizes 3D printed models with vital structures, such as Facial nerve, replaced with either a conductive alloy or fibre-optic material; inadvertent trauma alerts the user thus providing immediate feedback. The amount of structural damage and predicted patient deficits are noted, allowing residents to make mistakes on models rather than patients (28).

4. *Prostheses and reconstruction:* Another area where 3D printing may prove useful is in the synthesis of implantable structural tissues, especially in microtia. Customized 3D printed biomaterial implants for auricular reconstruction can be fabricated to reconstruct its cartilaginous framework (30). Studies report 3D printed tympanic membrane grafts which were found to better resist deformation than temporalis fascia and obviated the need for additional skin incisions and time for fascia harvesting (31). In a recent study, the same group 3D printed custom prostheses to successfully repair superior semicircular canal dehiscence in cadavers (32).

## BIOMATERIALS
### Nanotechnology

A nanoparticle is a particle ranging between 1 and 100 nm in size. They can exhibit significantly different physical and chemical properties to their larger material counterparts. Most nanoparticles are made up of only a few hundred atoms. Nanotechnology refers to the design, production and application of structures, devices and systems by controlled manipulation of nanoparticles. Nanotechnology has many applications in various fields, health care being one of them. A wide variety of its uses are currently in experimental stages and is expected to create revolutionary change in inner ear diseases.

One of the major applications of nanotechnology is to develop a safe delivery system of therapeutic agents into inner ear, whereby a drug molecule is loaded on to a nanoparticle and delivered to the inner ear. It has the dual challenge of delivering the therapeutic agent in effective quantity, while at the same time does not cause nanoparticle-induced cochlear toxicity. Effectiveness of nanoparticle drug delivery system to inner ear has been validated by many studies by measurement of concentration of drug delivered using high-performance liquid chromatography or fluorescence spectrophotometry. In one study, polyethylene glycol-coated polylactic acid (PEG-PLA) nanoparticles were used to deliver cisplatin to deafen guinea pigs after pre-treatment with administration of dexamethasone-loaded nanoparticles (33, 34). In both studies, administration of dexamethasone-loaded nanoparticles protected hearing in the 4 and 8 kHz frequencies. In a similar study, cisplatin-induced hearing loss was protected at 10, 14 and 16 kHz after administration of 6α-methylprednisolone was loaded onto nanoparticles using α-tocopherol derivatives (35).

On similar lines, it has been proved that nanoparticles can effectively deliver growth factors and genes into inner ear. Delivering a large macromolecule such as a growth factor remains challenging as intracochlear delivery requires surgery; therefore, it can only be attempted in completely deaf patients, such as for cochlear implant surgery. Intratympanic delivery is more useful because of easy clinical access. Gene delivery using nanoparticles is at its very nascent stage and several challenges must be addressed before it can be applied clinically, such as decreasing the particle size while stably integrating the gene into the particle and protecting the gene from degrading enzymes such as endonuclease (36).

## MOLECULAR BIOLOGY
### Proteomics

The word *proteome*, coined by Marc Wilkins in 1994, is a portmanteau of *protein* and gen*ome*. It is the overall protein signatures of a genome. Proteome is the entire set of proteins coded in the genome of a cell, tissue or an organism Proteomics, the identification and quantification of proteins of the proteome.

Proteomics is a rapidly growing field of molecular biology with applications for detection of various diagnostic markers, candidates for vaccine production, understanding pathogenicity mechanisms, alteration of expression patterns in response to different signals and interpretation of functional protein pathways in different diseases (37). Proteomics is exceptionally intricate and generates complex data. Bioinformatics, therefore, is integral to proteomics.

Proteomics have revealed the molecular biology of organ of Corti and has the potential in future to make our understanding of non-syndromic hearing loss amply clear. A regulatory complex consisting of two proteins – OCP1 and OCP2 – together with cullin-1 is believed to control an essential service system of the cochlea, the gap junction system. Their role in the removal of toxic waste, specifically the large amounts of K+ emanating in hair cells, is postulated to counteract the biological hardships imposed by a hostile electrochemical environment.

A proteomic profile from plasma of Ménière's disease affected individuals suggest potential use as an easily reproducible tool for early diagnosis and follow-up (38). In the context of BPPV, observation of the behaviour of the biochemical properties of Otoconin 90 of human otoconia prior to onset of degeneration should provide important insights into its patho-biologic mechanisms.

## INFORMATION TECHNOLOGY AND ARTIFICIAL INTELLIGENCE

Future of medical care is in the hands of digital technology. The paradigms of the current health care rewritten in the coming decades with AI and ML will make significant inroads into health sciences. Newer algorithms and information technology platforms will make the practice of medicine safer, efficient, accessible and cheaper than it is today. The future ENT surgeon needs to be familiarized to and equipped with the basics of the emerging technologies in medical care.

*Terminology:*

1. **Artificial Intelligence** is the use of ML algorithms to emulate human cognition in the analysis of complicated medical data and derive approximate conclusions without direct human input.

2. **Machine Learning** is a set of complex algorithms and statistical models used to perform specific tasks without using explicit instructions by relying on pattern recognition and using self-learning algorithms to develop automated inferences.

3. **Artificial Neural Networks** (ANN) or connectionist systems are computing systems that "learn" to perform tasks by considering examples, generally without being programmed with task-specific rules.

4. **Deep Learning** is a subset of ML in AI that has networks capable of learning unsupervised from data that is unstructured or unlabelled.

5. **Natural Language Processing** (NLP) is the subfield of AI that is focused on enabling computers to understand and process human languages.

6. There are in general two types of AI. The ability of a machine to represent the human mind and perform any intellectual task that a human can perform is termed **Artificial General Intelligence**. The ability of a machine to perform a single task extremely well is termed **Artificial Narrow Intelligence**.

Improving the diagnostic interpretation of electrophysiological tests such as ABR and OAE by using complex algorithms is one domain which has shown significant promise. Izworski et al. applied hybrid neural networks to enable automated detection of Wave V in ABR signals. Augmented with contextual information, 90% accuracy was achieved (39). Predictive capability of neuronal networks has been successfully used to predict impaired pure tone thresholds from Distortion Product Otoacoustic Emissions (DPOAEs) data using a feed-forward ANN with a back-propagation training algorithm. This research indicates the possibility of accurately predicting hearing ability within 10 dB in normal hearing individuals and in hearing-impaired listeners with DPOAEs and ANNs from 500–4000 Hz (40).

ML models and image processing techniques have been used for aiding otological diagnosis using otoscopy. Michelle et al. used various feature extraction techniques such as colour coherence vector, discrete cosine transform and filter bank to characterize the lesions on images of external auditory meatus and tympanic membrane achieving an average classification accuracy of 93.9%, average sensitivity of 87.8%, average specificity of 95.9% and average positive predictive value of 87.7% (41). This could be of immense use for the general practitioners for making better decisions prior to specialty referrals.

Expert systems which work on the concept of "Knowledge Base", whereby the machine helps the professional to infer solutions for clinical problems have been tested and found useful in various branches of health care. "Carrusel" is an expert system dealing with the diagnosis of vestibular disorders that achieves a success rate of 97% when compared to the human experts involved in its design (42). "ENT Diagnosis Expert System" (ENTDEx), using Bayesian networks, is a system developed to help ENT patients and non-patients to diagnose common adult ENT diseases based on the given symptoms. This application uses Bayesian networks, which is a probabilistic graphical model that represents a set of variables and their conditional dependencies in diagnosing the diseases. Based on a series of surveys and experiments conducted by the researchers, ENTDEx has a good feedback to its users as it provides the necessary information the users needed specifically in the field of otolaryngology (43).

Sudden Sensorineural Hearing Loss (SSNHL) is a multifactorial disorder with high heterogeneity, with significant variations in outcomes. ML tools have been used to prognosticate the outcome of SSH. In a study involving 1220 participants conducted at Setting, Chinese People's Liberation Army (PLA) hospital, Beijing, China, it was observed that an advanced deep learning technique, Deep Belief Network (DBN), together with the conventional Logistic Regression (LR), Support Vector Machine (SVM) and Multilayer Perceptron (MLP) were used to predict the dichotomized hearing outcome of SSNHL by inputting six feature collections derived from 149 potential predictors with accuracy of 77.58% (44).

Molecular basis for hearing loss still remains an enigma, thus rendering it difficult to design molecular and pharmacological treatment. A reliable biomarker is the key to improving the molecular diagnosis of inner ear disorders. Analysis of microRNAs (miRNA) in tissue and body fluid samples has gradually gained significant momentum as a diagnostic tool for a wide variety of diseases. miRNA profiling in inner ear perilymph is feasible and has been demonstrating distinctive miRNA expression profiles unique to different diseases. A first step in developing miRNAs as biomarkers for inner ear disease is linking patterns of miRNA expression in perilymph to clinically available metrics. ML has been used to build disease-specific algorithms that predict hearing loss using only miRNA expression profiles. This methodology not only affords the opportunity to understand what is occurring on a molecular level, but may also offer an approach to diagnosing patients with active inner ear disease (45).

A neural net is a "black box" information processing system that can be used for pattern matching, optimal prediction or functional approximation has been tested for optimal hearing aid fitting. For this purpose, a multilayer perceptron net was trained to generate an optimum match between a set of input pure tone audiograms and the corresponding best frequency response and gain for each subject. The feasibility of using neural nets to select hearing-aid response characteristics was tested using both simulated and real audiometric data. The simulation results indicate that a neural net can be successfully trained to reproduce a standard fitting rule and that a minimum of about 50 sets of audiometric response data are needed for the net to converge to a generalized solution. When used to predict, from the pure tone audiograms, the best frequency response characteristics determined for subjects having severe-to-profound hearing losses, the neural net was more accurate than the prescribed fitting procedure derived from the same data (46).

## SIMULATION

Generally, cadaveric temporal bones are used for dissection to develop surgical skills required for temporal bone surgery. However, it is difficult to get temporal bones in large numbers required for adequate training of surgeons. The temporal bone simulator, where the surgeons in training can practice their skills before taking on surgery in live patients solves this problem. Temporal bone simulator provides a viable alternative to cadaveric temporal bone dissection and is being used worldwide for training of surgeons. It provides real surgery like experience with feel of drilling and feedback, which is useful for surgeons in training. It can also be used to practise difficult/key surgical steps before starting the actual surgery so that chances of complications/ adverse events during actual surgical procedures can be reduced (47). With availability of surgical simulation, it is likely that there will be a paradigm shift in surgical training worldwide with development of well-structured and standardized training programmes (48).

## CONCLUSION

The field of medicine continues to make new headways and it is essential for the current generation of otologists to stay abreast with these new developments in order to stay relevant in practice of contemporary medicine. No part of patient care is untouched by the new technological developments and the role for new age technology in medicine is ever expanding. The modern-day medical practitioners have to adapt to all these changes and try to integrate the offerings of modern technology in their day-to-day practice.

## REFERENCES

1. Van de Water T, Staecker H. Basic Science and Clinical Review. New York: Thieme Medical Publishers, 2006.

2. Maiman TH. Stimulated optical radiation in ruby. Nature. 1960;187:493.

3. Sataloff J. Experimental use of laser in otosclerotic stapes. Arch Otolaryngol. 1967;85:614–6.

4. Hogberg L, Stahle J, Vogel K. The transmission of high powered ruby laser beam through bone. Acta Soc Med Ups. 1967;72:223–8.

5. Strunk CL, Quinn FB Jr, Bailey BJ. Stapedectomy techniques in residency training. Laryngoscope. 1992;102:121–4.

6. Vollrath M, Schreiner C. Influence of argon laser stapedotomy on inner ear function and temperature. Otolaryngol Head Neck Surg. 1983;91(5):521–6.

7. Buell BR, Schuller DE. Comparison of tensile strength in $CO_2$ laser and scalpel skin incisions. Arch Otolaryngol. 1983;109:465–7.

8. Perkins RC. Laser stapedotomy for otosclerosis. Laryngoscope. 1980;90:228–40.

9. Di Bartolomeo JR, Ellis M. The argon laser in otology. Laryngoscope. 1980;90:1786–96.

10. Escudero LH, Castro AO, Drumond M, et al. Argon laser in human tympanoplasty. Arch Otolaryngol. 1979;105(5):252–3.

11. Bartels W. KTP laser stapedotomy: is it safe? Otolaryngol Head Neck Surg 1990;103:685–92.

12. McGee TM, Diaz-Ordaz EA, Kartush JM. The role of KTP laser in revision stapedectomy. Otolaryngol Head Neck Surg. 1993 Nov;109(5):839–43.

13. Schwartz MS, Lekovic GP. Use of a flexible hollow-core carbon dioxide laser for microsurgical resection of vestibular schwannomas. Neurosurg Focus. 2018;44(3):E6.

14. Parkin JL, Dixon JA. Argon laser treatment of head and neck vascular lesions. Otolaryngol Head Neck Surg. 1985;93:211–6.

15. Escudero L, Castro A, Drummond M, Porto S, Bozinis D, Penna A, et al. Argon laser in human tympanoplasty. Arch Otolaryngol. 1979;105:252–3.

16. Palva T. Argon laser in otosclerosis surgery. Acta Otolaryngol. 1979;104:153–7.

17. Perkins R. Laser stapedotomy for otosclerosis. Laryngoscope. 1980;90:228–42.

18. Nissen R. Argon laser in difficult stapedotomy cases. Laryngoscope. 1998;108:1669–73.

19. Horn K, Gherini S, Griffin G. Argon laser stapedectomy using an endo-otoprobe system. Otolaryngol Head Neck Surg. 1990;102:193–8.

20. Vincent R, Bittermann A, Oates J, Sperling N, Grolman W. KTP versus $CO_2$ laser fiber stapedotomy for primary otosclerosis: results of a new comparative series with the otology-neurotology database. Otol Neurotol. 2012;33:928–33.

21. Jovanovic S, Schonfeld U, Scherer H. New developments in $CO_2$ laser stapedotomy. Med Laser Appl. 2002;17:202–13.

22. Young E, Mitchell-Innes A, Jindal M. Lasers in stapes surgery: a review. J Laryngol Otol. 2015;129:627–33.

23. Kiefer J, Tillein J, Ye Q, Klinke R, Gstoettner W. Application of carbon dioxide and erbium:yttrium-aluminum-garnet lasers in inner ear surgery: an experimental study. Otol Neurotol 2004;25(3):400–9.

24. Eskander A, Holler T, Papsin BC. Delayed Facial nerve paresis after using the KTP laser in the treatment of cholesteatoma despite inter-operative Facial nerve monitoring. Int J Pediatr Otorhinolaryngol. 2010;74:823–4.

25. Crafts TD, Ellsperman SE, Wannemuehler TJ, et al. Three-dimensional printing and its applications in otorhinolaryngology: head and neck surgery. Otolaryngol Head Neck Surg. 2017;156(6):999–1010.

26. Rose AS, Webster CE, Harrysson OL, Formeister EJ, Rawal RB, Iseli CE. Pre-operative simulation of pediatric mastoid surgery with 3D-printed temporal bone models. Int J Pediatr Otorhinolaryngol. 2015;79(5):740–44.

27. Da Cruz MJ, Francis HW. Face and content validation of a novel three-dimensional printed temporal bone for surgical skills development. J Laryngol Otol. 2015;129(Suppl 3):S23–9.

28. Hochman JB, Rhodes C, Wong D, Kraut J, Pisa J, Unger B. Comparison of cadaveric and isomorphic three-dimensional printed models in temporal bone education. Laryngoscope. 2015;125(10):2353–7.

29. Cohen J, Reyes SA. Creation of a 3D printed temporal bone model from clinical CT data. Am J Otolaryngol. 2015;36(5):619–24.

30. Bos EJ, Scholten T, Song Y, et al. Developing a parametric ear model for auricular reconstruction: a new step towards patient-specific implants. J Craniomaxillofac Surg. 2015;43(3):390–5.

31. Kozin ED, Black NL, Cheng JT, et al. Design, fabrication, and in vitro testing of novel three-dimensionally printed tympanic membrane grafts. Hear Res. 2016;340:191–203.

32. Kozin ED, Remenschneider AK, Cheng S, Nakajima HH, Lee DJ. Three-dimensional printed prosthesis for repair of superior canal dehiscence. Otolaryngol Head Neck Surg. 2015;153(4):616–9.

33. Sun C, Wang X, Chen D, Lin X, Yu D,Wu H. Dexamethasone loaded nanoparticles exert protective effects against cisplatin-induced hearing loss by systemic administration. Neurosci Lett. 2016;619:142–8.

34. Sun C, Wang X, Zheng Z, et al. A single dose of dexamethasone encapsulated in polyethylene glycol-coated polylactic acid nanoparticles attenuates cisplatin-induced hearing loss following round window membrane administration. Int J Nanomed. 2015;10:3567–79.

35. Saldana SM, Palao-Suay R, Trinidad A, Aguilar MR, Ramirez-Camacho R, San Román J. Otoprotective properties of 6α-methylprednisolone-loaded nanoparticles against cisplatin: in vitro and in vivo correlation. Nanomedicine. 2016;12(4):965–76.

36. Dong Kee K. Nanomedicine for inner ear diseases: a review of recent in vivo studies. Biomed Res Int. 2017;2017:3098230.

37. Aslam B, Basit M, Nisar MA, Khurshid M, Rasool MH. Proteomics: Technologies and Their Applications. J Chromatogr Sci. 2017;55(2):182–96.

38. Giuseppe C, Milena S, Domenica S, et al. Proteomics in Ménière disease. J. Cell. Physiol. 2012;227(7):308–12.

39. Izworski A, Tadeusiewicz R, Pasławski A. The utilization of context signals in the analysis of ABR potentials by application of neural networks. In: López de Mántaras R, Plaza E., editors. Machine Learning: ECML 2000 – 11th European Conference on Machine Learning Barcelona, Catalonia, Spain, May 3–June 2, 2000 Proceedings. Lecture Notes in Computer Science (Lecture Notes in Artificial Intelligence), vol 1810. Springer: Berlin, Heidelberg, 2000.

40. de Waal R, Maggi SJ, Johann JK. Predicting hearing loss from otoacoustic emissions using an artificial neural network. S Afr J Commun Disord. 2002;49:28–39.

41. Michelle V, Juan CM, Paul HD, Mariela T, Carlos S, Fernando AC. Computer-aided diagnosis of external and middle ear conditions: a machine learning approach. PLOS ONE. 2020;15(3):e0229226.

42. C Gavilan, J Gavlan. 'Carrusel': an expert system for vestibular diagnosis. Acta Otolaryngol. 1990;110(3–4):161–7.

43. Alonzo ALDC, Campos JJM, Layco LLM, Maratas CA, Sagun RA. ENTDEx: ENT diagnosis expert system using Bayesian networks IACSIT. J Adv Comput Netw. 2014;2(3):182.

44. Bing D, Ying J, Miao J, Wang Q. Predicting the hearing outcome in sudden sensorineural hearing loss via machine learning models. Clin Otolaryngol. 2019;43(3):868–74.

45. Shew M, New J, Wichova H, et al. Using machine learning to predict sensorineural hearing loss based on perilymph micro RNA expression profile. Sci Rep. 2019;9:3393.

46. JM Kates. On the feasibility of using neural nets to derive hearing-aid prescriptive procedures. J Acoust Soc Am. 1995;98(1):172–80.

47. Naik SM, Naik MS, Bains NK. Cadaveric temporal bone dissection: is it obsolete today? Int Archives of Otorhinolaryngology. 2014;18.63–7.

48. Alwani M, Baldani E, Larsen M, et al. Current state of surgical simulation training in otolaryngology: systematic review of simulation training models. Arch. Otorhinolaryngol. 2019;3(1):5.

# RECORD KEEPING IN OTOLOGY

# 17  Record Keeping in Otology

*Amit Sood and Dilip Raghavan*

## CONTENTS

## INTRODUCTION

'Verba volant, scripta manent' (spoken words fly away, written words remain)

**–Caius Titus**

Record keeping is an integral part of clinical practice, helping maintain records of patients, the procedures/surgeries conducted, the surgical outcomes achieved and any complications in the course of management. Record keeping not only helps us maintain a continuous data pool of the patients and the modalities offered, but also is a dynamic tool of help in audits and medico-legal aspects (if any arise).

## REVIEW OF LITERATURE

The word "record" means to write down for future reference (1). A medical record should document information regarding the patients, their illness and treatment administered. Meticulous record keeping helps both the clinician and the patient as these records may be evaluated at a later date for various purposes, including medical information, research and legal purposes (2). There are many instances where legal cases have been lost due to inadequate documentation or even illegible handwriting (3). In a surgical department, it is important that a system of review of cases is adopted so that any errors made may be identified and changes needed may be adopted for the benefit of patients. Records should indicate all relevant aspects of the case such as diagnosis, decision on surgery, preparation for surgery, choice of anaesthesia, postoperative care, complications, final results and follow-up if any (4, 5).

To ensure high quality of continuous medical care, accurate and legible clinical notes are essential, these records may be maintained in electronic form or on paper. Use of a standardized proforma helps to improve the content as well as legibility of notes (6–8).The standard of care is to record every activity and intervention that a patient receives in perioperative period.

This leads to fewer adverse patients related events and also fewer cases of litigation (9).

Surgery notes provide a comprehensive record of events inside an operation theatre. These include patient details, surgery details, findings, reconstruction technique used and complications if any. These details are crucial for patient management as well as for medico-legal purposes if need may arise. It has been noted that a proforma, including all essential details, helps in better record keeping and if used in electronic form, legibility issues are also taken care of (10–12).

With increase in use of computers, most of the institutes prefer record keeping in electronic format; however, in some conditions hard copy of records is mandatory (13):

1. Consent form

2. Referral to another doctor

3. Medico-legal cases

4. Certificate of fitness

Otology and neurotology are relatively narrow fields of medicine which are ideally suited for computerized/electronic record keeping. Various electronic templates can be developed for relatively common ontological problems and their management, including long-term follow-up, and this can help to create a data pool which is easily retrievable and more efficient as compared to hard copy of records (14).

There are various guidelines which must be adhered to in maintenance of records, their alteration, release to various authorities and destruction (15).

In recent times, litigation for malpractice or medical negligence has been on the rise; this is partly due to increased patient expectations, however in many cases claims for negligence are raised when there has been a known adverse effect of treatment/procedure. It is in these conditions that medical records assume great significance. A comprehensive written informed consent from the patient/guardian stating that the known adverse effects have been informed to them and patient has been counselled regarding the outcomes of treatment often come to the rescue of the clinician. In an analysis of litigation trends in otolaryngology in the UK, it was found that the commonest cause of litigation was delay/failure to reach a diagnosis, followed by complications of treatment/procedures (16).

## DISCUSSION

As seen above, record keeping is an essential part of clinical practice; these records achieve even greater significance in today's clinical practice as teams of doctors, nurses and paraclinical staff take care of patients in shifts and records are the only thing that can ensure continuation of highest level of care being provided. The medical records should be comprehensive regarding all aspects of patient care like

- Patient information
- Disease (complete diagnosis with ICD code)
- Treatment plan
- Foreseeable adverse effects
- Pre-procedure counselling
- Consent
- Procedure notes
- Post-procedure care
- Discharge instructions
- Referral to other doctors

In today's digital age, record keeping in digital format has assumed great importance and whenever possible digital records like video/still photography of clinical findings as well as findings during surgical procedures should be made. Such records are of great help in reviewing the progress of patients with therapy/surgery, academic discussions, conducting surgical audit of departments and are also helpful in cases of complications/litigation. All such records should be archived with details of patient in chronological order for easy retrieval and can also be forwarded to other practitioners in case a second opinion/referral is required. Procedures like otoscopy, video-nystagmography can be recorded in form of videos for future reference and reports of procedures like pure tone audiometry, objective tests of hearing and posturography can be obtained in standardized formats using various standard softwares like NOAH. In addition to being detailed, the clinical records should also be clearly legible so that no mistakes are made in interpretation of disease process, its treatment and follow-up. It is a good clinical practice to develop proformas/templates for commonly encountered conditions and common surgeries so that all essential parts of record keeping are covered and fewer mistakes are made in patient care.

Samples of few proformas being used in our department are being attached to provide reference in terms of their use (Figures 17.1–17.6). Individual hospitals/practitioners can develop their own proforma/templates for good record keeping. It is important to note that use of blanket proformas for consent is not recommended and consent form should be tailored for each procedure in order to reduce ambiguity and chances of confusion/litigation.

## PRE OP CLINIC NOTES

Date of Pre op clinic:-............

Date of Surgery:-.................

Name_____ Rank _____ Service no_____

Age_____Services _____ Unit/Ship _____

Diagnosis:

| | |
|---|---|
| Special Consent | [   ] |
| High Risk Consent | [   ] |
| ICU Bed availability | [   ] |
| Blood group and availability | [   ] |
| Alled specially | [   ] |

Pre Anesthesia check up:

Comordities:

Surgical plan:

Anesthesia plan:

Involment of other Dept/Spl instruments:

Discussion at pre op clinic

Signature of Resident:                                        Signature of Specialist

**Figure 17.1**   Pre-op clinic form.

## OTOLOGICAL SURGERY: DATA CARD

**PATIENT DETAILS:**

Name of pt:                          Age:          Sex:

Address:                                          Tele No.:

Diagnosis:

Pre-op findings:          (R)                              (L)

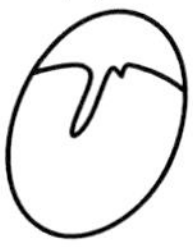

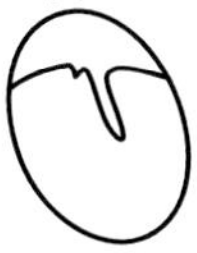

**TFT:**

Rinne                        Weber                          ABC

**PTA (4-tone average):**     (R)                          (L)

AC

BC

AB Gap

S/O–

**Surgery:**                                      **(Primary/Revision)**

**Date:**                        **Surgeon:**

**Intra-op Findings:**

**Ossicular status:**

**Reconstruction technique:**

**Special consent:**

   • Facial palsy: Yes/No
   • Hearing prognosis: Yes/No

**Figure 17.2**   Otology record card: COM.

## Post-op follow up:

**1st Visit**

Date:

Findings:                    (R)                                    (L)

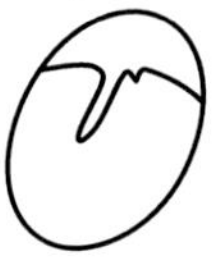

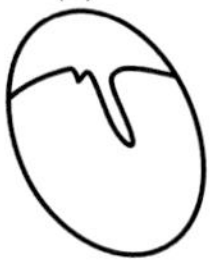

**TFT:**

Rinne                              Weber                              ABC

**PTA (4-tone average):**

**2nd Visit**

Date:

Findings:                    (R)                                    (L)

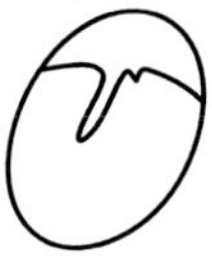

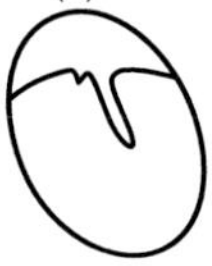

**TFT:**

Rinne                              Weber                              ABC

**PTA (4-tone average):**

**3rd Visit**

Date:

Findings:                    (R)                                    (L)

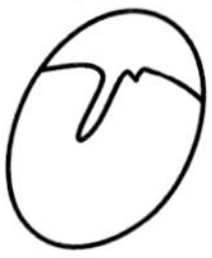

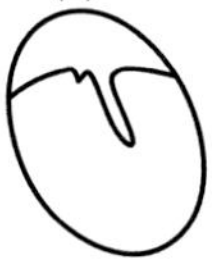

**TFT:**

Rinne                              Weber                              ABC

**PTA (4-tone average):**

**Figure 17.3**   Postoperative follow-up card.

## OTOSCLEROSIS: DATA CARD

**PATIENT DETAILS:**

Name of pt:                    Age:          Sex:         Relation:

Personal No.:                  Rank:         Name:

Address:                                     Tele No.:

Diagnosis:

Pre-op findings:        (R)                              (L)

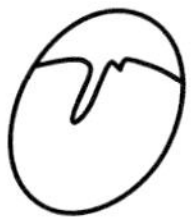

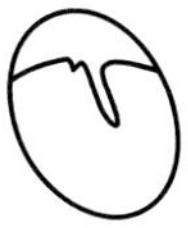

**TFT:**

Rinne                    Weber                          ABC

**PTA (4-tone average):**      (R)                      (L)

AC

BC

AB Gap

S/O–

**HRCT Temporal bone:** Symon's and Fanning Grade (Gd 0 / Gd 1 / Gd 2A / Gd 2B / Gd 2C / Gd 3)

Findings:

**Surgery:**                                      **(Primary/Revision)**

**Date:**                        **Surgeon:**

**Intra-op Findings:**

**Reconstruction technique:**

**Special consent:-**

- Facial palsy: Yes/No
- Giddiness: Yes/No
- Hearing prognosis: Yes/No

**Figure 17.4**   Otology record card: otosclerosis.

**History:**

DOB:

**Parental Details:**    Consanguinity:    Others:

**Risk Factors:**

**Previous evaluation & Treatment:**

Detection:

Hearing Aid fitting

Auditory Verbal Therapy:

**Other aspects:**

**Pre-op findings:**

**ENT:**

    Otological examination

    Oto-neurological examination:

**Paediatric:**

**Psychological Evaluation:**

**Investigations:**

**Audiological:**

    1. OAE (Dt:    ):

    2. Tympanogram (Dt:    ):

    3. ABR (Dt:    ):

    4. ASSR (Dt:    ):

    5. Behavioral Audiometry (Aided & Unaided, Dt:    ):

**Radiological:**

    1. MRI Brain (No:    ,Dt:    ):

    2. HRCT Temporal Bone (No:    ,Dt:    ):

Others: investigations:

**Diagnosis:**

    Comorbidities:

    Syndromic Association:

**Progress on AVT:**

**Candidacy Meeting Decision (Dt:    ):**

**Surgery:**

**Date:**    **Surgeon:**

**Intra-op Findings:**

**Date of Implant Switch-on:**

**Post-op Complications**

**AVT:**

**Speech Training:**

**Post-op Follow-up:**

**Figure 17.5**  Cochlear implant record card.

## SPECIAL CONSENT FOR TEMPORAL BONE SURGERY

Name:                                                      Reg No:

I, the undersigned, hereby declare that the following points have been explained to me in the language I understand best, and in adequate detail, unto my satisfaction.

The Nature of the surgery (Subtotal temporal bone Temporal bone resection which will involve accessing bone ,middle ear ,inner ear  and resecting the involved parts. This may involve removal of Middle ear inner ear ,allied bones, nerves which may pass through them and adjoining structures like the TM joint ,Parotid gland).

This surgery may involve many complications:
- Permanent damage to a cranial nerve especially facial nerve, which may result in paralysis of structures supplied by them, all of which have been explained to me.
- facial nerve paralysis will lead to deviation of angle of mouth ,facial asymmetry and inability to close the ipsilateral  eye completely
- Chances of infection of intracranial components, leading to meningitis.
- Chances of leakage of cerebrospinal fluid, which may take a long time to settle.

I have been explained the following possibilities:
R+ resection : The chances that after removal of all visible disease, microscopic disease may be left behind, or in some cases, where the disease is infiltrating some major structures, some disease may be left behind on the same. In case of such an R+ resection, post operatively, an additional modality of treatment will be required to control the disease.

Inoperability: On opening, if the disease is found to be widespread, and adherent to major structures which cannot be removed, the operation will be aborted and other modalities of treatment will be used for management of the disease.

Tracheostomy: An artificial opening into the windpipe, made in the neck, for breathing purpose may be required in some cases. Till the tracheostomy tube is present, voice will be completely gone, and will come back once the tube is removed. This tracheostomy may be temporary or permanent, depending on the condition for which it was done.

The chances of a prolonged ICU stay and ventilatory support.

The chances of excessive bleeding, and need for blood transfusion and its attendant hazards.

The chances of wound infection in the post operative period

The higher morbidity associated with this procedure, especially if associated co morbidities like hypertension, diabetes, heart disease etc. which increase the risk of surgery and anaesthesia considerably

The rare chance of mortality

Relative's signature                                    Patient's Signature

**Figure 17.6**   Consent for temporal bone surgery.

## REFERENCES

1. Oxford Advanced Learner's Dictionary, 14th ed., 2004; p. 1051.

2. Bali A, Bali D, Iyer N, Iyer N. Management of medical records: facts and figures for surgeons. *J. Maxillofac Oral Surg.* 2011;10(3):199–202.

3. Singh H, Vij K, Garg A, Dhattarwaal SK, Sandhu SS, Aggarwal D. Maintenance of records: how vital? *J Punjab Acad Forensic Med Toxicol.* 2012;12(2):10710.

4. Frazier CH. System of keeping surgical records. *Ann Surg.* 1916;347–8.

5. Grewal P. Surgical hospital audit of record keeping (SHARK): a new audit tool for the improvement in surgical record keeping. *J Surg Educ.* 2013;7(3):33–6.

6. Dexter SC, Hayashi D, Tysome JR. The ANKLe score: an audit of otolaryngology emergency clinical record keeping. *Ann R Coll Surg Engl.* 2008; 90:231–4.

7. Mathioudakis A, Rousalova I, Gagnat AA, et al. How to keep good clinical records. *Breathe.* 2016;12:371–5.

8. Diver AJ, Craig BF. Admission proforma significantly improves the medical record. *Scot Med J*. 2005; 50:101–2.

9. Pirie S. Documentation and record keeping. *Open Learning Zone*. 2011;21(1):22–8.

10. Ghani Y, Thakrar R, Kosuge D, Bates P. 'Smart' electronic operation notes in surgery: an innovative way to improve patient care. *Int J Surg*. 2014;12:30–2.

11. Singh R, Chouhan R, Anwar S. Improving the quality of general surgical operation notes in accordance with the Royal College of Surgeons guidelines: a prospective completed audit loop study. *J Eval Clin Pract*. 2012;18:578–80.

12. Payne K, Jones K, Dickenson AW. Improving the standard of operative notes within an oral and maxillofacial surgery department, using an operative note proforma. *J. Maxillofac Oral Surg*. 2011;10(3):203–8.

13. Behere SB Doctor & law. *Dr People*. 2010;2(7):11–14.

14. Green J, Postma D, Giddings N, Sapp K, Skinner T. Computerized medical record in a private neurotology practice. *Am J Otol*. 2000; 21(4):589–94.

15. Singh S, Sinha US, Sharma NK Preservation of medical records: an essential part of health care delivery. *IIJFMT*. 2005;3(4):1–8.

16. Savage JR, Weiner GM. Litigation in otolaryngology: trends and recommendations. *J Laryngol Otol*. 2006;120:1001–4.

# Index

Note: Locators in *italics* represent figures and **bold** indicate tables in the text.